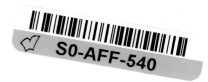
MEDICAL PARASITOLOGY
A Self-Instructional Text

FIFTH EDITION
Medical PARASITOLOGY
A Self-Instructional Text

Ruth Leventhal, PhD, MBA, MT (ASCP)
Provost and Dean Emerita
The Pennsylvania State University
Harrisburg, Pennsylvania, and
Emerita Professor of Biology
The Milton S. Hershey Medical Center
The Pennsylvania State University
Hershey, Pennsylvania

Russell F. Cheadle, MS, MT (ASCP)
Program Director, MLT
Professor of Medical Technology
University of Rio Grande
Rio Grande, Ohio

Illustrations by Elliot Hoffman

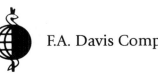

F.A. Davis Company • Philadelphia

F. A. Davis Company
1915 Arch Street
Philadelphia, PA 19103
www.fadavis.com

Printed in the United States of America

Last digit indicates print number: 10 9 8 7 6 5 4 3 2

Acquisitions Editor: Christa Fratantoro
Developmental Editor: Renee Gagliardi
Production Editor: Jack Brandt
Designer: Bill Donnelley
Cover Designer: Louis Forgione

As new scientific information becomes available through basic and clinical research, recommended treatments and drug therapies undergo changes. The author(s) and publisher have done everything possible to make this book accurate, up to date, and in accord with accepted standards at the time of publication. The authors, editors, and publisher are not responsible for errors or omissions or for consequences from application of the book, and make no warranty, expressed or implied, in regard to the contents of the book. Any practice described in this book should be applied by the reader in accordance with professional standards of care used in regard to the unique circumstances that may apply in each situation. The reader is advised always to check product information (package inserts) for changes and new information regarding dose and contraindications before administering any drug. Caution is especially urged when using new or infrequently ordered drugs.

Library of Congress Cataloging in Publication Data

Leventhal, Ruth.
  Medical parasitology : a self-instructional text / Ruth Leventhal, Russell F. Cheadle ;
illustrations by Elliot Hoffman.—5th ed.
    p. ; cm.
  Includes bibliographical references and index.
  ISBN 0-8036-0788-1
    1. Medical parasitology—Programmed instruction. I. Cheadle, Russell F. II. Title.
  [DNLM: I. Parasitology—Programmed instruction. QX 18.2 L657m 2002]
  QR251 .L38 2002
  616.9′6′0077—dc21

2001053881

To teachers and to scientists who labor in the field, whose work influences our knowledge and understanding, I gratefully appreciate your contributions to this text.

Ruth Leventhal

To my wife and best friend, Cathy, and daughter Valerie.

Russell F. Cheadle

PREFACE TO THE FIFTH EDITION

Since the publication of the first edition of this text in 1979, various phenomena have increased the incidence of parasitic diseases among North Americans. Increased world travel by U.S. residents and the influx of immigrants to this country from underdeveloped regions have brought increasing numbers of once seldom-encountered parasites to this country. Shifts in sexual behaviors in our society have altered the traditionally accepted epidemiology of infections such as giardiases and amebiasis. In addition, individuals with acquired immunodeficiency syndrome (AIDS) have acquired infections caused by previously rare opportunistic parasites and have suffered more severe symptoms from infections caused by usually less virulent organisms. Such situations lend an increased urgency to the correct diagnosis and treatment of parasitic diseases by American physicians and to the detection of these diseases by laboratory technologists. On a global basis, parasitic infections remain a most serious consideration. They affect the morbidity and mortality levels in every nation, affecting the countries with tropical and temperate climates very significantly. We believe, therefore, that now more than ever, all health professionals need a fundamental understanding of the diagnosis, treatment, and prevention of parasitic diseases. We have approached our revision with this belief in mind.

Medical Parasitology is designed to provide the reader with a concise, systematic introduction to the biology and epidemiology of human parasitic disease. The text is supported throughout by an array of carefully coordinated graphics. Many of the changes incorporated in this revision are based on responses from surveys of the users of the previous editions. The presentation of the symptomatology, pathology, and treatment of each parasitic disease has been expanded. New parasites have been added, most notably those associated with AIDS. Information concerning the role of arthropods as ectoparasites has been enhanced, and coverage of serologic testing has been strengthened. Resource lists for general and immunologic supplies have been added as well. Epidemiology and treatment topics have been reorganized and are expanded in the final chapter.

Enhancements to the graphic elements of the text have not been neglected. Line drawings and photographs of newly added parasites have been included and previous drawings modified as necessary. All laboratory procedures have been updated and expanded to conform to current quality control standards. Finally, pedagogical improvements include review questions within the text, all-new end-of-chapter post-tests, case studies, word puzzles, and thoroughly updated bibliographies.

Ruth Leventhal

Russell F. Cheadle

ACKNOWLEDGMENTS

The authors particularly wish to thank Lynne S. Garcia for her extensive review of the text and for generously permitting our use of table material in Chapters 5 and 7.

Ruth Leventhal wishes to thank her family and friends for their help and support.

Russell Cheadle wishes to especially thank his wife, Catherine, for her impeccable typing, for her critical front-end editing, and most of all, for her many years of support and devotion to this project.

PREFACE TO THE FIRST EDITION

There are many available textbooks about parasitology. Some of these treat the biology of parasites in great depth, while others are more graphic in nature. The laboratorian or clinician needs both kinds. This book was designed to provide a concise description of the biology and epidemiology of human parasites, coupled with an extensive series of color photographs and line drawings to facilitate visual recognition of parasites found in clinical specimens. Furthermore, several modes of graphic presentation have been incorporated in order to aid the various approaches to learning and mastering the requisites.

This book resulted from our recognition of the need for a self-instructional text in parasitology. Present formal course instruction in medical parasitology is often limited and generally is not designed to allow for different learning styles. Russell Cheadle conceptualized and wrote the original draft of this self-instructional text, while the research and writing thereafter became a truly collaborative effort. This product is, we believe, a useful learning tool for students in biology, medical technology, medicine, and public health, as well as an effective pictorial reference book for the clinical laboratory.

We wish to thank Catherine Cheadle, Mary Stevens, and Valerie Fortune for their kind assistance. Russell Cheadle would also like to thank Dr. Herbert W. Cox, his graduate advisor, for his encouragement.

Ruth Leventhal

Russell F. Cheadle

REVIEWERS

Stephen M. Johnson, MS, MT(ASCP)
Program Director
School of Medical Technology
Saint Vincent Health Center
Erie, Pennsylvania

Peter W. Pappas, PhD
Professor, Department of EEOB
Ohio State University
Columbus, Ohio

Phyllis Pacifico, EdD, MT(ASCP)
Program Director
Medical Technology
Wright State University
Dayton, Ohio

Lynn Shore Garcia, MS, CLS(NCA)
LSG & Associates
Santa Monica, California

Daniel P. deRegnier, MS, MT(ASCP)
Associate Professor
Clinical Laboratory Science
School of Allied Health
Ferris State University
Big Rapids, Michigan

Judith Schermond, MS, MT(ASCP)SM, CLS(NCA)
Clinical Assistant Professor
Medical Technology
University of Illinois at Chicago
Chicago, Illinois

CONTENTS

COLOR PLATES

The series of color photographs included with this text was selected to show clearly the morphologic and diagnostic characteristics of parasites of medical importance. A brief review of major disease symptoms, the life cycle of the parasite, and other pertinent information are included in the discussion of each photograph. Try to describe each diagnostic stage aloud, recalling the key features of each organism as labeled on the life cycle diagram, to assure yourself that you recall these features.

The Nematodes are a diverse group of roundworms, existing as both free-living and parasitic forms. They vary greatly in size from a few millimeters to over a meter in length. These organisms have separate sexes, and their body development is complex. Of the nematode species parasitic for humans, about half live as adults in the intestine, and the other half are tissue parasites in their definitive host. The pathogenicity in intestinal infections may be due to biting and blood sucking (e.g., hookworms, *Trichuris*), to allergic reactions caused by substances secreted from adult worms or larvae, or to migration through the body tissues. Tissue nematodes, the Filarioidea, live in various tissue locations in the host. These organisms require an arthropod intermediate host in their life cycle. The produced pathology varies with the location of the parasites in humans but may involve the occlusion of the lymphatics (*Wuchereria*, *Brugia*), localized subcutaneous swellings or nodules (*Onchocerca*, *Dracunculus*), or blindness (*Onchocerca*).

1,2. *Enterobius vermicularis* (pinworm). 1. Adult male (20 ×) and 2. female (10 ×). These mature in the anterior portion of the colon. The adult yellowish-white female worms are 8 to 13 mm and the male worms 2 to 5 mm in size. Each has a bulbar esophagus as well as finlike projections, called cephalic alae, about the anterior end. Male and female worms are further differentiated in that the male has a sharp curvature of the tail and small posterior copulatory spicule, whereas the female has a long, straight, sharply pointed tail. When the uterus is gravid with eggs, the female migrates from the colon (usually during sleeping hours of the host) to the perianal area, where she deposits her eggs and dies. The adult may also migrate to the appendix, where it can be found histologically. Pinworm disease is essentially an allergic reaction to the release of eggs and other secreted materials from the gravid female that causes severe rectal itching.

3. A higher-power view of the anterior end of the adult, clearly showing the alae.

4. Note the caudal curve and copulatory spicules of the male *Enterobius vermicularis*.

5. *Enterobius vermicularis* eggs (400 ×). Eggs may be recovered from the perianal folds by applying the sticky side of cellophane tape to the skin surfaces and then taping the cellophane, sticky side down, onto a microscope slide for examination. Eggs are rarely recovered in feces. The eggs are elongated (55 μm × 25 μm) and tend to be flattened on one side. The thick shell is transparent and colorless, and the folded larva may be seen within. Pinworm eggs are infective for the host within a few hours of being released. Scratching of the perianal region allows transfer of the eggs by hand to the mouth of the host. The eggs hatch soon after they are swallowed and develop to mature worms within 2 weeks. Bedding, night clothing, and even house dust may be sources of egg infection for others through ingestion or inhalation of airborne eggs. This is a very common parasitic infection in this country and spreads easily, so that those living with an infected individual are likely to become infected.

6. *Enterobius vermicularis* egg (900 ×). This view shows an egg under oil immersion; the developed larva can be clearly seen coiled inside the flattened shell.

7. *Enterobius vermicularis* egg (100 ×). A low-power view of the egg as seen on a cellophane tape preparation. Because of the transparency of the eggs, screening of the slides must be carefully performed, using low illumination.

8. *Trichuris trichiura* (whipworm) (4 ×). Adult female, measuring 35 to 50 mm. The anterior ends of both male and female worms are slender and threadlike, but the posterior one-third of the worm is wider. The posterior end of the female appears club-shaped and straight; the male has a 360-degree coiled posterior with two copulatory spicules. The adults in the intestine attach firmly by embedding a spearlike projection at their anterior end into the mucosa of the cecum and proximal colon. Distribution of this parasite is cosmopolitan, especially in moist, warm areas. This is the most commonly reported parasitic infection in this country. Light infections are usually asymptomatic, but heavy infections may cause enteritis and diarrhea with rectal prolapse.

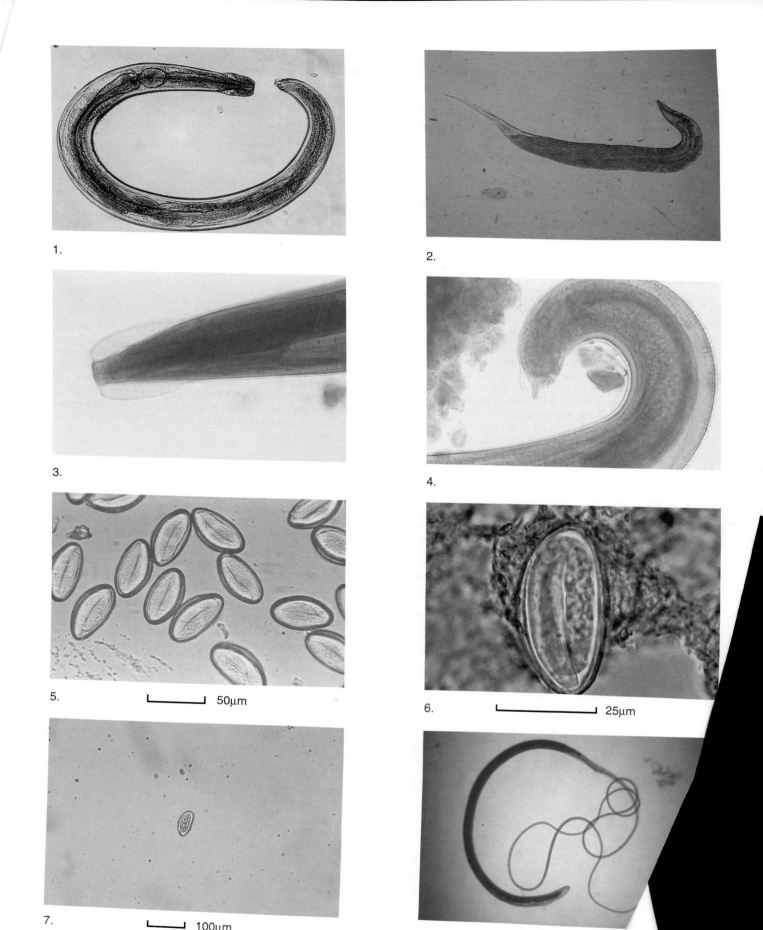

1.

2.

3.

4.

5. |⎯⎯⎯⎯⎯⎯| 50µm

6. |⎯⎯⎯⎯⎯⎯| 25µm

7. |⎯⎯⎯⎯| 100µm

8.

9. *Trichuris trichiura* egg (500 ×). Diagnosis: recovery of eggs in feces. Concentration technique needed to detect a light infection. The *Trichuris* egg is characteristically barrel-shaped and measures 20 μm × 50 μm. Note the undeveloped embryo; the clear, inner shell; the heavy, golden outer shell; and the transparent hyaline plugs at the ends of the egg. Eggs passed in feces must remain in a favorable soil environment for at least 10 days until larval development is complete; at this time the egg is infective. Ingestion of the egg from infected soil or contaminated food is followed by hatching in the intestines. The larva molts and develops in the intestines to become an adult. About 90 days are needed for a complete cycle from egg ingestion to egg output by the adults.

10. *Trichuris trichiura* egg. This view shows an egg at a magnification of 100 ×. (Note: Dog whipworm is an occasional zoonosis; egg is much larger [35 μm × 80 μm] and broader.)

11. *Ascaris lumbricoides*. Both male and female adults are shown. They are large, pinkish-white, and conically tapered at the anterior end. A female measures 22 to 35 cm in length by 3 to 6 mm in diameter and has a pinkish-white and straight tail. A male measures 10 to 31 cm by 2 to 4 mm and has a sharply curved tail with two copulatory spicules. The adults live in the small intestine and can survive for over a year. Females lay up to 250,000 eggs per day, which are passed in the feces and can be readily recovered by routine fecal examination. Passage of adult worms from the rectum is often the first indication of infection. Light infections are asymptomatic. Heavy infections may cause pneumonia early in the infection and, later, diarrhea, vomiting, or bowel obstruction. Complications such as perforation of the intestinal wall or appendix, with resultant peritonitis or obstruction of airways by vomited worms, may cause death. Known as the large intestinal roundworm.

12. An obstructed bowel from a heavily infected patient with *Ascaris lumbricoites*. Distribution of this parasite is worldwide, although it is more frequently found in tropical areas.

13. *Ascaris lumbricoides* egg (400 ×). Diagnosis: recognition of eggs (or adults) in feces. The fertilized egg measures 40 μm × 55 μm and contains an undeveloped embryo. This egg appears round, but *Ascaris* eggs are slightly oval. The outer coat is albuminous and mamillated; occasionally, eggs without coats may be found (decorticated). The thick, inner coat is of clear chitin. These characteristics are diagnostic. On reaching warm, moist soil, larvae develop within the egg shells in 2 to 3 weeks, and eggs are then infective for humans. Infection occurs by ingestion of these infective eggs in contaminated food or drink. It is not uncommon for *Ascaris* and *Trichuris* to coexist in the same person because of the same method of infection and the requirements for egg development in the soil. Eggs hatch in the intestine, and the *Ascaris* larvae rapidly penetrate the mucosal wall. They reach the liver and then the lungs via the blood circulation. Larvae emerge from the circulation into the lungs in about 9 days, migrate up the bronchi to the esophagus, and are swallowed. They mature in the intestine in about 2 months. In an immune individual, most larvae are destroyed in the liver.

14. *Ascaris lumbricoides* egg. This view shows an egg at a magnification of 100 ×. Ascarids of dogs and cats (*Toxocara* spp.) can undergo partial development and produce pathology in humans. After ingestion of an egg from soil, the *Toxocara* eggs hatch and the larvae penetrate the intestinal wall and enter the blood circulation but are unable to complete the migratory route. They lodge in tissues and cause inflammatory reactions leading to occlusions of capillaries of vital organs (e.g., eye, liver, brain, lungs). Symptoms vary, depending on the location of the parasite and the host's reaction to it. The disease is called visceral larval migrans. It is seen most commonly in children because they are more likely to ingest eggs from infected soil, such as at a playground where dogs are walked. High eosinophilia is a very common sign. Diagnosis is made serologically or by observing larvae in histopathologic sections. Species identification is difficult but can be done.

15. *Ascaris lumbricoides* egg (400 ×). An unfertilized egg. Note the elongated shape and the heavy, albuminous, mamillated coat. This type of egg is not uncommonly seen.

16. Adult male hookworm (10 ×). Adult hookworms are small, grayish-white nematodes. The anterior end is tapered and curved and has an open buccal capsule. The posterior end of the male terminates in a fan-shaped copulatory bursa and spicules. The raylike pattern of the chitinous supportive structure in the bursa is different for each species. Females (12 mm × 0.5 mm) are larger than males (9 mm × 0.4 mm). The female has a straight and pointed tail and produces 5000 to 10,000 eggs per day. She may live for up to 14 years.

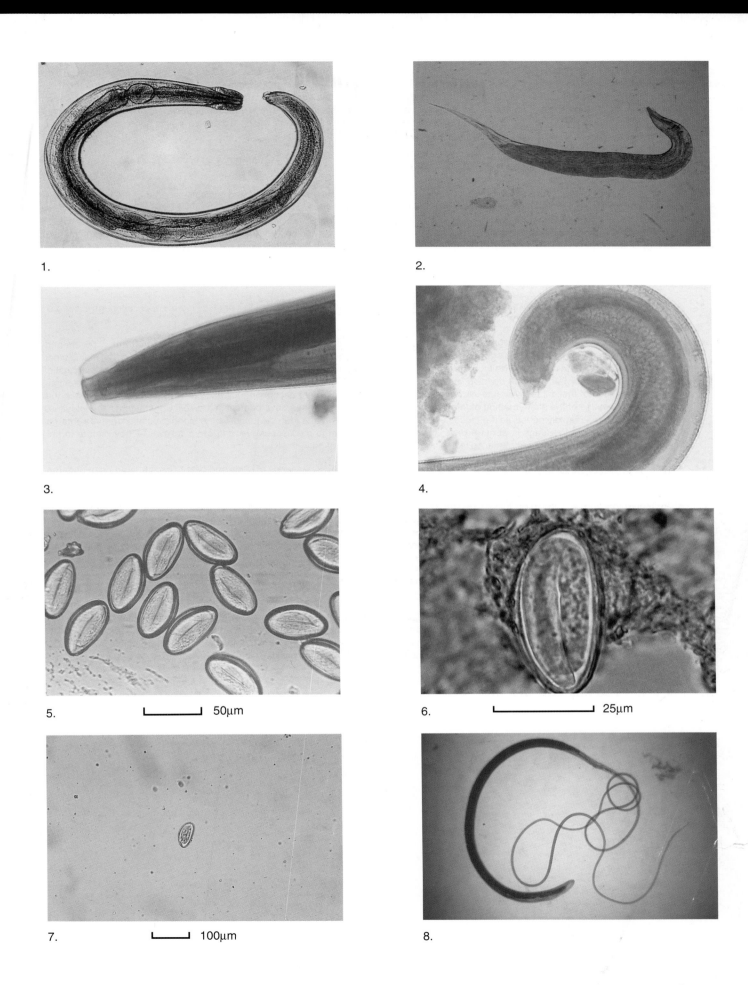

1.

2.

3.

4.

5. ⊢————⊣ 50μm

6. ⊢————⊣ 25μm

7. ⊢——⊣ 100μm

8.

9. *Trichuris trichiura* egg (500 ×). Diagnosis: recovery of eggs in feces. Concentration technique needed to detect a light infection. The *Trichuris* egg is characteristically barrel-shaped and measures 20 μm × 50 μm. Note the undeveloped embryo; the clear, inner shell; the heavy, golden outer shell; and the transparent hyaline plugs at the ends of the egg. Eggs passed in feces must remain in a favorable soil environment for at least 10 days until larval development is complete; at this time the egg is infective. Ingestion of the egg from infected soil or contaminated food is followed by hatching in the intestines. The larva molts and develops in the intestines to become an adult. About 90 days are needed for a complete cycle from egg ingestion to egg output by the adults.

10. *Trichuris trichiura* egg. This view shows an egg at a magnification of 100 ×. (Note: Dog whipworm is an occasional zoonosis; egg is much larger [35 μm × 80 μm] and broader.)

11. *Ascaris lumbricoides*. Both male and female adults are shown. They are large, pinkish-white, and conically tapered at the anterior end. A female measures 22 to 35 cm in length by 3 to 6 mm in diameter and has a pinkish-white and straight tail. A male measures 10 to 31 cm by 2 to 4 mm and has a sharply curved tail with two copulatory spicules. The adults live in the small intestine and can survive for over a year. Females lay up to 250,000 eggs per day, which are passed in the feces and can be readily recovered by routine fecal examination. Passage of adult worms from the rectum is often the first indication of infection. Light infections are asymptomatic. Heavy infections may cause pneumonia early in the infection and, later, diarrhea, vomiting, or bowel obstruction. Complications such as perforation of the intestinal wall or appendix, with resultant peritonitis or obstruction of airways by vomited worms, may cause death. Known as the large intestinal roundworm.

12. An obstructed bowel from a heavily infected patient with *Ascaris lumbricoites*. Distribution of this parasite is worldwide, although it is more frequently found in tropical areas.

13. *Ascaris lumbricoides* egg (400 ×). Diagnosis: recognition of eggs (or adults) in feces. The fertilized egg measures 40 μm × 55 μm and contains an undeveloped embryo. This egg appears round, but *Ascaris* eggs are slightly oval. The outer coat is albuminous and mamillated; occasionally, eggs without coats may be found (decorticated). The thick, inner coat is of clear chitin. These characteristics are diagnostic. On reaching warm, moist soil, larvae develop within the egg shells in 2 to 3 weeks, and eggs are then infective for humans. Infection occurs by ingestion of these infective eggs in contaminated food or drink. It is not uncommon for *Ascaris* and *Trichuris* to coexist in the same person because of the same method of infection and the requirements for egg development in the soil. Eggs hatch in the intestine, and the *Ascaris* larvae rapidly penetrate the mucosal wall. They reach the liver and then the lungs via the blood circulation. Larvae emerge from the circulation into the lungs in about 9 days, migrate up the bronchi to the esophagus, and are swallowed. They mature in the intestine in about 2 months. In an immune individual, most larvae are destroyed in the liver.

14. *Ascaris lumbricoides* egg. This view shows an egg at a magnification of 100 ×. Ascarids of dogs and cats (*Toxocara* spp.) can undergo partial development and produce pathology in humans. After ingestion of an egg from soil, the *Toxocara* eggs hatch and the larvae penetrate the intestinal wall and enter the blood circulation but are unable to complete the migratory route. They lodge in tissues and cause inflammatory reactions leading to occlusions of capillaries of vital organs (e.g., eye, liver, brain, lungs). Symptoms vary, depending on the location of the parasite and the host's reaction to it. The disease is called visceral larval migrans. It is seen most commonly in children because they are more likely to ingest eggs from infected soil, such as at a playground where dogs are walked. High eosinophilia is a very common sign. Diagnosis is made serologically or by observing larvae in histopathologic sections. Species identification is difficult but can be done.

15. *Ascaris lumbricoides* egg (400 ×). An unfertilized egg. Note the elongated shape and the heavy, albuminous, mamillated coat. This type of egg is not uncommonly seen.

16. Adult male hookworm (10 ×). Adult hookworms are small, grayish-white nematodes. The anterior end is tapered and curved and has an open buccal capsule. The posterior end of the male terminates in a fan-shaped copulatory bursa and spicules. The raylike pattern of the chitinous supportive structure in the bursa is different for each species. Females (12 mm × 0.5 mm) are larger than males (9 mm × 0.4 mm). The female has a straight and pointed tail and produces 5000 to 10,000 eggs per day. She may live for up to 14 years.

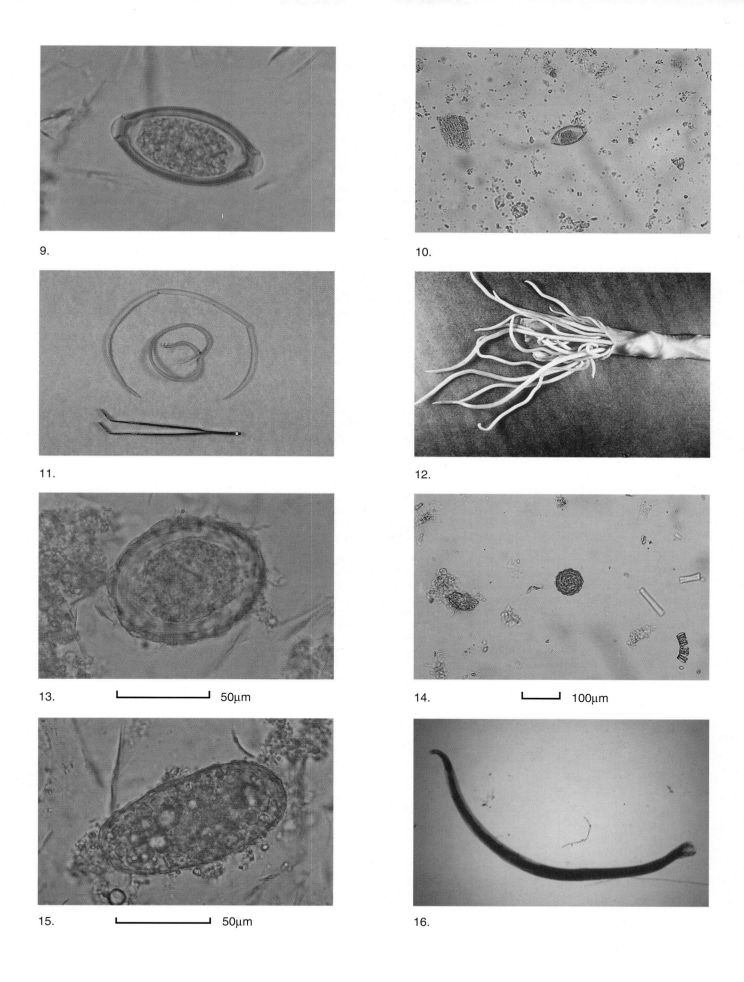

9.

10.

11.

12.

13.　　　⊢————————⊣　50µm

14.　　　⊢————⊣　100µm

15.　　　⊢————————⊣　50µm

16.

17. *Necator americanus* (New World hookworm). The anterior end of an adult worm. Species identification is helped by examining the buccal capsule. Note the pair of semilunar cutting plates in the upper side of the buccal cavity. There is also a second, smaller set of plates on the lower side.

18. *Ancylostoma duodenale* (Old World hookworm). The anterior end of an adult worm. Note the two pairs of teeth in the buccal cavity. The mouthparts of hookworms allow firm attachment to the mucosa of the small intestine and ingestion of blood. *N. americanus* is found throughout Africa and the southeastern United States; *A. duodenale* is found in southern Europe, northern Africa, the Far East, and the Mediterranean countries. Both are found in parts of Asia, Central and South America, and the South Pacific. Symptoms of the disease depend on the extent of the infection and the nutritional status of the patient and can appear clinically as a hypochromic microcytic anemia because of the bloodsucking activity of worms. Only a heavy infection causes the disease state.

19. Hookworm egg (500 ×). Note the definite but thin shell and the clear area around the embryo. Diagnosis of the presence of hookworms can be made upon recognition of the egg in feces, but adults must be examined for species identification because the eggs and larvae of these worms look alike. Eggs usually contain an immature embryo in the 4- to 8-cell stage of division if feces are promptly examined. Six cells are visible in this embryo. Eggs measure about 30 μm × 50 μm.

20. Hookworm eggs (500 ×). This view shows more mature eggs containing developing rhabditiform larvae. Eggs are shed in feces, and the embryo rapidly develops to a larva in 1 to 2 days. Eggs hatch to liberate rhabditiform larvae, which then further mature in the soil to become infective filariform larvae.

21. Hookworm rhabditiform larva, showing the anterior end of the first-stage larva (500 ×). Although these larvae are not normally seen in fresh fecal preparations, larvae may develop and hatch if feces are not promptly examined. This view has been included so that differential characteristics between hookworm larvae and *Strongyloides stercoralis* rhabditiform larvae may be studied. Note that the buccal cavity of a first-stage hookworm larva is slightly longer than the width of the head, appearing as two parallel lines extending back from the anterior edge of the larva. It has a longer buccal cavity than that of *S. stercoralis*; this is the primary characteristic differentiating the two (see Plate 25). In addition, the genital primordium is not obvious in hookworm larvae but is visible in *Strongyloides* larvae. The hookworm larva measures 250 μm × 17 μm.

22. Hookworm filariform larva (100 ×). Infection occurs when infective stage (filariform) larvae penetrate skin, especially between the toes. The larvae are carried throughout the body via lymphatic and blood circulation. Most larvae emerge from the circulation in the lungs, migrate up the bronchi to the esophagus, and are swallowed. They complete maturation in the intestine in about 2 weeks. Nonfeeding infective hookworm larvae in soil are ensheathed and have pointed tails. A short esophagus extending about one-quarter of the way down from the anterior end is another differentiating characteristic.

23. Infective filariform larvae of dog and cat hookworms, especially *Ancylostoma braziliense*, can invade human skin, producing an allergic dermatitis called creeping eruption or cutaneous larval migrans. Inasmuch as the human is an unnatural host for animal hookworms, further larval development does not occur. An itching, red papule is produced at the site of larval entry with development of a serpentine tunnel between the epithelial layers produced as the larva migrates. The larva moves several millimeters per day and may survive several weeks or months. This disease is widely distributed and is common in sandy areas on the Atlantic coast from New Jersey to the Florida Keys, along the Gulf of Mexico, and in many parts of Texas. It is also found in the midwestern United States.

24. *Strongyloides stercoralis* (threadworm) (400 ×). This view is of a rhabditiform larva (225 μm × 15 μm) seen in feces. Concentration techniques are helpful because numbers are low. The esophageal bulb is evident at the junction of the esophagus and intestine, which is about one-fourth of the parasite's length back from the anterior end. This is one diagnostic feature that may be used to differentiate hookworm and *Strongyloides* rhabditiform larvae, because this structure is not as prominent in hookworm larvae. Adult parthenogenic female worms (2.2 mm × 50 μm) live in the submucosa of the upper small intestine. Eggs pass through the mucosa, and the rhabditiform larvae hatch in the lumen of the intestine to be shed in feces. The larvae may develop in soil to become infective filariform larvae and penetrate the skin as do hookworm larvae. They may, however, also molt and become infective before they pass in feces and penetrate the mucosa of the colon to cause autoinfection, especially in debilitated or immunocompromised persons. In either case, they travel via the blood-lung route as do hookworm larvae, returning to the intestine to develop into adults. The life cycle of this parasite may also include a free-living cycle in the soil. In this case, rhabditiform larvae molt and develop in 2 to 3 days to become free-living mature adults. The sexually mature free-living male and female mate and produce eggs that develop into filariform larvae, which are infective to humans via skin penetration.

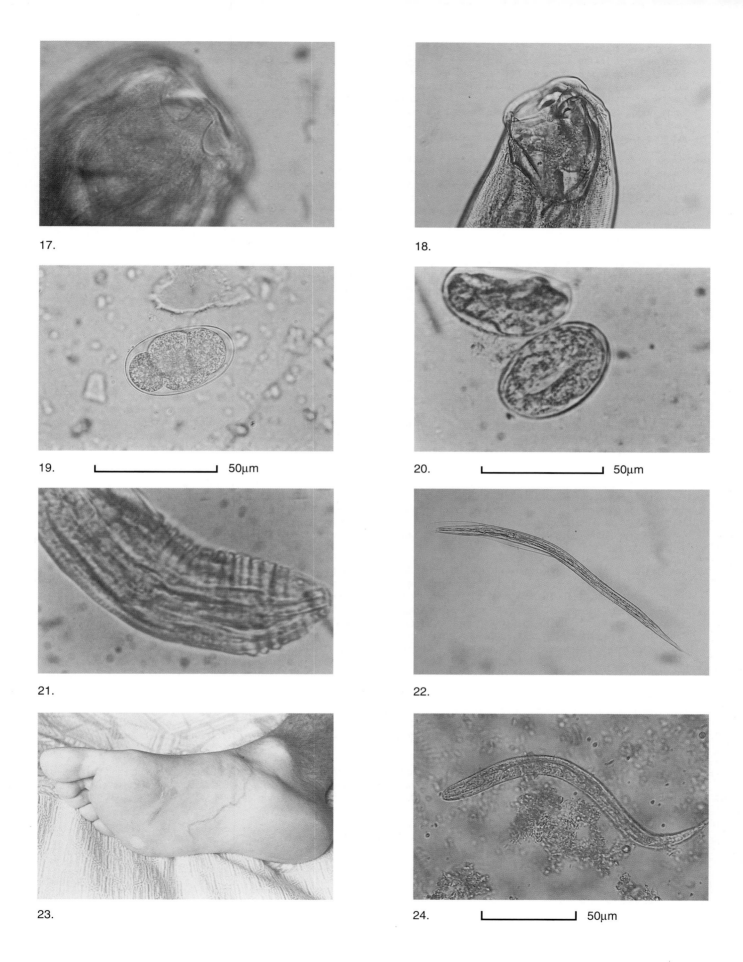

17.

18.

19.   ⊢————————⊣ 50µm

20.   ⊢————————⊣ 50µm

21.

22.

23.

24.   ⊢————————⊣ 50µm

25. *Strongyloides stercoralis* (500 ×). This view shows the short buccal cavity of the rhabditiform larva. The length is one-third to one-half the width of the head of the larva (compare with Plate 21). Diagnosis is based on the recovery of characteristic rhabditiform larvae from feces. The filariform (infective stage) larva of *Strongyloides* recovered from soil or cultured in the laboratory has a notched tail, whereas the filariform larvae of hookworms have pointed tails. This parasite is found worldwide, especially in warm climates. As with hookworm disease, there is a dermatitis at the site of repeated larval entry, and respiratory symptoms may result from the larvae as they migrate through the lungs. Abdominal symptoms vary with the extent of the infection, from mild epigastric pain to vomiting, diarrhea, and weakness with weight loss. Moderate eosinophilia is common. Untreated, the disease may last for many years because of autoinfection from larvae that develop in the colon and may cause death in immunosuppressed patients.

26. *Trichinella spiralis* (trichina worm). Encysted larva in muscle tissue (400 ×). Adult worms develop (in about 1 week) in the submucosal tissues of the small intestine. They are very small: the male measures 1.5 mm, and the female measures 3.5 mm. Larvae (1 mm) produced by the female pass into the mesenteric venules or lymphatics and are carried throughout the body. Within about 2 weeks they emerge from the blood to enter striated muscle cells or other tissue, although they survive only if they enter striated muscle cells (for instance, in the tongue or diaphragm). The 1-mm larvae become encysted in the muscle and calcify over time but remain alive for years. Many hundreds of larvae may be produced over the female's life span of 2 to 3 weeks. Infection occurs when undercooked pork or bear meat containing encysted larvae is ingested; the larvae develop into adults in the intestines in a few days. The disease state, trichinosis, is found worldwide among meat-eating populations (with the highest prevalence in Europe and North America) and presents a variety of symptoms, including gastric distress, fever, edema (especially of the face), and acute inflammation of muscle tissue. Daily study of blood smears showing increasing eosinophilia is a useful diagnostic aid. A history of eating undercooked meat, skin testing, and positive serologic tests are strongly suggestive of infection but are not conclusive. Definitive diagnosis depends upon demonstration of the encysted larvae in a muscle biopsy from the patient. Attempts at recovery of adult parasites from feces are usually futile. Light infections have vague symptoms, which may be missed.

27. *Trichinella spiralis*. A higher-power view of a stained section. Note the tissue inflammation around encysted larvae in the muscle "nurse cells."

28. *Wuchereria bancrofti* (Bancroft's filaria) microfilaria (400 ×). A thick, peripheral blood smear, stained with Giemsa stain, showing the sheathed embryo, which measures 250 μm in length. The ends of the sheath appear almost colorless and are noncellular, often staining poorly with Giemsa. The presence of a sheath and the pattern of cell nuclei, which can be seen in the posterior end of the microfilaria (upper center photograph), are diagnostic. In this species, a single column of cell nuclei extends only to near the tip of the tail, which has no nuclei. Microfilariae are most prevalent in the peripheral blood at night (nocturnal periodicity); therefore, they are best detected in blood specimens obtained between 9 PM and 3 AM. Blood concentration is helpful. Adult nematodes live in the lymphatics. Prolonged infections cause obstruction of lymph flow, resulting in elephantiasis of the lower extremities, genitalia, or breasts. Other symptoms include fever and eosinophilia caused by allergic reactions to the parasite. *Culex*, *Aedes*, *Mansonia*, and *Anopheles* mosquitoes serve as intermediate hosts of *W. bancrofti* and are found in tropical areas worldwide. Diagnosis: recovery of characteristic microfilariae in blood.

29. *Brugia malayi* (Malayan filaria) sheathed microfilaria (400 ×). The sheath stains pink with Giemsa. Note that the nuclei occur in groups to the end of the tail, with two nuclei in the tip (middle right of photograph). These features are diagnostic. The disease produced is essentially identical to *W. bancrofti* but is found primarily in Southeast Asia, India, and China. These microfilariae also exhibit nocturnal periodicity in the blood, and the mosquito vectors are species of *Mansonia*, *Aedes*, and *Anopheles*. Diagnosis: recovery of characteristic microfilariae in blood at night.

30. *Loa loa* (African eyeworm) microfilaria (400 ×). In this thick blood smear, the sheathed microfilaria can be seen, measuring 250 μm in length. Note that cell nuclei occur in groups through most of the body but are seen in a single line to the tip of the posterior end of the tail (upper right of photograph). This feature is diagnostic. In humans, adults migrate throughout the subcutaneous tissues, causing transient swellings called Calabar swellings. Adults may be seen migrating through the conjunctiva of the eye. Microfilariae are most prevalent in the blood during the day (diurnal periodicity), and the vector is the mango fly (*Chrysops*). The disease is chronic and relatively benign, although allergic reactions may occur, causing edema, itching, and eosinophilia. This parasite is found in West and Central Africa. Diagnosis: recovery of characteristic microfilariae in blood. The sheath does not stain with Giemsa.

31. Children with distinct fibrous nodules on their bodies, which contain adult worms and microfilariae of *Onchocerca volvulus*. The female discharges microfilariae that migrate through the skin but do not enter the blood. The disease is chronic and nonfatal. Allergic reactions to microfilariae cause local symptoms. If microfilariae reach the eye, blindness may occur. This parasite is a major cause of blindness (river blindness) in Africa. Diagnosis is made by excising a nodule with recovery of adult worms or by detecting microfilariae in a tissue scraping of the nodule or a skin snip. When present in the eye, microfilariae may be observed with an ophthalmic microscope. The vector is the blackfly, *Simulium*, which breeds in running water, and the disease is found in Central America, parts of northern South America, and west-central Africa.

32. *Onchocerca volvulus* microfilaria (100 ×) present in a tissue scraping of a skin nodule. The microfilariae are unsheathed and the pointed, often flexed tail contains no cell nuclei. Differentiate from *Mansonella streptocerca* microfilariae, which are also found in skin snips, by the tails, which, in *M. streptocerca*, are bent into button-hook shapes and have nuclei extending into the tips.

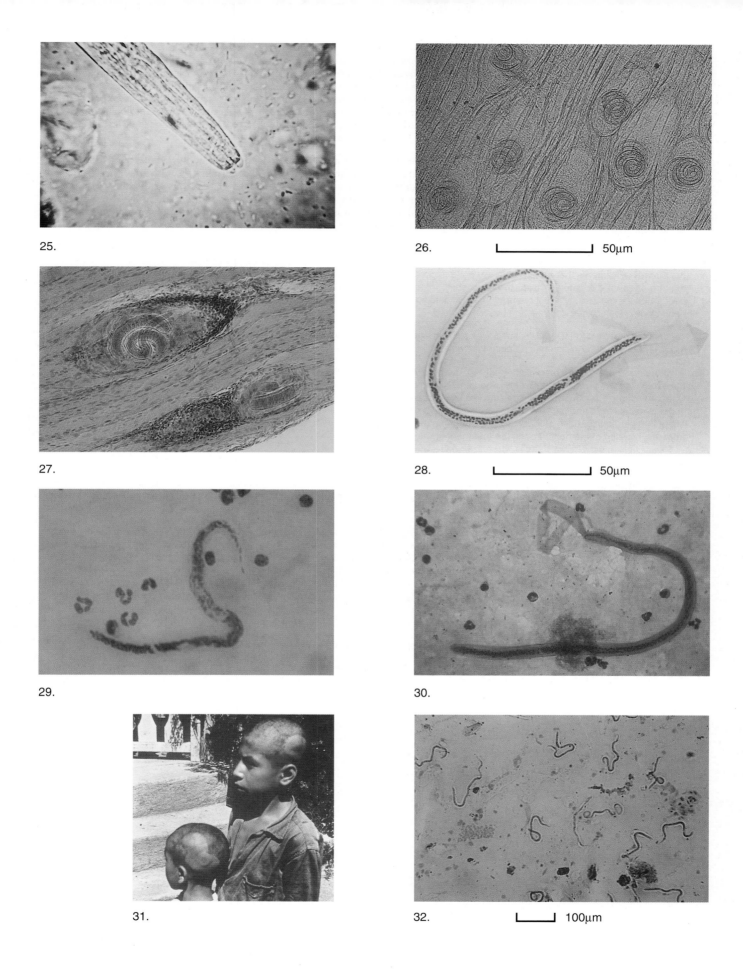

25.

26. ├─────────────┤ 50μm

27.

28. ├─────────────┤ 50μm

29.

30.

31.

32. ├───┤ 100μm

33. *Dracunculus medinensis* (Guinea worm). This view shows part of a female worm protruding from an ulcer and wrapped around a match stick. The female is 70 to 120 cm × 2 mm in length. These worms release larvae into water. Infection occurs when a human drinks water containing crustaceans of the genus *Cyclops* (the intermediate host) infected with a larva of *D. medinensis*. Larvae liberated from the copepods in the human small intestine migrate through the viscera to the subcutaneous tissues and become adults. In the subcutaneous tissues, the female induces an ulcer and releases larvae into water. Larvae released into fresh water penetrate the *Cyclops* intermediate host. The major clinical manifestation of this disease includes allergic symptoms, that is, fever, diarrhea, nausea, eosinophilia, and local symptoms caused by ulcer formation. This parasite is found in the Middle East, Central Africa, the West Indies, and the Guianas. Species that parasitize animals have been found in North America. Diagnosis: detection of the adult in local lesions.

The Cestoda are a subclass of endoparasitic Platyhelminthes (flatworms); the cestodes are commonly known as the tapeworms. The adults live in the intestinal tract of vertebrates, whereas larval forms inhabit tissues of vertebrates or invertebrates. The head (scolex) is modified by suckers and sometimes hooks for attachment to the intestinal wall, and the segments (proglottids), containing both male and female sex organs, bud from the posterior end of the scolex to form the body of the tapeworm (the strobila). The length of tapeworms varies from 2 to 3 mm up to 10 meters. Infection in humans produces primarily intestinal symptoms. Transmission to humans occurs (depending on the species) when insufficiently cooked food containing larvae is eaten or when eggs are ingested.

34. *Hymenolepis nana* (dwarf tapeworm) egg (400 ×). Diagnosis: recovery of characteristic clear, spherical, 30 to 47 μm eggs in feces. Note the threadlike filaments that radiate from two polar thickenings into the area between the embryo and outer shell. Three pairs of hooklets may be seen on the embryo inside the inner shell. Infection is by ingestion of the egg, which hatches in the duodenum. The embryo penetrates the mucosa, where it matures to a cysticercoid larva in the intestinal wall. The larva emerges in a few days and develops to an adult worm. No separate intermediate host is required.

35. *Hymenolepis nana* egg (100 ×). A low-power view of another egg. The rat tapeworm (*H. diminuta*) may also infect humans; the egg is much larger (70–85 μm) and has no polar filaments.

36. *Hymenolepis nana* mature proglottids (100 ×). The proglottid contains a bilobed ovary and three round testes. The testes are visible, but the ovary is not easily seen in this view. Segments are tiny and usually disintegrate in the intestine before passage in the feces. The whole worm measures 2.5 to 4 cm and is the smallest tapeworm to parasitize humans. Multiple infections are common because eggs can hatch in the intestinal tract and cause an immediate autoinfection as the larvae enter the mucosa. The body of the worm (the strobila) contains about 200 proglottids. Each of these flattened segments contains complete male and female reproductive organs. All nutrient is absorbed from the intestine of the host through the tegument of the tapeworm.

37. *Hymenolepis nana* scolex (100 ×). The small scolex bears four suckers and a retractable rostellar crown with one row of 20 to 30 hooklets. These structures provide for firm attachment to the intestinal mucosa. Light infections may be asymptomatic, but heavy infections produce diarrhea, vomiting, weight loss, and anal irritation. This parasite is found in India and South America and is common in children in the southeastern United States. Autoinfection may occur if eggs hatch inside the host, but usually reinfection is caused by hand-to-mouth transfer of eggs after scratching the irritated anal region.

38. *Taenia* species egg. *Taenia solium* (pork tapeworm) or *T. saginata* (beef tapeworm) egg (400 ×). *Taenia* eggs (30 to 45 μm) are diagnostic for the genus only. Notice the thick, yellow-brown outer shell with its radial striations. The hexacanth embryo inside the eggshell bears six chitin hooklets. The six hooklets are not visible in this view. Eggs of *T. solium* are infective for both pigs and humans. If eggs are accidentally ingested by humans, they hatch, just as they do in pigs, in the small intestine. Larval forms (*Cysticercus cellulosae*) develop in the subcutaneous tissues, striated muscles, and other tissues of the body. Symptoms vary with the location of the cyst. Eggs of *T. saginata* are not at all infective for humans. The source of human infection with the adult pork or beef tapeworm is ingestion of insufficiently cooked pork or beef containing encysted *Cysticercus* larvae. After being digested free, the scolex in the *Cysticercus* everts and attaches to the small intestine, and the larva grows to become an adult in 6 to 10 weeks.

39. *Taenia* spp. eggs (100 ×). This view shows four eggs at low power. Pollen grains may resemble eggs under low power.

40. *Taenia solium* (pork or "armed" tapeworm) scolex (100 ×). Four suckers and a rostellum bearing 20 to 30 large hooks are set in two rows at the anterior end of the scolex. *T. saginata* can be differentiated from *T. solium* because the *T. saginata* scolex does not have hooks, only four suckers, and is therefore said to be "unarmed."

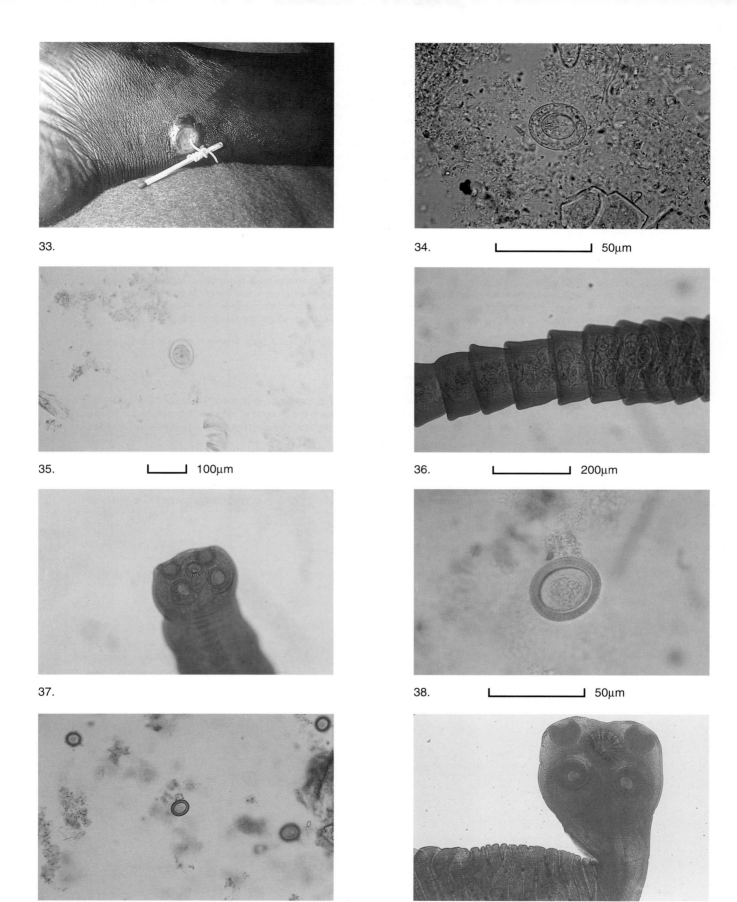

33.

34.   ⊢————————⊣ 50μm

35.   ⊢——⊣ 100μm

36.   ⊢————⊣ 200μm

37.

38.   ⊢————⊣ 50μm

39.   ⊢——⊣ 100μm

40.

41. *Taenia saginata* (beef tapeworm) scolex (100 ×). This is the unarmed tapeworm; the scolex bears only four large, cup-shaped suckers and no hooks.

42. *Taenia solium* gravid proglottid (5 ×). The adult worm measures 2 to 8 meters in length, usually with fewer than 1000 proglottids. The gravid proglottid has 7 to 13 (usually 9) lateral uterine branches (here stained dark brown) filled with eggs, which is diagnostic for the species when recovered in the feces. Gravid proglottids of *Taenia* species must burst open to release eggs because they have no uterine opening. (Note: Handle with care because eggs are infective.)

43. *Taenia saginata* (beef tapeworm) gravid proglottid (5 ×). The adult measures 5 to 10 meters in length and has 1000 to 2000 proglottids. Each gravid proglottid has 15 to 30 lateral uterine branches containing about 80,000 eggs, which is diagnostic for the species when recovered in feces. The life cycle of both worms requires that the eggs be ingested by the appropriate intermediate host (the pig or cow). The eggs hatch in the small intestine after ingestion by the intermediate host, and the six-hooked embryos penetrate the mucosal wall. They are carried by the circulation (blood and lymphatic) to various tissues, where they encyst. Undercooked or raw beef or pork containing *Cysticercus* larvae, when ingested, allow larvae to develop into adults. Toxic metabolites and irritation at the site of scolex attachment in the intestine by adult worms cause the human clinical symptoms. These are variable and frequently vague and include abdominal distress, weight loss, and neuropathies.

44. *Diphyllobothrium latum* (broad fish tapeworm) egg (400 ×). *D. latum* eggs (56 to 76 μm × 40 to 50 μm) are operculated (have a lid) and may be differentiated from operculated eggs of other helminths by the polar knob seen opposite the operculum, the large size, and the undeveloped embryo seen within. Diagnosis is made when these eggs are recovered in stool specimens. Undeveloped eggs discharged from segments of the adult tapeworm must reach fresh water, where they mature and hatch, and the embryo infects the first intermediate host (copepods). Fish ingest infected copepods (water fleas) and serve as the second intermediate host. Humans and dogs acquire the infection by eating raw or undercooked parasitized fish containing the infective larval stage, the plerocercoid.

45. *Diphyllobothrium latum* egg (400 ×). The operculum (eggshell cap) of this egg is open. A polar knob is evident at the opposite end of the shell.

46. *Diphyllobothrium latum* egg (100 ×). A low-power view of the same egg.

47. *Diphyllobothrium latem* scolex (5 ×). The scolex of this species does not have hooks or cup-shaped suckers but is characterized by two grooved suckers (bothria), one on each side of the scolex. This worm attaches to the mucosa of the small intestine by the bothria and can grow to 20 meters in length. Eggs develop in cold, clear lakes in temperate regions, including the Great Lakes in North America.

48. *Diphyllobothrium latum* proglottid (10 ×). The mature segment is much wider than it is tall and contains a rosette-shaped uterus. There is a uterine pore through which eggs are discharged. This parasite is found worldwide in areas around fresh water. In the United States, it is found in Florida, the Great Lakes region, and Alaska. The disease is often asymptomatic or is accompanied by vague, digestive disturbances. Some patients develop a macrocytic anemia of the pernicious anemia type because the worm successfully competes with the host for dietary vitamin B_{12} and absorbs it before it can enter the host's circulation. Chains of proglottids may be found in feces.

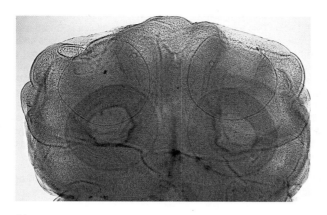

41.

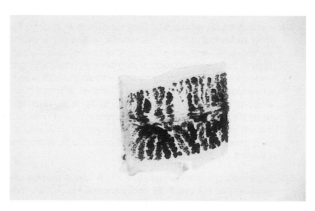

42.

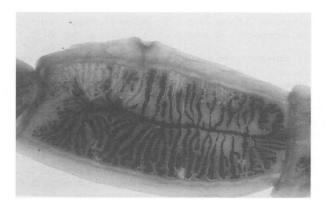

43.

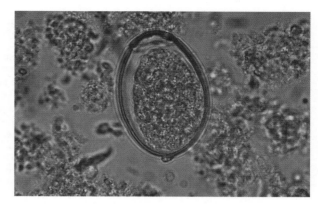

44. |⊢——————⊣| 50µm

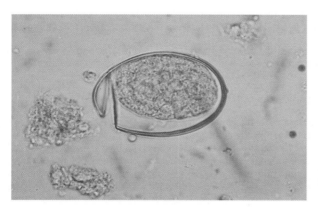

45. |⊢——————⊣| 50µm

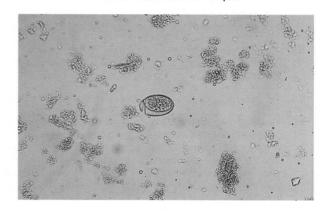

46. |⊢——⊣| 100µm

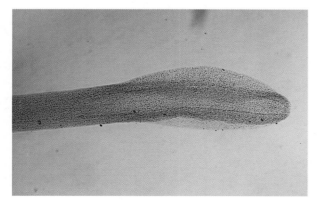

47.

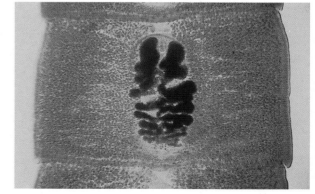

48.

49. *Echinococcus granulosus* (dog tapeworm or hydatid cyst tapeworm) adult (5 ×). This view shows the entire worm, which is 3 to 6 mm long and is found only in the small intestine of the canine host. The dog or wolf is the definitive host and harbors the sexually mature adult parasites. Sheep and other ruminants are natural intermediate hosts and harbor the asexual stage of the parasite in the tissues, but a human can be an accidental intermediate host for *E. granulosus.* Infection of sheep or humans occurs when eggs are ingested in contaminated food or water or by hand-to-mouth transfer from objects soiled with dog feces. Eggs hatch in the small intestine, and larvae migrate to various organs (usually liver or lung) to produce cysts. Dogs and other wild carnivores become infected by eating raw meat containing a hydatid cyst, thus completing the cycle. In humans the produced disease varies with the location of the cyst. There may be no symptoms, or death may result if vital organs are involved. The parasite is found worldwide. Although rare in Europe and most of the United States, except in sheep-raising areas, it is common in Alaska and Canada. Diagnosis in humans is by history of possible exposure; by radiology; by immunodiagnostic skin testing or serologic testing; and by observing hooklets, scolices, and larval cyst membranes in histopathologic sections or other body fluids.

50. *Echinococcus granulosus* (100 ×). A tissue section showing the wall of the hydatid cyst and three brood capsules containing scolices growing into the cyst fluid from germinal tissue that underlies the outer cyst wall.

51. *Echinococcus granulosus* (500 ×). A higher magnification of a single cyst. Each scolex clearly shows the suckers and crown of hooks. Each scolex in a hydatid cyst will grow to an adult tapeworm after ingestion by a dog.

52. *Echinococcus granulosus* cysts. This view shows several small cysts taken from the vertebral column of a patient with spinal cord compression. Cysts in humans can be in any tissue, including bone, but are more common in liver, lung, or central nervous system (CNS).

The Digenea (flukes) are known as flatworms because they appear flat, elongated, and leaf-shaped. Both male and female sex organs are found in each adult fluke that parasitizes the intestine, bile duct, or lungs. The blood flukes (genus *Schistosoma*), however, are unisexual but live paired together in the blood vessels. Attachment is by the oral and ventral cup-shaped suckers; moreover, the tegument of the flukes may bear small spines that aid attachment. These parasites vary in size from less than 1 mm to several centimeters in length. All trematodes require specific species of snail intermediate hosts, and infection of humans occurs either by direct penetration of the skin by a free-swimming cercaria (schistosome species) or by ingestion of an encysted metacercaria (infective larva) of hermaphroditic flukes. Adult flukes live many years.

53. *Fasciola hepatica* (sheep liver fluke) adult (2 ×). This parasite is found in sheep- and cattle-raising areas worldwide, including the United States. Encysted metacercariae on aquatic vegetation, eaten by humans, sheep, or cattle, excyst, burrow through the intestinal wall, migrate to the liver, and work their way through the parenchyma until they enter the proximal bile duct, where they become adults (3 cm × 1.3 cm). Visible structures include the anterior cone, the oral and ventral suckers located at the anterior end, the compact uterus (dark brown) adjacent to the ventral sucker, Mehlis' gland (a round structure centered beneath the uterus), and the testes, occupying the central portion of the fluke. The vitellaria (finely branching, yolk-producing glands) extend from top to bottom toward the outer edges of the parasite and partially cover the testes over the posterior one-third. Disease symptoms reflect traumatic damage, with tissue necrosis and toxic irritation to the liver, bile duct, and gallbladder. Diarrhea, vomiting, irregular fever, jaundice, and eosinophilia are characteristic symptoms.

54. *Fasciola hepatica* egg (400 ×). Diagnosis: by recovery of this large, operculated egg in feces and by clinical signs. This egg is very similar to that of *Fasciolopsis buski* (see Plate 57). Differentiation of eggs of these two parasites is very difficult. Eggs of *F. hepatica* measure 140 μm × 70 μm.

55. *Fasciola hepatica* egg (100 ×). A low-power view of the large *F. hepatica* egg in the midst of naturally occurring fecal debris.

56. *Fasciolopsis buski* (large intestinal fluke) (2 ×). *F. buski* (2 to 7.5 cm × 1 to 2 cm) is found primarily in Asia. Encysted larvae (metacercariae) on vegetation eaten by humans or pigs mature to become adults and attach to the mucosa of the small intestine. Identifiable and differential structures include the unbranched intestinal ceca running laterally from top to bottom toward the outer edges; the two suckers of unequal size (round structures at the top of the organism); the uterus (a dark canal centered under the ventral sucker, branching laterally); Mehlis' gland with attached ovary centered approximately one-third of the way posterior to the ventral sucker; and the testes, branching laterally from the center, beneath the ovary. The anterior end tapers to form the oral sucker, which is visible in this view. Disease symptoms caused by toxic products absorbed into the host's circulation include general edema, diarrhea, vomiting, anorexia, and, possibly, malabsorption syndrome. Slight anemia and eosinophilia occur in severe infections.

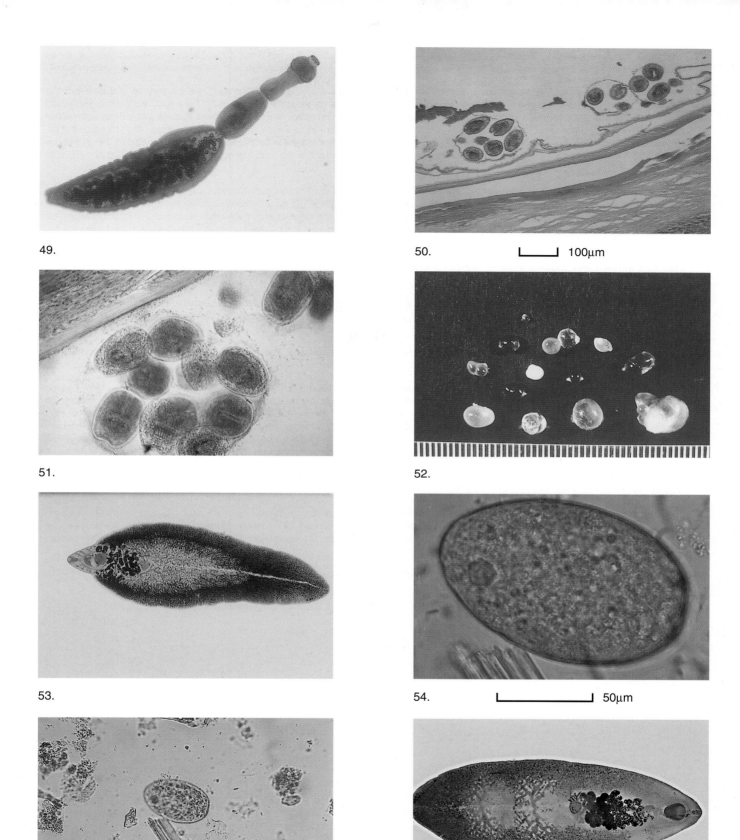

49.

50. |⊢———⊣| 100μm

51.

52.

53.

54. |⊢————⊣| 50μm

55. |⊢——⊣| 100μm

56.

57. *Fasciolopsis buski* egg (400 ×). Recovery of this large, thin-shelled, operculated egg (140 μm × 70 μm) is diagnostic. The operculum (lid) is visible here, open at the right end of the egg. This egg is empty; it was previously incubated, and the larva has hatched out of the shell.

58. *Fasciolopsis buski* egg (100 ×). Immediately below this large egg appears a *Trichuris trichiura* egg; this is a very good example of the difference in size between the eggs of the two organisms. The operculum is visible at the left end of the fluke egg, and the material inside of it is yolk. Most of the trematode eggs are undifferentiated when found in fecal specimens. Eggs of all species must reach fresh water before further development occurs. After full development, the first larval form (miracidium) hatches and penetrates the soft tissues of an appropriate intermediate host, the snail. The miracidia develop through several stages to produce free-swimming cercariae, which then (in this species) encyst on aquatic vegetation as metacercariae, which are infective when the vegetation is eaten by a human. *Fasciola hepatica* eggs look identical.

59. *Clonorchis sinensis* (Oriental liver fluke) (4 ×). This adult measures 1 to 2.5 cm × 3 to 5 mm. Humans are infected by eating raw fish, the second intermediate host, containing encysted metacercariae. Larvae excyst in the small intestine and migrate to the bile ducts, where they develop into adult worms. Visible structures include the oral sucker at the anterior end, the ventral sucker one-quarter posteriorly to the oral sucker, the uterus (a dark, branching structure extending downward from the ventral sucker to the ovary), and the testes, immediately below the large, oval Mehlis' gland. The ceca extend from top to bottom toward the outer edge. The vitellaria are parallel to the uterus. This parasite is found throughout the Orient and causes obstructive liver damage with extensive biliary fibrosis. Symptoms result from local irritation and systemic toxemia. Loss of appetite, diarrhea, abdominal pain, and eosinophilia (5 to 40 percent) are common symptoms.

60. *Clonorchis sinensis* egg (500 ×). Eggs (15 μm × 30 μm) are deposited in the bile duct and are evacuated in feces. Diagnosis: recovery of this small, bile-stained egg in feces. Note the thick shell, the characteristic bell shape, and the thickened opercular rim (the shoulders). There is usually a polar knob opposite the operculum.

61. *Clonorchis sinensis* egg (100 ×). A low-power view of a developed *C. sinensis* egg. The eggs are difficult to differentiate from those of other genera (e.g., *Opisthorchis*).

62. *Paragonimus westermani* (lung fluke) (4 ×). This lung-dwelling adult measures 0.8 to 1.2 cm × 4 to 6 mm. Humans are infected by eating raw crab or crayfish, the second intermediate host, containing encysted metacercariae. Larvae excyst in the small intestine; burrow through the mucosa; and migrate through the peritoneal cavity, the diaphragm, and the pleural cavity to the lungs, where they develop into adult worms. Visible structures include the oral sucker at the anterior end; the ovary, which is immediately below the ventral sucker about midway down in the organism; the dark-staining uterus to the left of the ovary; and the testes, located in the clear space beneath the ovary. The branching vitellaria are visible along the outer edges of the parasite. This parasite is found throughout the Orient and parts of Africa. It causes a chronic tuberculosis-type disease with fibrous capsules forming around the adults. Eggs are coughed up in sputum and are visible as orange-brown flecks. Clinical signs resemble those of tuberculosis, including cough with bloody sputum. Adults may invade other organs. Symptoms vary with the location of the adult fluke.

63. *Paragonimus westermani* egg (300 ×). Diagnosis: recovery of this operculated egg (80 to 120 μm × 50 to 60 μm) in sputum or feces. Eggs can be found in fecal specimens when sputum containing eggs is swallowed. Skin testing may provide better evidence of infections than do fecal examinations. Notice the thin shell and the thickened rim around the operculum. The shell also thickens at the end opposite the operculum.

64. *Paragonimus westermani* egg (100 ×). A low-power view of the egg in the center of fecal debris.

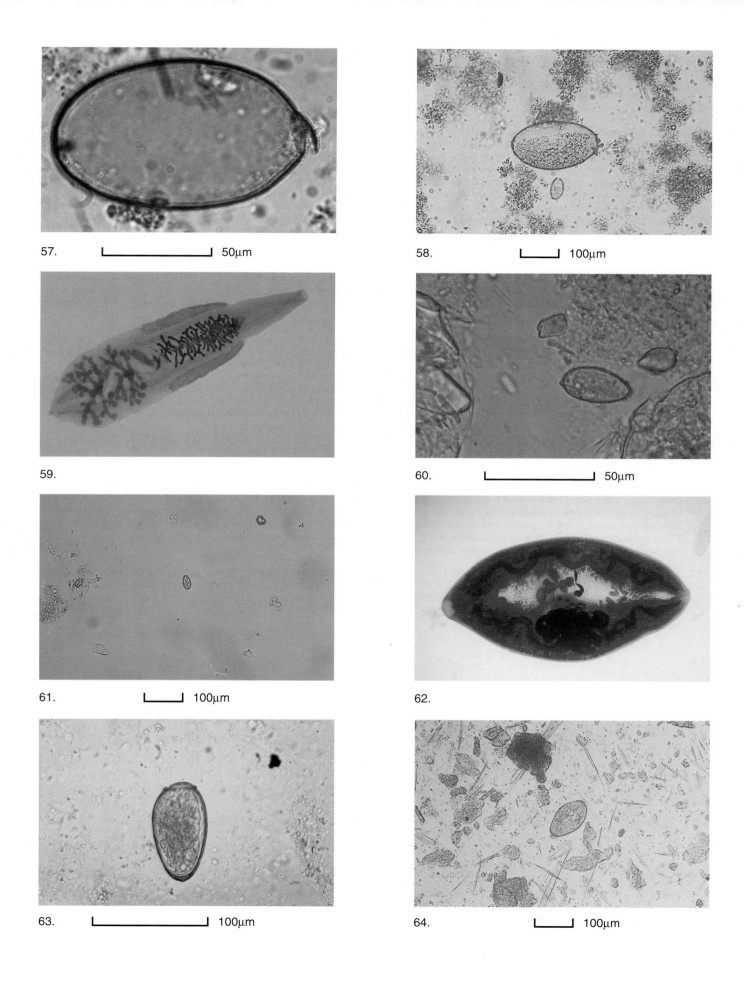

57. ├─────────────┤ 50μm

58. ├───┤ 100μm

59.

60. ├─────────┤ 50μm

61. ├───┤ 100μm

62.

63. ├─────────┤ 100μm

64. ├───┤ 100μm

65. *Schistosoma* species (blood flukes). Adults are in copula. The female (15 to 30 mm × 0.2 mm) is seen lying inside the gynecophoral canal of the male. These unisexual worms have a cylindroidal shape and live in pairs, surviving for many years. Infection occurs when free-swimming, fork-tailed cercariae escape from the snail intermediate host; burrow into the capillary bed of feet, legs, or arms of humans; and are carried to the blood vessels of the liver, where they develop into adults. From there, *S. mansoni* and *S. japonicum* migrate to mesenteric veins around the colon. *S. haematobium* migrates to pelvic veins around the urinary bladder.

66. *Schistosoma mansoni* egg (400 ×). Diagnosis: recovery of eggs in feces. Unlike the other trematodes, schistosome eggs do not have an operculum. Note the large size (115 to 175 μm × 50 to 70 μm) and the conspicuous lateral spine protruding from the side near one pole. A ciliated miracidium is indistinct but visible inside this egg, but in fresh specimens it is generally distinct and motile, with active cilia and flame cells. Eggs are deposited into venules, eventually rupture the wall to effect passage into the lumen of the intestine, and are evacuated in the feces. Many eggs are caught in tissues of the liver and intestine, and a granuloma forms around each egg in response to toxic enzymes released by the miracidium. Clinical manifestations include high eosinophilia (up to 50%), gastrointestinal bleeding, rectal polyps, and hepatic cirrhosis. This parasite is found in Africa, the Middle East, parts of South America, the West Indies, and Puerto Rico. Infected persons can frequently be found in immigrant populations living in North American urban centers.

67. *Schistosoma mansoni* egg (100 ×). A low-power view of several eggs. Note the lateral spines on the eggs.

68. *Schistosoma japonicum* egg (400 ×). Diagnosis: recovery of eggs in feces. This egg measures 70 to 100 μm × 50 to 60 μm. A small lateral spine on the eggshell is characteristic for this species. A ciliated miracidium is seen inside the egg. The produced disease is similar to that of *S. mansoni*. Because *S. japonicum* produces 10 times as many eggs as *S. mansoni*, the disease is more severe. Many eggs are swept back into the bloodstream to the liver and are trapped, causing fibrosis and cirrhosis of the liver. Toxic symptoms are severe. This parasite is found in the Orient.

69. *Schistosoma japonicum* eggs (100 ×). A low-power view of several eggs. The lateral spine is barely visible in some eggs. *S. mekongi* eggs are similar but small (50 to 75 μm × 40 to 65 μm). These eggs are often coated with fecal debris and are more difficult to notice.

70. *Schistosoma haematobium* egg (400 ×). Diagnosis: recovery of eggs in urine. This egg measures 115 to 175 μm × 40 to 70 μm. A pointed terminal spine is characteristic for this species. A ciliated miracidium is visible inside. Egg deposition by *S. haematobium* causes local traumatic damage to the rectum and the urinary bladder. Bladder colic is a cardinal symptom. Blood, pus cells, and necrotic tissue debris are passed during urination. Systemic symptoms are less severe than those produced by the other schistosomes. There is a high correlation with bladder cancer in infected persons. This parasite is found in Africa, the Middle East, and Portugal.

71. *Schistosoma haematobium* egg (300 ×). A high-power view of the egg, showing a differently shaped terminal spine. Urine should be concentrated to aid detection. Eggs are most often in the last few drops expelled from the bladder.

Amebae are unicellular protozoa, some of which may be parasitic in humans. These organisms are found worldwide, and some can live as parasitic or commensal trophozoites (the motile, feeding, reproductive stage) in the lower gastrointestinal tract of humans. Most intestinal protozoa form a cyst stage (a dormant, protective stage for the parasite in unfavorable environments after being evacuated in the host's feces) and in the cyst form may remain viable for long periods in warm, moist conditions. Transmission of intestinal amebic diseases is from ingested cysts in fecally contaminated food, soil, or water. Cysts are most commonly passed in feces by asymptomatic carriers.

72. *Entamoeba histolytica* trophozoite (10 to 60 μm) (1000 ×). This ameba is pathogenic for humans. It can invade the intestinal mucosa, causing flask-shaped lesions and bloody diarrhea. The trophozoite releases lytic enzymes and can also spread to other tissues, such as the liver, and cause amebic ulceration. Notice the nucleus, which has a light chromatin ring at the edges, surrounding a centrally located karyosome (compare with *Entamoeba coli*, Plate 78). The cytoplasm is finely granular as compared with that of *E. coli*. This is a trichrome-stained organism.

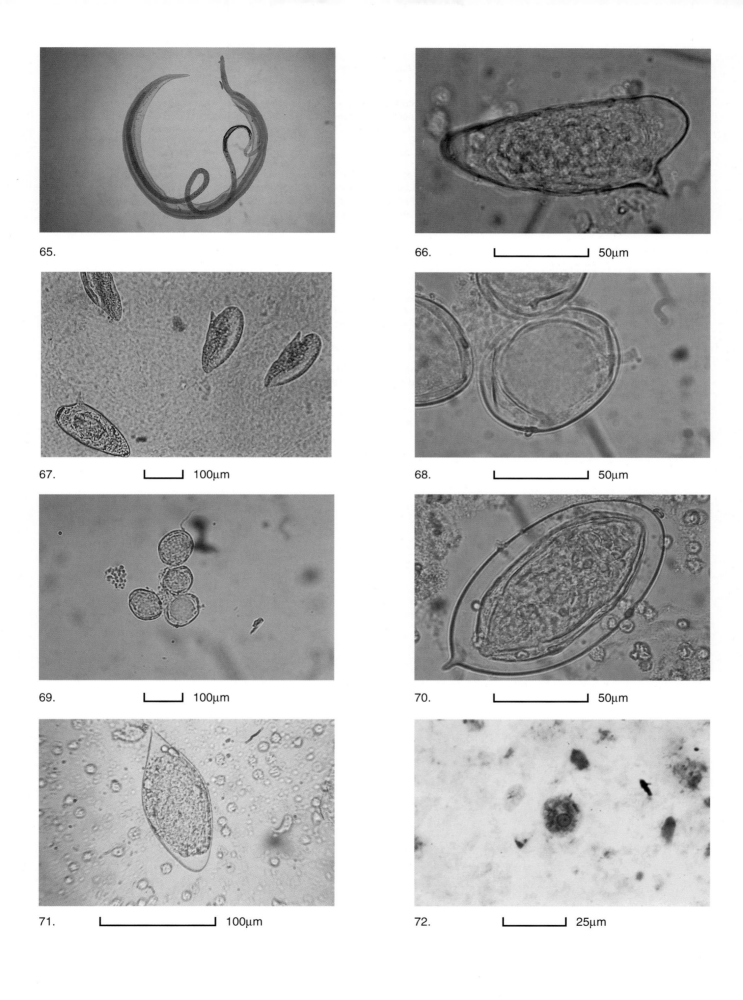

65.

66. |⸻| 50μm

67. |⸻| 100μm

68. |⸻| 50μm

69. |⸻| 100μm

70. |⸻| 50μm

71. |⸻| 100μm

72. |⸻| 25μm

73. *Entamoeba histolytica* (1000 ×). This trophozoite in feces contains five engulfed red blood cells, the presence of which is a diagnostic feature, inasmuch as no other ameba contains these. In saline solution, the trophozoite exhibits progressive, active motility, with thin, finger-like pseudopodia.

74. *Entamoeba histolytica* cyst (1000 ×). Cysts of *E. histolytica* are over 10 μm in size (10 to 20 μm). There are up to four typical nuclei in the mature cyst. One nucleus is clearly visible here. The nuclear structure is identical in both trophozoites and cysts. The dark bars are chromatoid bodies, generally cigar-shaped, which may be found in cysts. These are crystalline RNA. Iron hematoxylin stain.

75. *Entamoeba histolytica* cyst (1000 ×) showing four nuclei. Iodine stain.

76. *Entamoeba hartmanni* trophozoite (1000 ×). Note the morphologic similarity between the nucleus of this commensal and that in Plate 72. This organism was previously identified as *E. histolytica* but is now known as *E. hartmanni*. It is not pathogenic, but morphologically resembles *E. histolytica*, differing only in size; it is less than 10 μm in size. This characteristic is important because correct diagnosis depends upon the careful measurement of the parasite. A trophozoite or cyst resembling *E. histolytica* that is less than 10 μm in diameter is classified as *E. hartmanni*.

77. *Entamoeba hartmanni* cyst (1000 ×). The cyst (5 to 10 μm) resembles that of *E. histolytica* but is classified as *E. hartmanni* because of its small size, the upper limits being 10 μm. This cyst is stained with iodine. It can have up to four nuclei. It is important to differentiate *E. histolytica* from this and other nonpathogenic amebae to ensure correct treatment of the patient.

78. *Entamoeba coli* trophozoite (1000 ×). This is a common commensal, and care must be taken to differentiate it from *E. histolytica*. Notice the nucleus, which has a dark, irregularly thickened chromatin ring around the membrane and a large, eccentrically located karyosome. This parasite is often larger than *E. histolytica* (15 to 60 μm) and has coarser cytoplasm and sluggish motility, with blunt pseudopodia.

79. *Entamoeba coli* trophozoite (1000 ×). This trophozoite has a very large karyosome located next to the chromatin ring.

80. *Entamoeba coli* cyst (1000 ×). Five nuclei are visible in the cyst (10 to 30 μm). *E. coli* is differentiated from *E. histolytica* by the nuclear morphology and by the fact that the cyst may contain up to eight nuclei, rather than four. Chromatoid bars in stained cysts are splinterlike, with pointed ends.

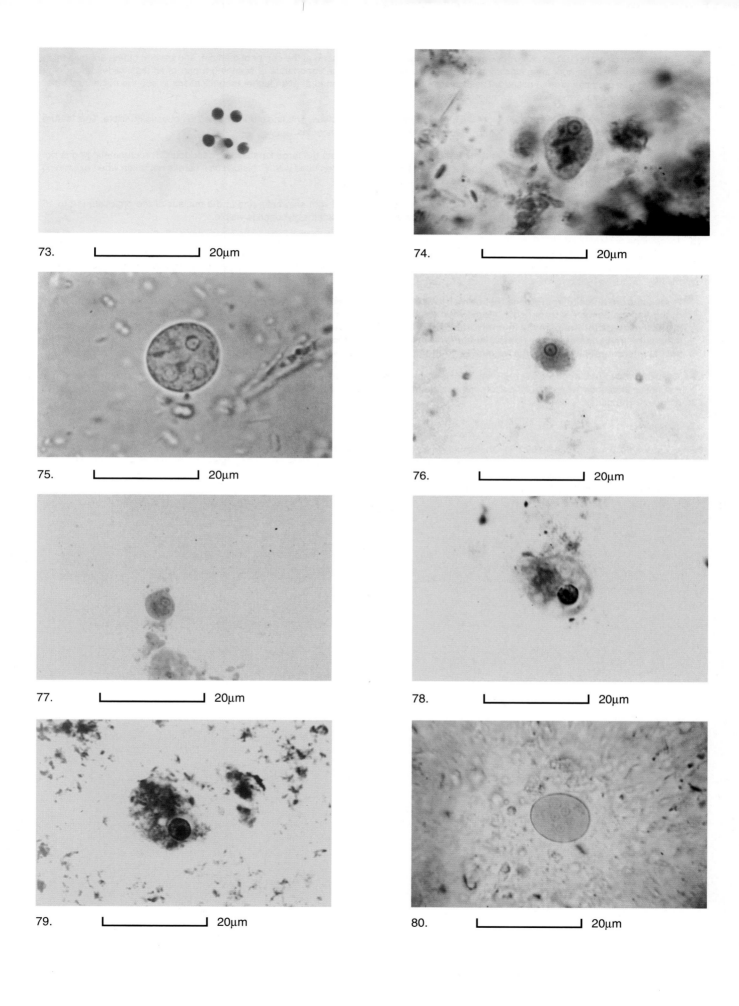

73. |⎯⎯⎯⎯⎯⎯⎯| 20μm

74. |⎯⎯⎯⎯⎯⎯⎯| 20μm

75. |⎯⎯⎯⎯⎯⎯⎯| 20μm

76. |⎯⎯⎯⎯⎯⎯⎯| 20μm

77. |⎯⎯⎯⎯⎯⎯⎯| 20μm

78. |⎯⎯⎯⎯⎯⎯⎯| 20μm

79. |⎯⎯⎯⎯⎯⎯⎯| 20μm

80. |⎯⎯⎯⎯⎯⎯⎯| 20μm

81. *Entamoeba coli* cysts (100 ×). A low-power view of several cysts. One is seen at the center of the field, and several others are evident in the lower left area, all appearing as dark dots. This view demonstrates the importance of scanning a part of all fecal slides under high power so that protozoa are not missed. These cysts also should be examined at even higher magnifications to see the nuclei and other features for correct diagnosis of the parasite species.

82. *Endolimax nana* trophozoite (1000 ×). Note the large karyosome in the nucleus. The fine chromatin ring is not usually visible. This feature is diagnostic for this commensal (6 to 12 μm). Note also the cytoplasmic vacuoles.

83. *Endolimax nana* cyst (2000 ×). The ovoid mature cyst has four nuclei. Note the large karyosome (dark dots). The chromatin ring is not visible. These features are diagnostic. This parasite (8 to 10 μm) may be confused with *E. histolytica* if care is not taken when examining the nuclear structure and the cyst shape.

84. *Iodamoeba bütschlii* trophozoite (1000 ×). Note the large karyosome and light chromatin ring in the nucleus of the organism (12 to 15 μm). The cytoplasm is coarsely granular, and a small, light vacuole that contains glycogen is visible.

85. *Iodamoeba bütschlii* cyst (1000 ×). Note the large karyosome in the single nucleus of this trichrome-stained cyst (5 to 20 μm). A large vacuole from which glycogen has been removed by the staining process is visible (clear area inside cyst), which is diagnostic for this commensal. The glycogen vacuole stains dark brown when an iodine wet mount is used. The nucleus of this species does not stain with iodine.

Flagellates are unicellular protozoa that move by means of flagella (motile fibrils extending from the body of the organism). Many of the flagellates have a trophozoite stage, which is the active, feeding, motile form, and also a cyst stage, which is a dormant, protective stage for the parasite in unfavorable environments outside the host's intestine. Transmission of the intestinal flagellates is by ingestion of fecally contaminated food or drink; *Trichomonas vaginalis* trophozoites are directly transmitted during sexual intercourse; and the hemoflagellates (found in the blood or tissues) are transmitted by arthropod intermediate hosts.

86. *Dientamoeba fragilis* trophozoite (1000 ×). This flagellate (5 to 12 μm) does not form cysts. Note that it has two nuclei. This feature is diagnostic inasmuch as no other ameboid trophozoite has more than one nucleus. This organism may be pathogenic and may cause diarrhea in humans.

87. *D. fragilis.*

88. *Giardia lamblia* trophozoites (1000 ×). These flagellates (10 to 20 μm × 15 μm) live in the duodenum and often do not produce disease. When present in large numbers, they may cause epigastric pain and diarrhea. Note the smiling face–like appearance of the trophozoite, which is bilaterally symmetric with two anterior nuclei, a central axostyle, and four pairs of flagella. In fresh fecal wet-mount preparations, the motile trophozoite moves like a leaf falling from a tree.

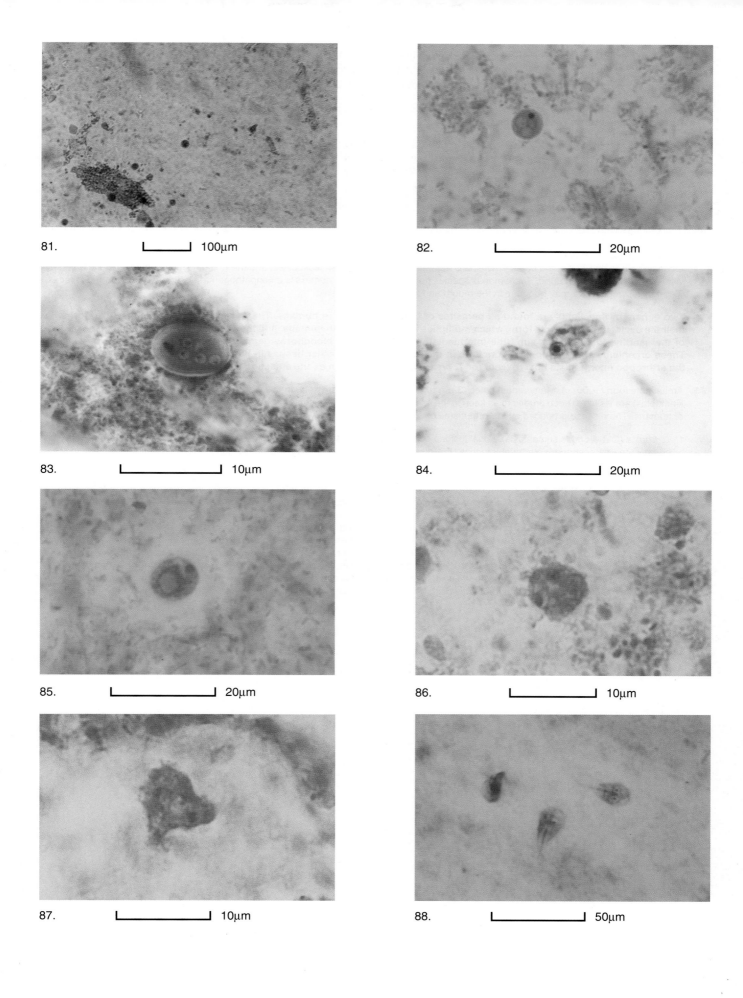

81.   100µm

82.   20µm

83.   10µm

84.   20µm

85.   20µm

86.   10µm

87.   10µm

88.   50µm

89. *Giardia lamblia* cyst (1000 ×). Diagnosis: recovery of trophozoites or cysts (8 μm × 10 μm) in feces. The mature cyst has four nuclei, although the immature cyst may have only two. Three are visible in the upper cyst in this view.

90. Unusual sight of *Entamoeba coli* trophozoite containing several ingested *Giardia lamblia* cysts (1000 ×).

91. *Giardia lamblia* trophozoites (1000 ×). This stained section of duodenal mucosa shows two trophozoites adhering. Note the two nuclei visible in the trophozoite centered in the field.

92. *Chilomastix mesnili* trophozoite (1000 ×). This commensal flagellate (7 μm × 20 μm) lives in the upper large intestine and does not produce disease. Note the single prominent nucleus at the rounded anterior end. The posterior is tapered with a noticeably angled projection. There are four anterior flagella and a distinct longitudinal spiral groove. Viable trophozoites move in a spiral path.

93. *Chilomastix mesnili* cyst (1000 ×). Diagnosis: recovery of cysts (5 μm × 8 μm) in feces. There is a single, large nucleus in this lemon-shaped cyst. Correct diagnosis is important so that this is not confused with *Giardia* or other pathogenic infection.

94. *Trichomonas vaginalis* trophozoite (1000 ×). This parasite (18 μm × 25 μm) is recovered in urine or in urethral or vaginal mucosal scrapings. Symptoms in women vary from mild irritation to painful itching, with a frothy, yellowish vaginal discharge. Infected men are usually asymptomatic carriers. There are four anterior flagella, a large nucleus, and an undulating membrane (not visible in this view) extending along one-half of the body. *T. vaginalis* appears slightly larger than leukocytes, and the whipping motion of the flagella is clearly visible in fresh, unstained urine. *Trichomonas* species do not form cysts. *T. hominis* is a nonpathogenic intestinal flagellate found in feces; *T. gingivalis* trophozoite may be found in the mouth and is also nonpathogenic.

Two genera of flagellates are found as parasites of blood and tissue in humans. The *Leishmania* parasites have two forms in their life cycle: the amastigote form, which multiplies in macrophages in humans, and the promastigote form found in the midgut of the sandfly, *Phlebotomus* spp. (the intermediate host). The other bloodborne genus parasitic in humans is *Trypanosoma*. These organisms are in trypomastigote form in the bloodstream and other tissues in humans, and in the epimastigote form in the arthropod intermediate host (except for *T. cruzi*, which is also seen as the amastigote form in human heart muscle).

95. Amastigote form (1000 ×). Many amastigotes (3 μm to 5 μm in diameter) are seen in this view. The nucleus and the smaller, bar-shaped kinetoplast are visible in each organism as seen in the center of this field. The leishmania invade reticuloendothelial cells and macrophages of humans. The disease produced by the organisms of each species is as follows:

1. *L. tropica* (Old World leishmaniasis). Local lesions occur at the site of the sandfly bite, followed by focal necrosis. Although it may be complicated by secondary bacterial infection, the disease is usually self-limiting and produces life-long immunity to reinfection. This parasite is found in Africa, India, and the Middle East.
2. *L. braziliensis* (New World leishmaniasis). The primary lesion is local, as with *L. tropica*, but the ulcer heals slowly. Erosion of soft tissues, especially of the nose, mouth, ears, and cheeks, often occurs years later, inasmuch as this organism tends to migrate to secondary sites, often complicated by bacterial invasion followed by local and systemic symptoms. This parasite is found in Central and South America.
3. *L. donovani* (kala-azar). The local primary lesion is usually not reported. The amastigotes gain access to the bloodstream or lymphatics and eventually spread to fixed tissue macrophages in the viscera. Sites of this invasion are the liver, spleen, and bone marrow, where multiplication usually proceeds unchecked. Anemia usually follows because of increased production of macrophages and decreased erythropoietic activity. The acute phase of the systemic disease is characterized by double spiking fever fluctuating daily (between 90°F and 104°F). There is moderate erythrocytopenia, absolute monocytosis, and neutropenia. Massive hepatosplenomegaly occurs because of parasite multiplication, and death frequently occurs if the patient is untreated. This parasite is widely distributed, except in the United States.

96. *Leishmania donovani* (1000 ×) seen multiplying in a macrophage in a press preparation of spleen tissue.

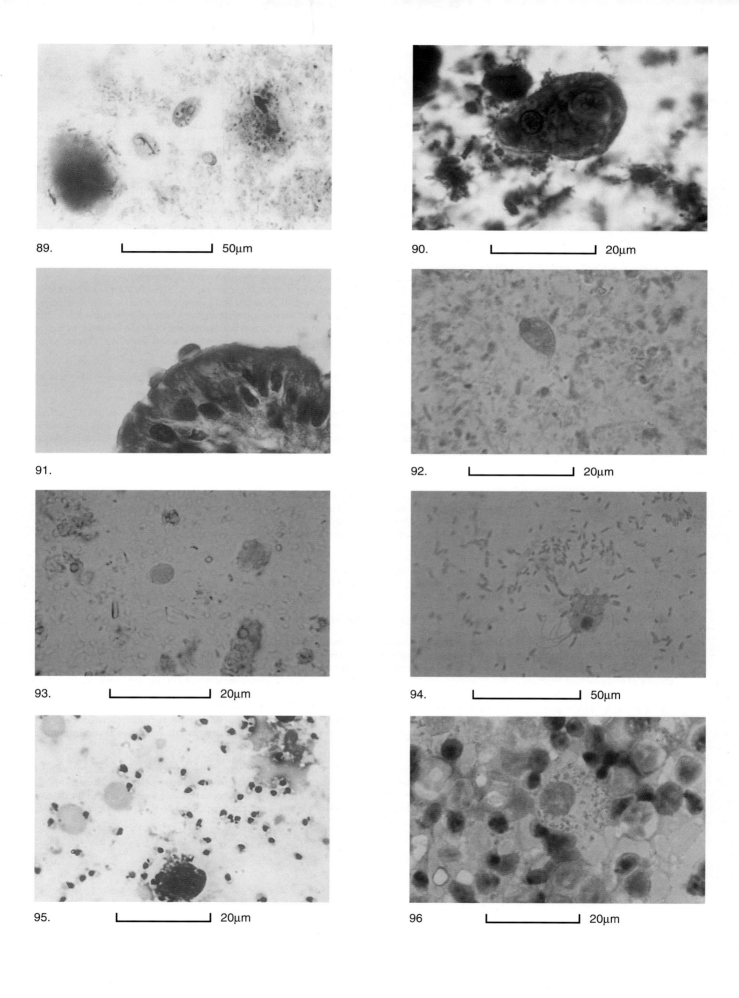

89. |⊢———⊣| 50μm

90. |⊢————————⊣| 20μm

91.

92. |⊢————————⊣| 20μm

93. |⊢————————⊣| 20μm

94. |⊢————————⊣| 50μm

95. |⊢————————⊣| 20μm

96 |⊢————————⊣| 20μm

97. Leishmaniasis. A typical skin lesion caused by *L. braziliensis.* Note the open ulcer on the man's forehead.

98. Promastigote form (100 ×). This stage is found in the midgut and proboscis of the sandfly, *Phlebotomus.* It is the infective form of leishmaniasis and is transferred to humans by the biting fly. The large nucleus, bar-shaped kinetoplast, and flagellum are visible. Note the relative position of these structures.

99. Trypomastigote form (1000 ×). The trypanosome is found extracellularly, free in the blood. It is the infective form transferred to humans by the biting arthropod vector (intermediate host). Trypanosome species are not readily differentiated in peripheral blood. Visible structures include the flagellum, the large central nucleus, and the undulating membrane that is attached to the kinetoplast at the posterior end of the organism. The diseases produced by these organisms are as follows:

1. The sleeping sickness diseases produced by *T. rhodesiense* and *T. gambiense* are similar, differing primarily in the severity of the second stage, which is so severe with *T. rhodesiense* infections that death rapidly results. The disease begins with local inflammation at the site of the fly bite (tsetse fly). This subsides as the trypanosomes enter the blood. They migrate to the lymph nodes, where severe inflammation occurs because of rapid multiplication. Toxic metabolites and occlusion of vascular sinuses by the proliferating organisms may cause death at this stage. Enlarged lymph nodes, myocarditis, fever episodes, edema, and rapid weight loss are cardinal symptoms for *T. rhodesiense.* Trypanosomes invade the central nervous system in the third stage to produce sleeping sickness and eventually death. *T. gambiense* usually proceeds to this stage. The posterior cervical lymph nodes in the neck are invaded and undergo massive swelling. This is called Winterbottom's sign. Other nodes may be invaded, producing weakness, pain, and cramps.

2. *T. cruzi* (Chagas' disease). The primary lesion at the bite site of the reduviid bug intermediate host is often near the eye, producing unilateral edema of the eyelid (Romaña's sign). Next, primary parasitemia with S- or C-shaped trypanosomes with a large kinetoplast (as seen in this view) occurs in the blood, causing fever and toxic conditions resembling typhoid fever (may be fatal in children). The chronic disease is characterized by leishmanial forms multiplying in tissue macrophages, and symptoms of tissue invasion, including enlargement of the spleen, occur. Cardiac and central nervous system pathology occurs as tissue destruction continues. There may be fever episodes and parasitemia when trypanosomes are free in the blood.

Diagnosis of these diseases is confirmed when parasites are recovered in blood or seen in tissue specimens. Trypanosomes are 15 to 30 μm in length.

100. *Trypanosoma cruzi* (amastigote form) in cardiac tissue (1000 ×). The trypomastigote in reduviid bug feces is pushed into the bite wound when the host scratches at the bite site, and these circulate in the blood until phagocytized, or they invade tissue macrophages, after which they change to the amastigote form. Note the nest of multiplying amastigote forms in the heart muscle. Trypomastigote forms can be found in blood.

The Ciliata

101. *Balantidium coli* trophozoite (400 ×). This organism (40 μm × 60 μm) is a ciliate that is characterized by having many short cilia on the surface of both the motile and encysted trophozoite. *B. coli* is the only ciliate pathogenic for humans. The disease is characterized by invasion of the intestinal submucosa with inflammation and ulcer formation. There may be fulminating diarrhea in heavy infections or an asymptomatic carrier state in light infections. This organism has two nuclei: a large, kidney bean–shaped macronucleus and a small, round micronucleus not visible in this view.

102. *Balantidium coli* cyst (400 ×). This large, round cyst (50 μm) is characterized by the presence of macronuclei and micronuclei; the latter are rarely seen, but when present, generally appear as small dots near the concavity of the macronucleus. Cilia are evident around the inside edge of the cyst on the organism. This form, or the trophozoite, is diagnostic when recovered in feces or seen in intestinal tissue.

103. *Balantidium coli* cyst (100 ×). A low-power view of the cyst. This large parasite is easily recognized even at this magnification.

Sporozoa are protozoa that have both a sexual and an asexual phase in their life cycle. The genus *Plasmodium* includes the malaria parasites. The asexual phase is found in the human intermediate host, and the sexual phase occurs in the definitive host, the *Anopheles* mosquito. Sporozoites are injected into the blood by the biting mosquito and then invade liver cells. The asexual stages of malaria first multiply in the liver and later in peripheral blood. Asexual schizogony results in release of merozoites that may either invade new red blood cells and develop into new schizonts or develop to become male and female gametocytes. If the mosquito ingests gametocytes while feeding, these will develop throughout the sexual cycle to produce new sporozoites, the infective form for humans. The clinical symptoms vary with the species of parasite, but all cause anemia (because of destruction of the red blood cells by the schizont form), headaches, general weakness, and a characteristic repetitive fever and chills syndrome.

104. *Plasmodium vivax* (benign tertian malaria). This drawing shows the erythrocytic stages of *P. vivax.* The prominent feature is the presence of Schüffner's dots. These appear as red spots on infected red blood cells on a stained blood smear and are seen in all developmental stages after the early trophozoite stage. The infected red blood cell is larger than normal red blood cells because the parasites preferentially invade reticulocytes, the larger, immature blood cell. The trophozoite divides to form a schizont containing 16 to 18 merozoites, which is a differentiating characteristic for *P. vivax.*

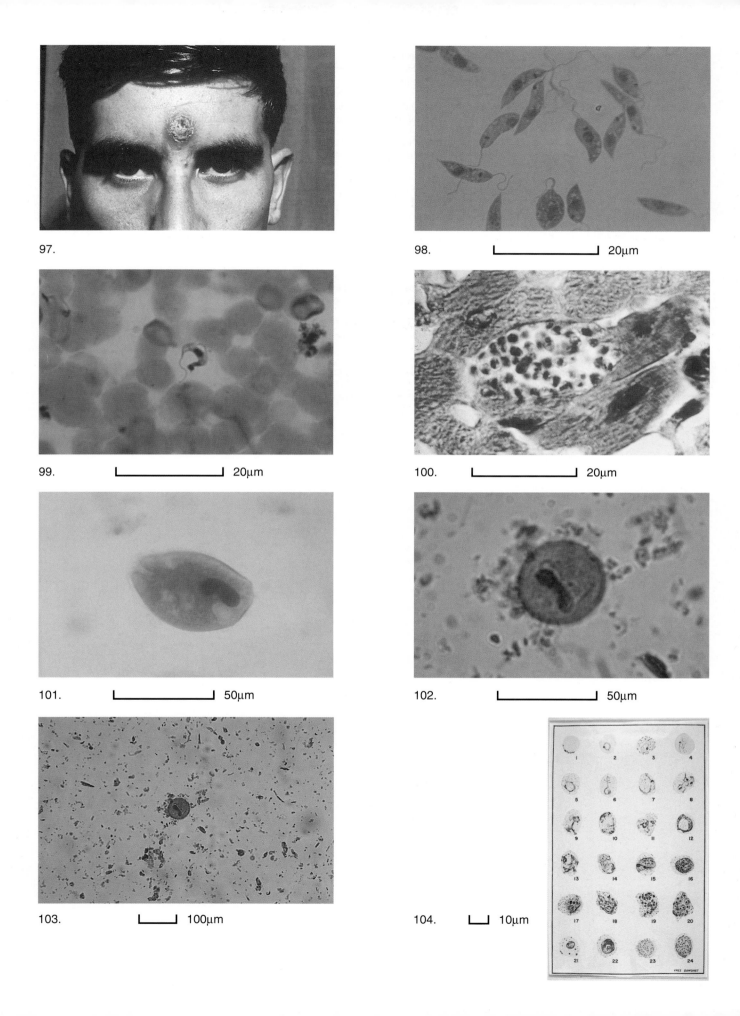

97.

98. |⊢————————⊣| 20μm

99. |⊢————⊣| 20μm

100. |⊢————⊣| 20μm

101. |⊢————⊣| 50μm

102. |⊢————⊣| 50μm

103. |⊢——⊣| 100μm

104. |⊢⊣| 10μm

105. *Plasmodium vivax* (100 ×). A trophozoite is clearly visible in the center of the field. Note the red Schüffner's dots. Note also the ring (blue) and the chromatin dot (red) of the trophozoite. Each ring form (about one-third of the cell diameter in size) represents one parasite; multiple parasites in a red cell are not commonly seen in this species.

106. *Plasmodium vivax* (1000 ×). An older trophozoite than that in the previous plate is seen in the center of the field. Note the larger size of the red cell, the bizarre ameboid shape of the motile trophozoite, and the characteristic Schüffner's dots.

107. *Plasmodium vivax* (1000 ×). An older trophozoite than that in the previous plate is shown. This cell is enlarged and Schüffner's dots are evident. The trophozoite is clearly ameboid in its movements. Plates 104 to 109 clearly illustrate the maturation of the trophozoite stage of *P. vivax*.

108. *Plasmodium vivax* (1000 ×). Developing schizont. Many merozoites are seen inside the cell. A trophozoite appears in the upper right of the field.

109. *Plasmodium vivax* (1000 ×). Mature schizont. Fourteen merozoites are visible inside the cell. Characteristically, the schizont divides to form 16 to 18 merozoites. Development from the invasion of the red blood cell by the trophozoite to the fully mature schizont occurs in 48 hours.

110. *Plasmodium vivax* (1000 ×). Mature schizont. Eighteen merozoites are visible inside the cell. The red blood cell ruptures, releasing the merozoites, which may invade new red blood cells to repeat the asexual erythrocytic cycle. Some merozoites invade red cells and become male or female gametocytes, which are part of the sexual cycle in the mosquito after the gametocytes are ingested in a blood meal.

111. *Plasmodium ovale*. This view shows the erythrocytic stages of *P. ovale*. The red blood cells are enlarged and oval in shape. This parasite is rare in humans and may be confused with *P. malariae* when Schüffner's dots are not present or with *P. vivax* when Schüffner's dots are present.

112. *Plasmodium ovale* trophozoites (1000 ×). This parasite is similar to *P. vivax* because Schüffner's dots are visible. It also resembles *P. malariae* because the mature schizont usually contains 8 to 12 merozoites. The diagnostic characteristic, when present, is the ragged, irregular appearance and oval shape of the host red blood cell, as can be seen here.

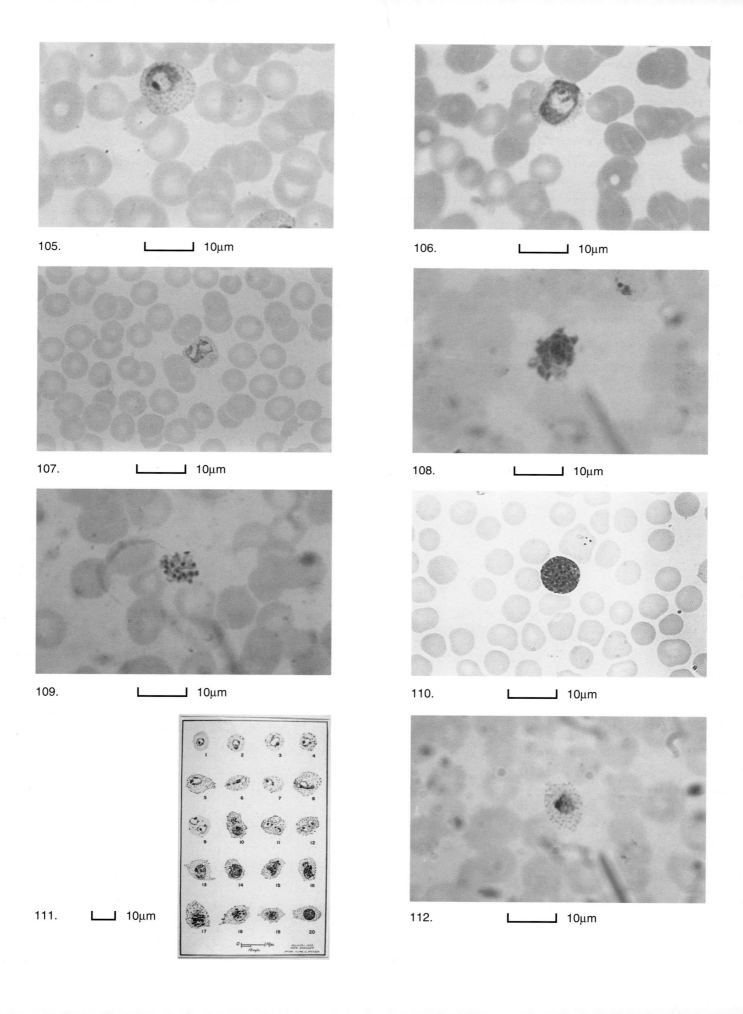

105.   10μm

106.   10μm

107.   10μm

108.   10μm

109.   10μm

110.   10μm

111.   10μm

112.   10μm

113. *Plasmodium ovale* trophozoites (1000 ×). This parasite is similar to *P. vivax* because Schüffner's dots are visible. It also resembles *P. malariae* because the mature schizont usually contains 8 to 12 merozoites. The diagnostic characteristic, when present, is the ragged, irregular appearance and oval shape of the host red blood cell, as can be seen here.

114. *Plasmodium malariae* (quartan malaria). This view depicts erythrocytic stages of *P. malariae*. The trophozoite measures about one-third of the diameter of the red blood cell. The prominent features include a large ring form; the band form of the early schizont with coarse, dark granules; and the mature schizont, containing 8 to 12 merozoites, assuming a characteristic rosette shape with malaria pigment deposited in the center of the rosette.

115. *Plasmodium malariae* trophozoite (1000 ×). The band-form trophozoite across the red cell is characteristic during the early development of the schizont.

116. *Plasmodium malariae* schizont (1000 ×). A schizont containing seven merozoites is seen in the upper left corner. By 72 hours after the trophozoite enters the red blood cell, the mature form contains 8 to 10 merozoites and assumes the characteristic rosette shape. Two young trophozoites are also seen in this view.

117. *Plasmodium malariae* schizont (1000 ×). Another view of a maturing schizont.

118. *Plasmodium malariae* gametocyte (1000 ×). This form is similar to that of *P. vivax* but is smaller and contains less pigment.

119. *Plasmodium falciparum* (malignant subtertian malaria). This plate demonstrates the erythrocytic stages of *P. falciparum*. The prominent features are small ring forms with double chromatin dots, multiple rings in the same cell, and crescent-shaped gametocytes. Other stages in schizont formation are not seen in peripheral blood because these (other) stages of maturation occur in the capillaries of internal organs.

120. *Plasmodium falciparum* ring forms (1000 ×). Note the small ring size and multiple infections, not seen with *P. vivax* or *P. malariae*.

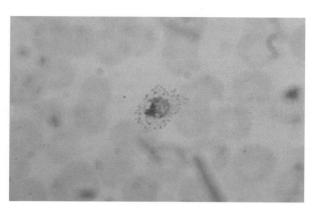

113. |⊢——⊣| 10µm

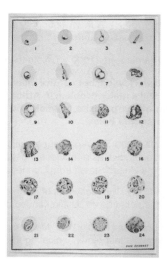

114. |⊢——⊣| 10µm

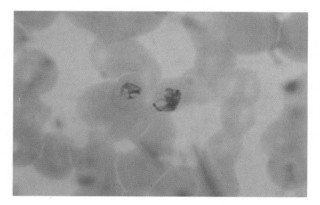

115. |⊢——⊣| 10µm

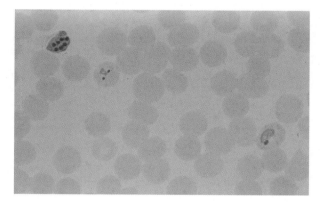

116. |⊢——⊣| 10µm

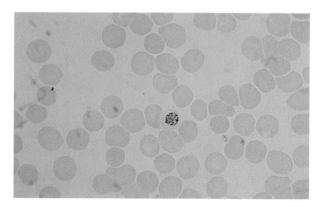

117.

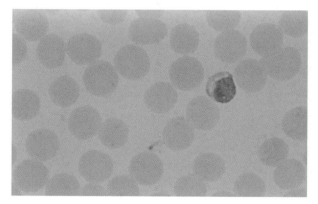

118. |⊢——⊣| 10µm

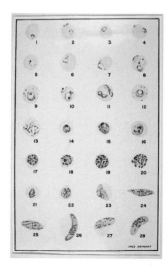

119. |⊢——⊣| 10µm

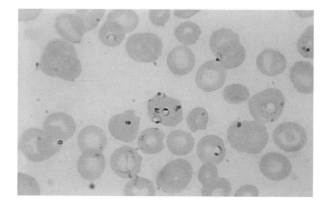

120. |⊢————⊣| 20µm

121. Double malaria infection (1000 ×). A *P. vivax* trophozoite is shown in the center of the field. The small ring form seen at upper left has a double chromatin dot, a diagnostic feature of *P. falciparum* rings.

122. *Plasmodium falciparum* gametocyte (1000 ×). Note the characteristic crescent or banana shape of this form.

Malaria has been found worldwide, but control measures have essentially eliminated the disease from many countries, including the United States. It is still a major problem in Africa, Asia, Central and South America, and the South Pacific. Diagnosis: clinical signs and observation of the parasite in thick and thin blood films obtained ideally during the fever cycle. Other important sporozoan parasites are noted below.

123. *Babesia microti* ring forms (1000 ×). A pair of parasitic forms. Note the rings lie at right angles to each other. When four rings are present they may form a tetrad known as a "maltese cross." This parasite is transmitted by ixodid ticks. Most cases are found in Europe and along the East Coast of the United States from Connecticut to Nantucket.

124. *Isospora belli* oocyst (400 ×). This oocyst containing one sporoblast is stained using the modified acid-fast stain. Note that the oocyst wall does not stain but it is noted as an outline caused by precipitated stain.

125. *Toxoplasma gondii* trophozoites (1000 ×). *T. gondii* trophozoites viewed by fluorescence microscopy in the indirect fluorescent antibody test (IFAT). This is a negative test result, indicating that patient's serum, previously incubated with these organisms, has no detectable antibody to *T. gondii*. No green fluorescence is observable.

126. *Toxoplasma gondii* trophozoites (1000 ×). This is a positive IFAT result for the detection of antibodies to *T. gondii* in serum. Note the green fluorescence over the entire body of the organisms, indicating the presence of antibodies bound to the surface.

127. *Toxoplasma* pseudocyst (400 ×). A dormant pseudocyst filled with bradyzoites of *T. gondii* as seen in a brain section. Immunosuppression of the host would allow these trophozoites to emerge and successfully invade new host cells and to continue multiplication. Brain pseudocysts are also infective if ingested by the definitive host (cats) from mouse brains.

128. *Sarcocystis* spp. (1000 ×). A stained section of muscle tissue in which one can see a sarcocyst filled with potentially infective organisms. These are infective if ingested by the definitive host.

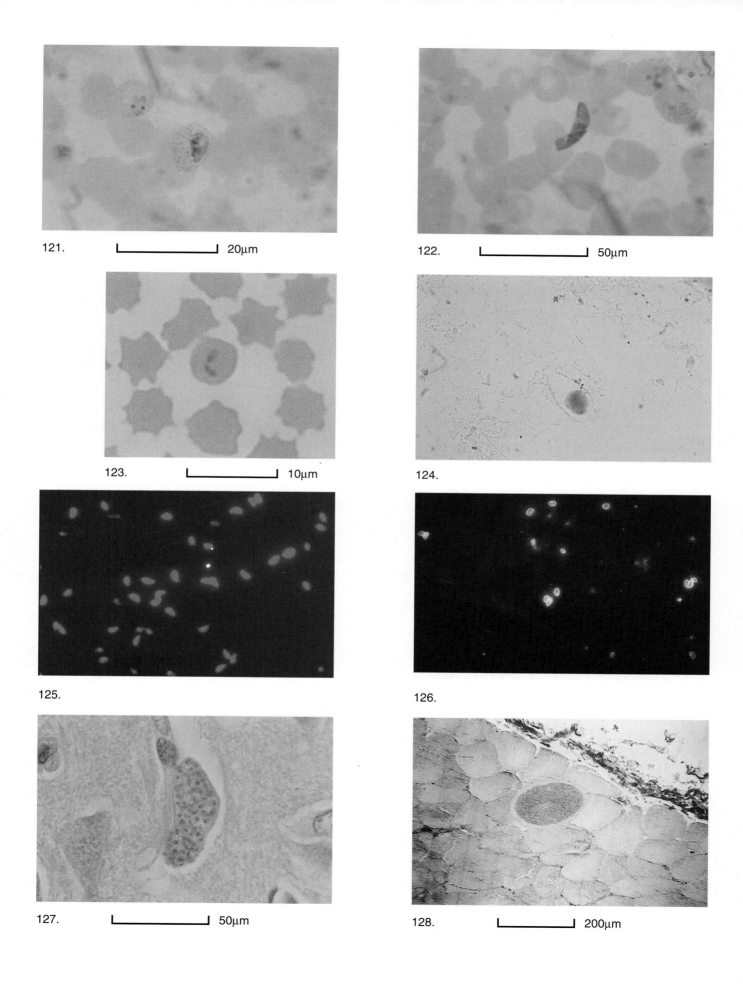

121. |⎯⎯⎯⎯⎯⎯⎯| 20μm

122. |⎯⎯⎯⎯⎯⎯⎯| 50μm

123. |⎯⎯⎯⎯⎯⎯⎯| 10μm

124.

125.

126.

127. |⎯⎯⎯⎯⎯⎯⎯| 50μm

128. |⎯⎯⎯⎯⎯⎯⎯| 200μm

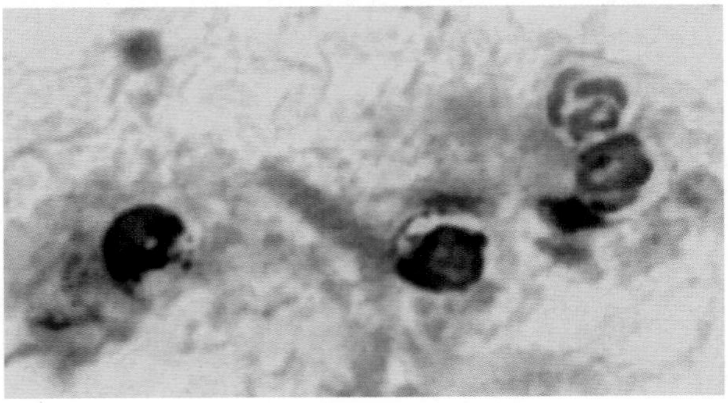

129.

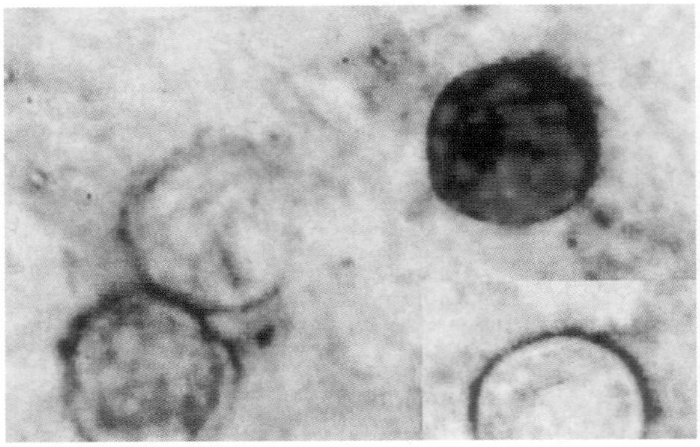

130. 10µm

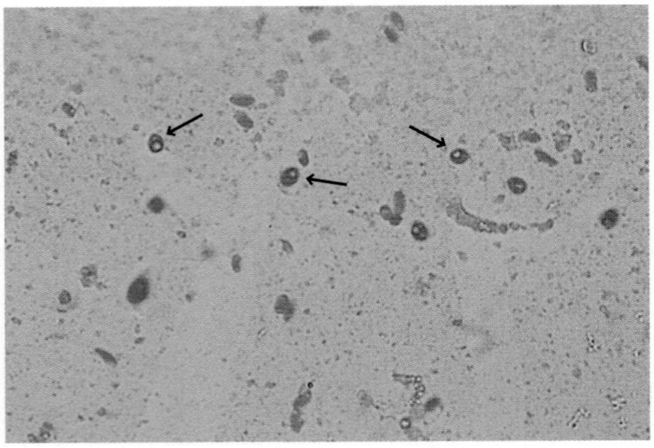

131. 10µm

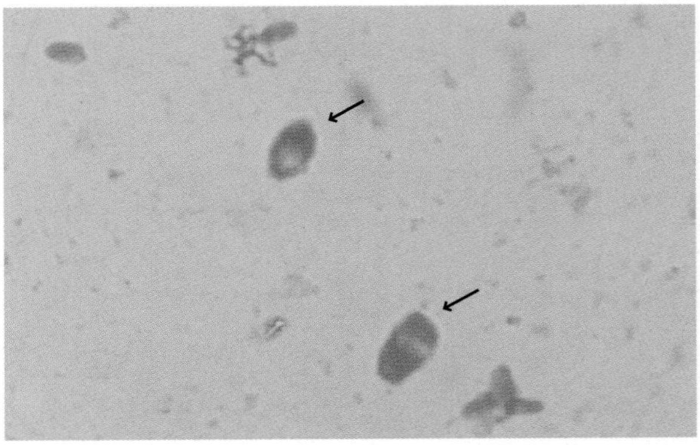

132. 5µm

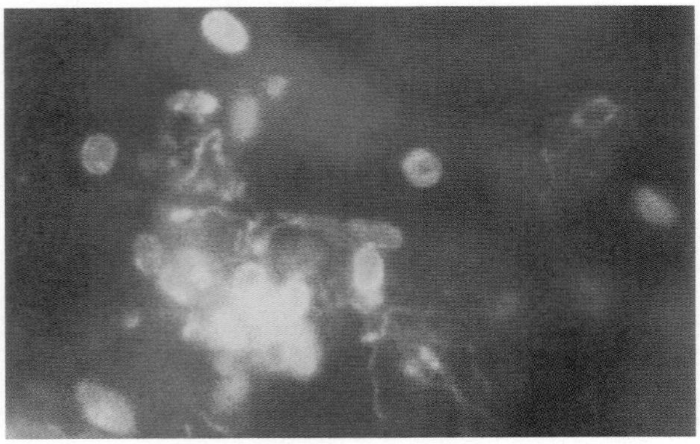

133. 5µm

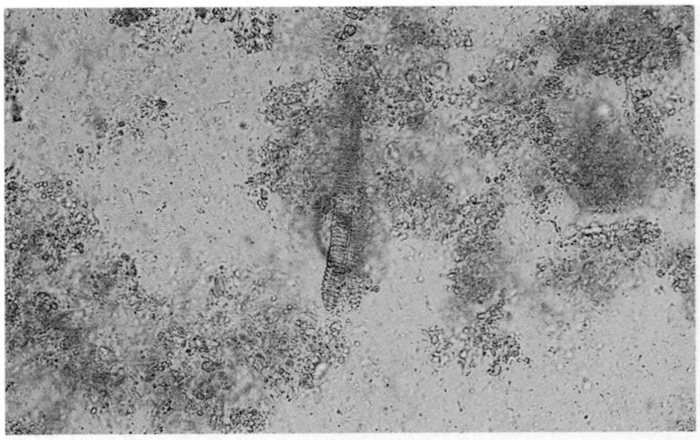

134.

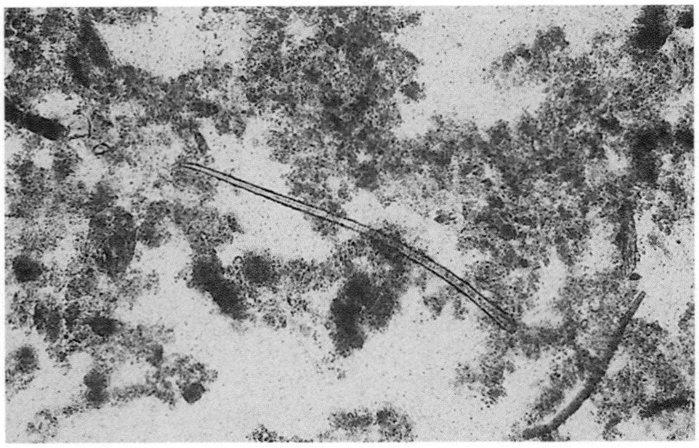

135.

129. *Cryptosporidium parvum* oocysts (1000 ×). The oocysts measuring 4-6 μm stain red (acid-fast stain) against the blue-green background. Sporocysts are visible in the two oocysts on the right side of figure.

130. *Cyclospora* spp. oocysts (1000 ×). Note the variable staining and wrinkled appearance of these oocysts (8-10 μm) preserved in 10% formalin and stained using acid-fast technique.

131. *Enterocytozoon* spp. Spores (0.7-1.0 × 1.1-1.6 μm). Several acid-fast spores are visible in this view (400 ×).

132. *Enterocytozoon* spp. Spores. This view illustrates spores as seen at 1000 × magnification.

133. *Encephalitozoon hellem.* Spores. These spores were recovered in a bronchoalveolar lavage sample from a 30-year-old patient with AIDS. This view (1000 ×) illustrates a monoclonal antibody-based immunofluorescent identification technique. Polar tubules are visible as fluoresent strands extending from the spores.

134. Artifacts (400 ×). Many fecal artifacts may be confused with parasitic forms to the untrained. A vegetable spiral in the center of the field is superimposed over a form that may resemble a nematode egg.

135. Artifacts (500 ×). The most notable artifact in this view is a plant hair that resembles a nematode. Hairs usually have one blunt end and one tapered end, while nematodes have one tapered end and one round end, usually with visible formed mouth structures.

Color Plate Credits
Clay Adams: 1, 6, 9, 13, 15, 24, 26, 27, 29, 32, 41, 48, 51, 59, 60, 67, 75, 86, 89, 91, 93, 97, 104, 105.
David M. Wright, M.D.: 90, 95, 123, 124.
Herman Zaiman, M.D.: 3, 4, 5, 12, 19, 23, 28, 30, 31, 33, 40, 42, 43, 49, 52, 72, 79, 83, 88, 94, 96, 99, 106, 109, 115, 116, 118, 125, 126.
Centers for Disease Control: 25, 73, 76, 77, 78, 80, 84, 87, 92, 129, 130, 133.
National Institutes of Health: 103, 110, 113, 117.

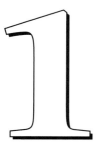

INTRODUCTION

Academic Objectives

ON COMPLETION OF THIS SELF-STUDY TEXT, THE STUDENT WILL BE ABLE TO:

1 State definitions of general terms used in parasitology.

2 Recall the scientific and common names for each parasite studied.

3 State the general geographic distribution of each parasite.

4 State the parasitic form that causes disease in humans and its location in the body.

5 Describe the means by which each infection occurs.

6 State the name of the disease produced and its most common symptoms and pathology.

7 State the appropriate body specimen to examine for the diagnostic stage of each parasite, and list other laboratory tests useful in its diagnosis.

8 Recognize and draw the diagnostic stage of each parasite.

9 Demonstrate graphically the life cycle of each parasite.

10 Discuss the procedures used to identify parasites (including concentration, culture, and staining techniques), as well as potential sources of error involved and quality-control procedures.

11 Identify potentially successful methods for the epidemiologic control of parasitism.

12 Given sufficient case history information, identify the most probable helminth or protozoan causing the symptoms and the body specimen of choice for study.

Practical Objectives

ON COMPLETION OF THIS SELF-STUDY TEXT AND WITH APPROPRIATE EXPERIENCE IN THE LABORATORY, THE STUDENT WILL:

1 Be able to perform appropriate and satisfactory microscopic and macroscopic examination of body specimens—such as blood, urine, or feces—to detect and identify parasites. (NOTE: Acceptable performance is the identification of at least 80% of the parasites present in specimens. In actual clinical settings, accuracy should be 100%.)

2 Have mastered two fecal concentration techniques (one for sedimentation and one for flotation) as demonstrated by satisfactory performance of these techniques and correct identification of recovered parasites.

3 Be able to prepare and stain slides of fecal material and blood satisfactorily as demonstrated by the correct diagnosis of at least 80% of the parasites contained therein.

4 Be able to perform a variety of other tests satisfactorily, including a blood concentration test for microfilaria and serodiagnostic testing for various parasites.

GLOSSARY

accidental (or incidental) host. Infection of a host other than the normal host species. A parasite may or may not continue full development in an accidental host.

apical complex. Polar complex of secretory organelles in sporozoan protozoa.

carrier. A host harboring a parasite but exhibiting no clinical signs or symptoms.

commensalism. The association of two different species of organisms in which one partner is benefited and the other is neither benefited nor injured.

definitive host. The animal in which a parasite passes its adult existence, sexual reproductive phase, or both.

differential diagnosis. The clinical comparison of different diseases that exhibit similar symptoms; designed to determine which disease the patient has.

disease. A definite morbid process having a characteristic train of symptoms.

ectoparasite. A parasite established on or in the body of its host.

endoparasite. A parasite established within the body of its host.

epidemiology. A field of science dealing with the relationships of the various factors that determine the frequency and distribution of an infectious process or disease in a community.

facultative parasite. An organism capable of living an independent or a parasitic existence; not an obligatory parasite, but potentially parasitic.

generic name (or scientific name). The name given to an organism consisting of its appropriate genus and species title.

genus (pl. genera). A taxonomic category subordinate to family (and tribe) and superior to species, grouping those organisms that are alike in broad features but different in detail.

host. The species of animal or plant that harbors a parasite and provides some metabolic resources to the parasitic species.

in vitro. Observable in a test tube or other nonliving system.

in vivo. Within the living body.

infection. Invasion of the body by a pathogenic organism (except arthropods), with accompanying reaction of the host tissues to the presence of the parasite.

infestation. The establishment of arthropods on or within a host (including insects, ticks, and mites).

intermediate host. The animal in which a parasite passes its larval stage or asexual reproduction phase.

Metazoa. A subkingdom of animals consisting of all multicellular animal organisms in which cells are differentiated to form tissue. Includes all animals except protozoa.

obligatory parasite. A parasite that cannot live apart from its host.

parasitemia. The presence of parasites in the blood (e.g., malaria schizonts in red blood cells).

parasitism. The association of two different species of organisms in which the smaller species lives on or within the other and has a metabolic dependence on the larger host species.

pathogenic. Production of tissue changes or disease.

pathogenicity. The ability to produce pathogenic changes.

reservoir host. An animal that harbors a species of parasite that is also parasitic for humans and from which a human may become infected.

serology. The study of antibody-antigen reactions in vitro, using host serum for study.

species (abbr. spp.). A taxonomic category subordinate to a genus. A species maintains its classification by not interbreeding with other species.

symbiosis. The association of two different species of organisms exhibiting metabolic dependence by their relationship.

transport host. An animal that harbors a parasite that does not reproduce; it carries the parasite from one location to another to infect a new host.

vectors. Any arthropods or other living carriers that transport a pathogenic microorganism from an infected to a noninfected host. A vector may transmit a disease passively (mechanical vector) or may be an essential host in the life cycle of the pathogenic organism (biological vector).

zoonosis (pl. zoonoses). A disease involving a parasite that has accidentally infected a human; the normal host for the parasite is an animal.

North Americans do not suffer from a multitude of harmful parasites, largely because of general good health; high standards of education, nutrition, and sanitation; a temperate climate; and the absence of necessary **vectors**. Parasitic **infections** do exist in the United States, however, and are still far from eradicated. Increased travel throughout the world and the general low level of understanding about parasitic infections have added to the problem of **disease** transmission in the United States. Many other parts of the world have high levels of parasite-induced morbidity and mortality among humans and animals, as well as significant parasitic damage to crops. These problems place great drains on manpower and food productivity, thus affecting the international economy. In recognizing this problem, the World Health Organization (WHO) named five parasitic diseases (malaria, leishmaniasis, trypanosomiasis, onchocerciasis, and schistosomiasis) as among the six most harmful infective diseases afflicting humanity today. More than 4.5 billion people harbor parasites.

A worldwide survey of common helminth infections was attempted in the 1940s. Global prevalence of *Ascaris lumbricoides*, hookworm, and *Trichuris trichiura* infections at that time were estimated to be 24%, 24%, and 17%, respectively. A similar survey performed again in the early 1990s found the same relative percentages for these parasitic infections. When one adds to these numbers that 489 million people have malaria, killing 1.5 million people each year (including at least 1 million children younger than 5 years of age), it becomes evident that parasitic infections greatly affect the health and welfare of the world's population. Table 1–1 summarizes these data.

The real significance of these numbers is the realization that at least 25% of the world's population (about 1.5 billion people) suffer from the consequences of parasitic infections, such as malnutrition, iron deficiency anemia, and other parasite-specific chronic health effects, with periodic acute disease symptoms (e.g., malaria). The economic consequences are staggering. To overcome the effects of parasitic infections, water and sewage treatment, changes in behavior due to improved health education, and overall improvement in the economic standards of living are required. These are serious challenges, especially in poor countries.

Although the incidence of indigenous (endemic) infection is low in the United States and other developed nations, parasitic infections affect poor people more seriously than they affect the more wealthy inhabitants of the same countries. Other infections are brought into these countries by immigrants from tropical areas and by travelers and military personnel returning with "exotic" diseases from foreign endemic areas. "New" disease-causing agents are emerging as opportunistic infections in immunocompromised individuals, and increasingly, waterborne and foodborne parasites such as *Cryptosporidium* are being found in healthy people. Continuing surveillance of parasitic diseases by the Centers for Disease Control and Prevention (CDC), the WHO, and others is necessary to ensure the future health of citizens of the United States and other parts of the world.

TABLE 1–1 □ ESTIMATE OF GLOBAL MORBIDITY AND MORTALITY RATES FROM MAJOR HELMINTH INFECTIONS AND MALARIA

Parasitic Disease	Number of Infections (in millions)	Morbidity (%) (of world population affected)	Mortality (number of deaths—1997) (% of infected population)
Ascaris	1,472	23	60,000 0.004
Hookworm infections	1,298	12	65,000 0.005
Lymphatic filariasis	120	37	N.A.
Onchocerciasis	18	4.2	45,000 0.25
Schistosomiasis	200	10	20,000 0.01
Trichuriasis	1,049	21	10,000 0.001
Malaria	489	3	1,500,000 0.3

Adapted from data presented in Crompton, 1999.

● *What Is Parasitology?*

Parasitology is a study of a particular relationship among certain **species**. **Symbiosis** means "living together" and generally refers to a positive relationship between members of different species. Mutualism is usually an obligatory relationship in which both organisms benefit. An example of mutualism is the termite and its intestinal flagellate fauna. The termite benefits because it could not digest its cellulose-containing food without the flagellate, and the intestinal organism benefits by having a secure habitat in which to live and a good source of food. **Commensalism** is usually not obligatory, but it is a relationship in which one species of organism benefits and the other neither benefits nor is harmed. Humans can harbor several species of amoeba with no ill effects to the **host** but with benefit to the amoebae. **Parasitism** is a relationship in which one species of organism lives on or with another organism, with the parasite living at the expense of and often causing harm to the host. Most parasites inflict varying degrees of harm depending on the general health and nutritional status of the host, the size of the parasite, the number of parasites present, and the parasites' location or migration path within the host.

Types of Parasites

A parasite that lives inside the host is called an **endoparasite;** one that lives on or in the skin is called an **ectoparasite.** Most parasites are obligate; that is, they must spend part or all of their life cycle within a host to survive. A **facultative parasite** is usually a free-living organism that can become parasitic if it is accidentally ingested or enters a wound or other body opening. *Naegleria fowleri,* an amoeba, enters through a person's nose when he or she is swimming in contaminated water. Ectoparasites can be insect forms that interact temporarily or permanently with a human host.

Accidental parasites are those that normally live in or on a host other than humans, and these parasites do not survive long in an unnatural human host. The **accidental (or incidental) host** may or may not experience symptoms. Larvae of dog and cat hookworms and roundworms that accidentally penetrate human skin are an example. Another term used to describe this problem is **zoonosis.**

Hosts

Hosts can be characterized as definitive, intermediate, transport, or reservoir. A **definitive host** is one in which the parasite reaches sexual or reproductive maturity. An **intermediate host** is one that harbors asexual reproduction. Sometimes both types of hosts are required in a parasite's life cycle.

A **transport host** is one that harbors a parasite that does not reproduce but merely goes on to infect a new host. The transport host serves only to carry the parasite from one location to another. For example, a house fly might passively transfer an amoeba on its feet from contaminated feces to a cooking utensil in a kitchen. A new host could then ingest the parasite stage, producing a new infection. A **reservoir host** may harbor a parasite that is also infective for humans. For example, the bush buck antelope often harbors the protozoa that causes sleeping sickness in humans, but the antelope suffers no ill effects.

● *Classification of Parasites*

I. The **metazoan** helminths—wormlike invertebrates. (Only those parasitic for humans are included in this text.) The following are considered:
A. Phylum Nemathelminthes
1. Class Nematoda: roundworms (body round in cross-section)
B. Phylum Platyhelminthes: flatworms
1. Class Cestoda: tapeworms (body flattened and segmented)
2. Class Digenea: trematodes, flukes (body flattened, leaf-shaped, and nonsegmented)
II. Protozoa*—unicellular eukaryotic microorganisms. The following are considered:
A. Phylum Sarcomastigophora
1. Class Lobosea: organisms that move by means of pseudopodia
2. Class Zoomastigophorea: organisms that move by means of flagella

*Classification derived from scheme adopted by Society of Protozoologists (Cox, 1993).

B. Phylum Ciliophora
  1. Class Kinetofragminophorea: organisms that move by means of cilia
C. Phylum Apicomplexa
  1. Class Sporozoea: organisms with both sexual and asexual reproductive cycles; **apical complex** can be seen with electron microscope
III. Arthropods—possess a hard exoskeleton and jointed appendages. Only those that are parasitic to humans and those that transmit parasitic diseases are included.
  A. Phylum Arthropoda
    1. Class Insecta: flies, mosquitoes, bugs, lice, fleas
    2. Class Arachnida: ticks, mites

● *How to Use This Text*

To function as a competent practitioner, prepared to aid in accurate diagnosis of parasitic infections, you must exhibit knowledge and skills in both clinical and academic areas. This self-study text is designed to help you reach that goal.

To prepare you to identify organisms that parasitize humans, this book explains parasitism as a biological concept and introduces specific parasites of medical importance. It also includes the information necessary to assist in the diagnosis of infection. The life cycles of parasites of major medical importance are displayed graphically and pictorially to help you understand how transmission and control of the spread of infection can occur and how the location of each parasite stage in the human body correlates with clinical symptoms and pathology. Knowing the life cycle helps you understand which parasite stage will be seen in body specimens, such as blood, urine, feces, or sputum; this is the key to diagnosis.

For a substantive review of the biology of any particular parasite, you are referred to a variety of texts and specific journal articles, as noted in the bibliography of each chapter. The bibliographies include both classic references in the field plus newer findings of importance. Pertinent references have been included in the bibliography to guide you toward in-depth studies in various areas of parasitology, such as the biochemistry, treatment, pathology, or immunology of parasitic infections.

Six glossaries of important terms appear in this text. In addition to the basic terms defined in the glossary at the beginning of this chapter, separate glossaries are included in the chapters on the Nematoda, Cestoda, Digenea, Protozoa, and Arthropoda. Study and master all of the words in each of the glossaries. It is recommended that the glossaries be used in conjunction with the boldfaced terms appearing in the text. Before taking each post-test, review again the glossary included in the chapter.

Throughout the text you will find words in bold type (e.g., **vector**) that are defined in the glossary of that chapter; a medical dictionary, however, will be helpful to you in your studies. This text is best used in conjunction with a course that includes supplementary hands-on laboratory experiences. By the time you have worked through studying the helminths (which are presented first in the text), your practice with microscopic and other techniques will have made you more effective and efficient in locating and identifying the small protozoa and in differentiating them from other formed, unicellular structures or artifacts present in body specimens.

Recommended treatments (e.g., drugs or surgery) are also included for each organism that can infect humans. New regulatory requirements related to reagent and specimen handling, as well as new findings and classifications of parasites, have mandated this newest edition. In addition to comprehensive presentations of each parasite, an extensive descriptive key with accompanying color photographs is also included and is located at the front of the book. These descriptions and pictures have been chosen carefully to provide important information on each parasite discussed. The photographs and descriptive key are arranged in the same sequence as the species presented in the text and should be studied as part of each chapter.

The pre-test in this section is designed to allow you to evaluate your general knowledge of medical parasitology. The test answers are at the back of the book, starting on page 221. Following each chapter, a brief post-test enables you to judge your mastery of that particular area. Learning objectives at the beginning of each chapter should guide your study and help prepare you for the tests.

After reading the chapter objectives, you should review the words found in the glossary at the beginning of each chapter. The chapters contain word puzzles that you can use to review each chapter. Each chapter also contains review questions that emphasize important points. You should respond in writing to each question, and then check the accuracy of your answers by rereading the chapter.

Review each chapter and its corresponding color plates and plate key until you have successfully completed your learning tasks, as determined by a satisfactory score on the chapter post-test. A final examination at the end of the text allows you to evaluate your overall self-paced learning accomplishment. A score of 80% correct must be achieved to demonstrate minimally satisfactory completion of each chapter, but you are encouraged to review difficult-to-grasp material and use supplementary reading materials until you are satisfied that you have learned the material completely.

Twelve practice case studies are also found in this text. Answers for the cases and the word puzzles are included at the end of the book.

Word Puzzle

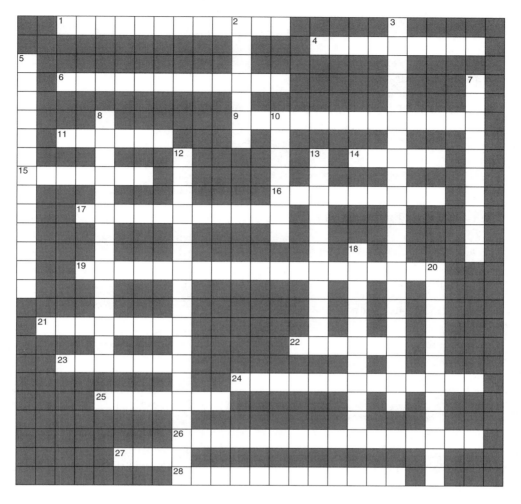

Across

1. A parasite established on or in the body of its host
4. The association of two different species of organisms exhibiting metabolic dependence by their relationship
6. The association of two different species of organisms in which one partner is benefited and the other is neither benefited nor injured
9. An animal that harbors a species of parasite that is also parasitic for humans and from which a human may become infected (2 words)
11. Any arthropod or other living carrier that transports a pathogenic microorganism from an infected to a noninfected host
14. A taxonomic category subordinate to family (and tribe) and superior to species, grouping those organisms that are alike in broad features but different in detail
15. A host harboring a parasite but exhibiting no clinical signs or symptoms
16. Invasion of the body by a pathogenic organism (except arthropods), with accompanying reaction of the host tissues to the presence of the parasite
17. The name given to an organism consisting of its appropriate genus and species title (2 words)
19. An organism capable of living an independent or a parasitic existence; not an obligatory parasite, but potentially parasitic (2 words)
21. The study of antibody-antigen reactions in vitro, using host serum for study
22. Within the living body (2 words)
23. A subkingdom of animals consisting of all multicellular animal organisms in which cells are differentiated to form tissue; includes all animals except protozoa

24. The ability to produce pathogenic changes
25. A definite morbid process having a characteristic train of symptoms
26. The animal in which a parasite passes its larval stage or asexual reproduction phase (2 words)
27. The species of animal or plant that harbors a parasite and provides some metabolic resources to the parasitic species
28. A parasite established within the body of its host

Down

2. Observable in a test tube or other nonliving system (2 words)
3. The clinical comparison of different diseases that exhibit similar symptoms; designed to determine which disease the patient has (2 words)
5. Polar complex of secretory organelles in sporozoan protozoa (2 words)
7. Production of tissue changes or disease
8. Infection of a host other than the normal host species (2 words)
10. A taxonomic category subordinate to a genus; a species maintains its classification by not interbreeding with other species
12. A parasite that cannot live apart from its host (2 words)
13. The establishment of arthropods upon or within a host (including insects, ticks, and mites)
18. The presence of parasites in the blood (e.g., malaria schizonts in red blood cells)
20. Field of science dealing with the relationships of the various factors that determine the frequency and distribution of an infectious process or disease in a community

Pre-Test

*The following questions will help you evaluate your general knowledge of parasitology. Allow 30 minutes for completion of the test. The multiple-choice questions are worth **6 points** each; questions 11 and 12 are worth **20 points** each. Write your answers on separate sheets of paper.*

1. Pinworm disease may be diagnosed by which procedure?
   a. Direct fecal smear
   b. Cellophane tape test
   c. Fecal concentration methods
   d. Egg-count technique

2. *Taenia solium* tapeworm infection occurs when:
   a. Undercooked beef is eaten
   b. Eggs are ingested from contaminated soil
   c. Larvae invade the skin of the feet
   d. Undercooked pork is eaten

3. The most common helminth infection in the United States is:
   a. *Necator americanus*
   b. *Ascaris lumbricoides*
   c. *Enterobius vermicularis*
   d. *Schistosoma mansoni*

4. The definitive host for *Plasmodium vivax* is a:
   a. Flea
   b. Human
   c. Mosquito
   d. Fish

5. *Clonorchis sinensis* is commonly known as the:
   a. Beef tapeworm
   b. Hookworm
   c. Chinese liver fluke
   d. Bladder worm

6. The most pathogenic amoeba in humans is:
   a. *Entamoeba histolytica*
   b. *Entamoeba coli*
   c. *Giardia lamblia*
   d. *Balantidium coli*

7. Which of the following may be used to culture amoebae in the laboratory?
   a. Horse serum
   b. Wheatley trichrome
   c. Loose moist soil
   d. Balamuth fluid

8. Xenodiagnosis is used for which parasite?
   a. *Schistosoma mansoni*
   b. *Trypanosoma cruzi*
   c. *Loa loa*
   d. *Wuchereria bancrofti*

9. Diptera is an order of insects including which of the following?
   a. Mosquitoes
   b. Lice
   c. Fleas
   d. Bugs
   e. Ticks

10. The common name for *Necator americanus* is:
    a. Pinworm
    b. Trichina worm
    c. Hookworm
    d. Fish tapeworm

11. Match the disease in the left column with the correct causative parasite in the right column:

    ____ a. Dwarf tapeworm disease
    ____ b. Threadworm disease
    ____ c. Traveler's diarrhea
    ____ d. Liver rot
    ____ e. Whipworm disease

    1. *Giardia lamblia*
    2. *Fasciola hepatica*
    3. *Hymenolepis nana*
    4. *Trichuris trichiura*
    5. *Strongyloides stercoralis*

12. Define or explain the following terms:
    a. Vector
    b. Host
    c. Proglottid
    d. Definitive host
    e. Operculum

The answer key to all tests starts on page 221.

BIBLIOGRAPHY

American Society of Medical Technology Staff: Clinical Diagnostic Parasitology, ed 3. Kendall-Hunt, Dubuque, Iowa, 1992.

Ash, LR, and Orihel, TC (eds): Atlas of Human Parasitology, ed 4. ASCP Press, Chicago, 1997.

Benke, JM (ed): Parasites, Immunity and Pathology: The Consequences of Parasitic Infection in Mammals. Taylor and Francis, New York, 1990.

Campbell, WC, and Rew, RS (eds): Chemotherapy of Parasitic Diseases. Plenum Press, New York, 1986.

Chan, MS: The global burden of intestinal nematode infections—fifty years on. Parasitology Today 13:438–443, 1997.

Cheng, TC, et al: Parasitic and Related Diseases: Basic Mechanisms, Manifestations and Control. Plenum Press, New York, 1985.

Cook, GC: Parasitic Disease in Clinical Practice. Springer-Verlag, London, 1990.

Cox, FEG (ed): Modern Parasitology, ed 2. Blackwell Scientific Publication, Oxford, England, 1993.

Cox, FEG, et al (eds): Parasitology, Vol. 5. In Collier, L, et al (eds): Topley & Wilson's Microbiology and Microbial Infections. Arnold, London, 1998.

Crompton, DW: How much human helminthiasis is there in the world? J Parasitol 85(3):397–403, 1999.

Daws, B (ed): Advances in Parasitology. Academic Press, London, volumes published annually since 1962.

Esh, GW, and Fernandez, J: Functional Biology of Parasitism: Ecological and Evolutionary Implications. Chapman and Hall, New York, 1993.

Faust, EC, et al: Animal Agents and Vectors of Human Disease, ed 4. Lea & Febiger, Philadelphia, 1975.

Garcia, LS: Diagnostic Medical Parasitology, ed 4. ASM Press, Washington, DC, 2001.

Garcia, LS: Practical Guide to Diagnostic Parasitology. ASM Press, Washington, DC, 1999.

Gibbons, A: Researchers fret over neglect of 600 million patients. Science 256:1135, 1992.

Goldsmith, R, and Hayneman, D: Tropical Medicine and Medical Parasitology. Appleton & Lange, Norwalk, Conn., 1989.

Guerrant, RL, et al (eds): Tropical Infectious Diseases: Principles, Pathogens, and Practice. Churchill Livingstone, Philadelphia, 1999.

Hopkins, DR: Homing in on helminths. Am J Trop Med Hyg 46:626–634, 1992.

Leach, RM, and Jeffery, HC: Atlas of Medical Helminthology and Protozoology, ed 3. Churchill, New York, 1991.

MacLeod, C (ed): Parasitic Infections of Pregnancy and the Newborn. Oxford University Press, New York, 1988.

Markell, EK, et al: Medical Parasitology, ed 8. WB Saunders, Philadelphia, 1999.

Parasitology. Science 264(5167):1857–1886, 1994.

Peters, W, and Gilles, HM: A Color Atlas of Tropical Medicine and Parasitology, ed 4, Mosby-Wolfe, London, 1995.

Schmidt, GD, and Roberts, LS: Foundations of Parasitology, ed 4. Mosby, St. Louis, 1981.

Soulsby, EJL (ed): Immune Responses in Parasitic Infections: Immunology, Immunopathology and Immunoprophylaxis, 4 Vols. CRC Press, Boca Raton, Fla., 1987.

Stoll, NR: This wormy world. J Parasitol 33:1–18, 1947.

Strickland, GT (ed): Hunter's Tropical Medicine, ed 7. WB Saunders, Philadelphia, 1991.

Sun, T: Color Atlas and Textbook of Diagnostic Parasitology. Igaku-Shoin, Tokyo, New York, 1988.

Symons, LE: Pathophysiology of Parasitic Infections. Academic Press, New York, 1989.

Taylor, AER, and Baker, JR (eds): In Vitro Methods for Parasite Cultivation. Academic Press, New York, 1988.

Guerrant, RL, et al (eds). Tropical Infectious Diseases: Principles, Pathogens, and Practice. Churchill Livingstone, Philadelphia, 1999.

Wakelin, D: Immunity to Parasites: How Parasitic Infections Are Controlled. Cambridge University Press, Cambridge, England, 1996.

Warren, KS. Immunology and Molecular Biology of Parasitic Infections, ed 3. Blackwell Scientific Publications, Oxford, England, 1992.

Warren, KS, and Mahmoud, AAF: Tropical and Geographical Medicine, ed 2. McGraw-Hill, New York, 1990.

Wyler, DJ (ed): Modern Parasite Biology: Cellular, Immunological and Molecular Aspects. WH Friedman, New York, 1990.

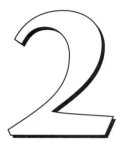

NEMATODA

LEARNING OBJECTIVES

ON COMPLETION OF THIS CHAPTER AND STUDY OF THE SUPPLEMENTARY COLOR PLATES AS DESCRIBED, THE STUDENT WILL BE ABLE TO:

1 Define terminology specific for **Nematoda.**

2 State the scientific and common names of all intestinal nematodes for which humans serve as the usual definitive host.

3 State the body specimen of choice to be used for examination to help diagnose nematode infections.

4 State the geographic distribution and relative incidence of medically important nematode infections.

5 Describe the general morphology of an adult nematode.

6 Describe the life-cycle development of parasitic intestinal nematodes from egg through adult stages.

7 Differentiate the adult parasitic intestinal Nematoda by structure and location.

8 Given an illustration or photograph or an actual specimen (if given adequate laboratory experience), identify the diagnostic stages of intestinal Nematoda.

9 Differentiate microfilariae found in infected human blood by the staining patterns of cells in the tail and by the presence or absence of an embryonic sheath.

10 Discuss zoonotic nematode infections of humans and symptoms thereof.

11 Differentiate and discuss methods by which the Nematoda infect humans. Include the scientific name of any required intermediate host and the infective stage for humans.

12 Perform generic identification of parasitic infections by detecting, recognizing, and stating the scientific name of parasites present in biological laboratory specimens (given appropriate laboratory experiences, as described in Chap. 7).

13 Use these learning objectives as guides for your acquisition of knowledge. Assure yourself that you have acquired the information necessary to accomplish each learning task described before you attempt a chapter post-test.

GLOSSARY

autoreinfection. Reinfecting oneself. In the pinworm life cycle, infected individuals may reinfect themselves via hand-to-mouth transfer from scratching the perianal region after the female worm has deposited eggs. In other life cycles, infective eggs may hatch inside the host and then develop into an adult (e.g., *Strongyloides stercoralis, Hymenolepis nana*).

buccal capsule (cavity). Oral cavity of roundworms. (In the case of hookworms, the cavity contains species-specific cutting plates or cutting teeth.)

bursa (pl. bursae). Fan-shaped cartilage expansion at the posterior end of some male nematodes (e.g., hookworms) that holds onto the female during copulation.

copulatory spicules. Needlelike bodies possessed by some male nematodes; spicules lie in pouches near the ejaculatory duct and may be inserted in the vagina of the female worm during copulation.

corticated. Possessing an outer, mamillated, albuminous coating, as on the eggs of *Ascaris lumbricoides*.

cutaneous larval migrans. A disease caused by the migration of larvae of *Ancylostoma* spp. (dog or cat hookworm) or other helminth larvae traveling under the skin of humans. Larval migration is marked by thin, red papular lines of eruption. Also termed creeping eruption.

cuticle. The surface of roundworms; a tough protective covering that is resistant to digestion.

dermatitis. Inflammation of the skin.

diagnostic stage. A developmental stage of a pathogenic organism that can be detected in human body secretions, discharges, feces, blood, or tissue by chemical means or microscopic observations. Identification serves as an aid in diagnosis.

diurnal. Occurring during the daytime.

edema. Unusual excess fluid in tissue, causing swelling.

elephantiasis. Overgrowth of the skin and subcutaneous tissue in limbs or genitalia resulting from obstructed circulation in the lymphatic vessels; can occur in the presence of some long-term chronic filaria infections (e.g., *Wuchereria bancrofti*).

enteritis. Inflammation of the intestine.

eosinophilia. High levels of circulating eosinophils in the blood.

fecundity. Reproductive capacity.

filaria (pl. filariae). A nematode worm of the order Filariata; requires an arthropod intermediate host for transmission of infection to humans.

filariform larva. Infective, nonfeeding, sheathed, third-stage larva; larva has a long, slender esophagus.

gravid. Pregnant; female has developing eggs, embryos, or larvae in reproductive organs.

immunosuppression. Depressed immune response system; can accompany various diseases or can be induced by drugs.

incubation period. The time from initial infection until the onset of clinical symptoms of a disease.

infective stage. The stage of the life cycle at which the parasite is capable of entering and continuing development within the host.

intermediate host. A species of animal that serves as host for only the larval or sexually immature stages of parasite development. Required part of the life cycle of that parasite.

larva (pl. larvae). An immature stage in the development of a worm before becoming a mature adult. Nematodes molt several times during development, and each subsequent larval stage is increasingly mature.

life cycle. Entrance into a host, growth, development, reproduction, and subsequent transmission of offspring to a new host.

microfilaria (pl. microfilariae). The embryo stage of a filaria parasite; usually in the blood or tissue of humans; can be ingested by the arthropod intermediate host in which the microfilaria will develop to the infective stage.

molt. A process of replacement of the old cuticle with an inner, new one and subsequent shedding of the old, outer cuticle to allow for the growth and development of the larva; the actual shedding of the old cuticle is termed ecdysis.

Nematoda. A class of the animal phylum Nemathelminthes—the roundworms.

occult. Hidden; not apparent.

parthenogenic. Capable of unisexual reproduction; no fertilization is required (e.g., *Strongyloides stercoralis* parasitic female).

pathognomonic. Indicative of disease; characteristic symptoms suggest the disease.

periodicity. Recurring at a regular time period.

pica. Habit of eating dirt or other unusual substances, such as chalk or plaster. Seen most often in children or in adults with anemia.

prepatent period. The time elapsing between initial infection with the immature parasite and reproduction by the adult parasite.

pruritus. Intense itching. *Pruritus ani* refers to anal itching, as in enterobiasis.

rectal prolapse. Weakening of the rectal musculature resulting in a "falling down" of the rectum; occasionally seen in heavy whipworm infections, particularly in children.

rhabditiform larva. Noninfective, feeding, first-stage larva; the larva has an hourglass-shaped esophagus.

tropical eosinophilia. A disease syndrome associated with high levels of blood eosinophils and an asthmalike syndrome. Caused by zoonotic filaria (or other nematode) infections in which no microfilariae are detectable in peripheral blood in most cases.

visceral larval migrans. A disease in humans caused by the migration of the larval stage of the roundworm *Toxocara canis* or *T. cati* through the liver, lungs, or other organs. The normal host of these ascarids is the dog or cat. The disease is characterized by hypereosinophilia and hepatomegaly and often by pneumonia. Migrating **larvae** can invade ocular spaces and cause retinal damage. This migration is called ocular larval migrans (OLM).

● *Nematodes*

The class Nematoda includes both metabolically independent free-living species and parasitic species that have a metabolic dependence on one or more host species to continue their life cycles. As a group, the nematodes are referred to as roundworms because they are round when viewed in cross-section. The different species vary in size from a few millimeters to more than 1 meter in length. There are separate sexes, with the male generally being smaller than the female. The male often has a curved or coiled posterior end with **copulatory spicules** and, in some species, a **bursa.** The adult anterior end may have oral hooks, teeth, or plates in the **buccal capsule (cavity)** for the purpose of attachment. It also may have small body surface projections, known as setae or papillae, which are thought to be sensory in nature. Body development is fairly complex. The exterior resistant surface of the adult worm is called the **cuticle;** this is underlain with several muscle layers. The internal organ systems include a complex nerve cord; a well-developed digestive system (oral buccal capsule, muscular esophagus, gut, and anus); and complete, tubular, coiled reproductive organs, which are proportionally very large and complex. In the male, reproductive organs include the testes, vas deferens, seminal vesicle, and ejaculatory duct. The female reproductive organs include two ovaries, oviducts, uterine seminal receptacle, and vagina. A female can produce from several hundred up to millions of offspring, depending on the species. **Fecundity** is usually proportional to the complexity of the life cycle of the parasite—those involving direct-contact transmission to a new host produce the fewest offspring; those requiring multiple hosts often produce the most.

Humans are the definitive host for the roundworms of medical importance because humans harbor the reproducing adult roundworms. Depending on the species, the adult female nematode produces either fertilized eggs or **larvae** that may be infective to a new host by one of three routes: (1) Eggs may be immediately infective by being ingested, (2) eggs or larvae may require a period of external development to reach the infective stage, or (3) an insect may transmit eggs or larvae to a new host. Developing larvae generally go through a series of four **molts** during the **incubation period.**

Most often it is the third-stage larva (the filariform stage) that is infective. Infection of humans with different species of roundworms is by ingestion of the infective stage egg or larva, by larval penetration through the skin of the host, or via transmission of larvae by the bite of an insect. The development of a parasite to the infective stage, the manner in which humans become infected, and the life cycle are different for each parasite species.

Of the species of nematodes that are parasitic for humans, about half reside as adult worms in the intestinal tract; the other species are found as adults in various human tissues. The pathogenicity of intestinal nematodes may be due, in part, to migration of adults or larvae through human tissues such as liver or lungs, piercing of the intestinal wall, bloodsucking activities of adult worms, or allergic reactions to substances secreted or excreted by either adult worms or larval stages. This can be serious in heavy infections. Pathogenicity induced by the tissue-dwelling adult roundworms primarily results from immune and nonspecific host responses to the parasite secretions and excretions and to degenerating parasite material. In some cases it may result from circulating larval stages. Migrating nematodes are usually associated with blood or tissue **eosinophilia.** Most infected persons have low worm burdens and modest symptoms.

Diagram 2–1 is a generalized example of a **life cycle** that illustrates the key points to study while learning about any parasite. Understanding the life cycle is the key to understanding how to break the cycle in nature and thereby control the transmission of parasitic diseases. Minimally, the five parts noted on the sample diagram of a life cycle must be known:

1. Location of the parasite stage in a human host (e.g., adults in intestinal tract or in tissue site).
2. The means by which parasite stages leave the human host (e.g., eggs in feces; feeding insect ingests larval stage from tissue). Usually, the parasite stage that is seen and identified in the laboratory is found when examining a fecal or tissue specimen from an infected human. A parasite stage that is routinely recognized in a biological specimen and thus serves as a key to diagnosis is termed the **diagnostic stage.**

DIAGRAM 2-1

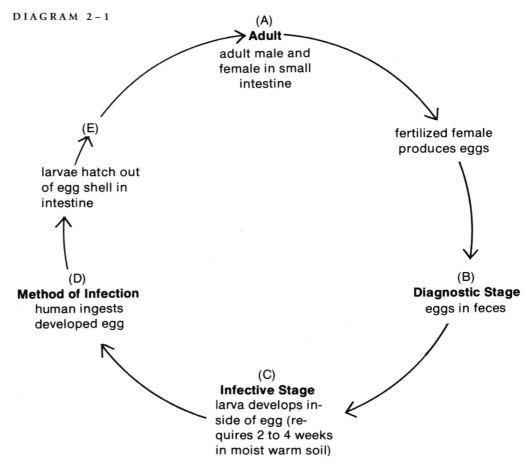

An example of a life cycle

3. When the parasite is infective. The parasite stage that is infective to humans (e.g., the third-stage larva) is termed the **infective stage.** To understand how the potential spread of the disease can be halted, you must know if external development is required for the parasite to reach infectivity (e.g., eggs develop in the soil) or if it spends a part of the life cycle in another host.
4. The means by which a new human host is infected (e.g., egg is ingested; larvae enter through skin).
5. Sites of development and maturation of the parasite in humans (e.g., it migrates through the intestinal wall, liver, and lungs and then is coughed up and reswallowed into the intestinal tract).

Intestinal Nematodes

Table 2-1 lists the scientific (genus and species) names and the common names for the intestinal roundworms of medical importance that are included in this section. On the following pages are the life-cycle diagrams, disease names, some of the major pathology and symptoms caused by infection with these roundworms, distribution, and other points of diagnostic importance. Also see Color Plates 1 to 27 and their accompanying descriptions. When you complete the study of each organism, you should be able to write:

1. The scientific name
2. The common name
3. The location of the adults in humans
4. The diagnostic stage and body specimen of choice for examination
5. The method of infection of humans
6. Other specific information pertinent to the diagnosis of each parasitic infection

Proper pronunciation of the scientific name is given beneath each name in Table 2–1. Practice pronouncing the scientific name aloud and spelling it on paper. In addition to the life-cycle charts, Table 2–2 (p. 30) will help you review the pertinent information for each parasite, including the epidemiology and the major disease manifestations that these parasites cause. The second section of this chapter covers the tissue nematodes in the same manner as the intestinal nematodes, and the third section discusses nematode zoonoses. While learning the text material, be sure to also study the corresponding pictures and descriptive key found in the color section at the front of the book.

All other chapters of this book follow the same format. When you think you have mastered these chapter materials (as outlined in the learning objectives), you will be ready to take the post-test on the section. The directions for each test are included on the test pages, and the answer key begins on page 221.

TABLE 2–1 □ INTESTINAL ROUNDWORMS

Order	Scientific Name (genus and species)	Common Name
Ascaridida	*Enterobius vermicularis* (en"tur-o'bee-us/vur-mick-yoo-lair'is)	pinworm, seatworm
Trochocephalia	*Trichuris trichiura* (Trick-yoo'ris/trick"ee-yoo'ruh)	whipworm
Ascaridida	*Ascaris lumbricoides* (as-kar-is/lum-bri-koy'deez)	large intestinal roundworm
Strongylida	*Necator americanus* (ne-kay'tur/ah-merr"I-kay'nus)	New World hookworm
Strongylida	*Ancylostoma duodenale* (An"si-los'tuh'muh/dew'o-de-nay'lee)	Old World hookworm
Rhabditida	*Strongyloides stercoralis* (Stron"ji-loy'-deez/stur"ko-ray'lis)	threadworm
Trichocephalida	*Trichinella spiralis* (trick"i-nel'uh/spy-ray'lis)	trichina worm

Enterobius vermicularis (pinworm, seatworm)

DIAGRAM 2-2

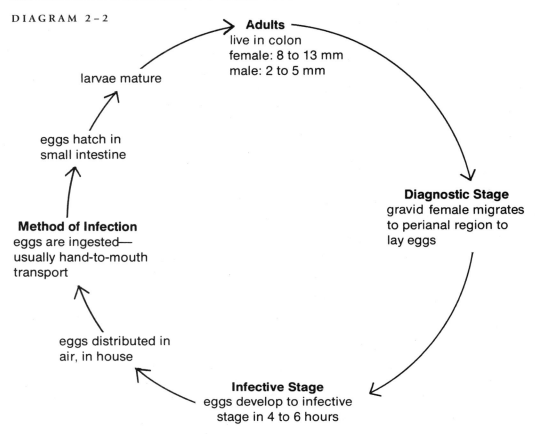

Enterobius vermicularis (pinworm, seatworm)

METHOD OF DIAGNOSIS

Recover eggs or yellowish white female adult from perianal region with a cellophane tape preparation taken early in the morning when the patient first wakes (see Chap. 7, p. 176).

DIAGNOSTIC STAGE

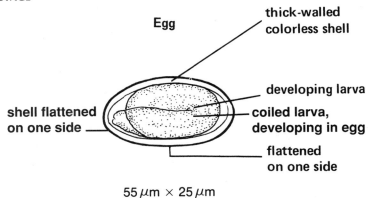

55 μm × 25 μm

DISEASE NAMES

- Enterobiasis
- Pinworm or seatworm infection

MAJOR PATHOLOGY AND SYMPTOMS

1. Many cases are asymptomatic. Occasionally, severe clinical problems develop.

2. Rarely, the disease causes serious lesions, which are usually limited to minute ulcers and mild inflammation of the intestine. About half of all patients report abdominal pain.
3. Other symptoms are associated with the migration of the **gravid** female out from the anus to lay her eggs on the perianal region at night.
   a. Cardinal feature: hypersensitivity reaction from **autoreinfection** causing severe perianal itching; eggs get on hands from scratching and are ingested; **pruritus** ani is **pathognomonic**
   b. Mild nausea or vomiting
   c. Loss of sleep and irritability
   d. Slight irritation to intestinal mucosa
   e. Vulval irritation in girls from migrating worms entering vagina

TREATMENT

Mebendazole or pyrantel pamoate; warm tap-water enemas; may need to treat the whole household because eggs are easily spread in the environment.

DISTRIBUTION

Distribution is worldwide, but it is more prevalent in temperate climates. *E. vermicularis* is the most common helminth infection in the United States. It is a group infection, especially common among children.

OF NOTE

1. Humans are the only known host. Infection is generally self-limiting.
2. Each female produces up to 15,000 eggs. Most eggs become infective within 4 hours of release and remain infective for only a few days. Cleaning eggs from the environment and treating all persons in the household are important to break the life cycle.
3. Eggs are rarely found in fecal samples because release is external to the intestine. Adult females occasionally can be recovered on cellophane tape preparation used to find eggs on perianal area.
4. Hatched larvae on perianal area may migrate back into rectum and large intestine and develop into adults (retroinfection), or autoreinfection (ingestion of eggs) can occur.

 FOR REVIEW

1. *Write the scientific name for seatworm:* _____
2. *Draw and label a picture of the diagnostic stage for this parasite.*
3. *The diagnostic test for this parasite is the* _____ *test and is best performed in the* A.M. _____ *or* P.M. _____.
4. *This infection can be increased in the host by* _____ *or* _____.

Trichuris trichiura (whipworm)

DIAGRAM 2–3

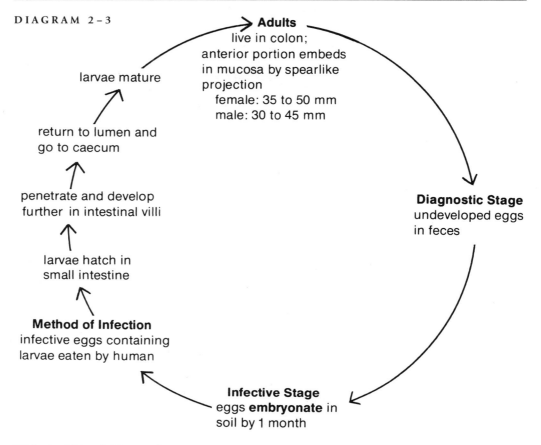

Adults
live in colon;
anterior portion embeds
in mucosa by spearlike
projection
    female: 35 to 50 mm
    male: 30 to 45 mm

larvae mature

return to lumen and
go to caecum

penetrate and develop
further in intestinal villi

larvae hatch in
small intestine

Method of Infection
infective eggs containing
larvae eaten by human

Diagnostic Stage
undeveloped eggs
in feces

Infective Stage
eggs **embryonate** in
soil by 1 month

Trichuris trichiura (whipworm)

METHOD OF DIAGNOSIS

Recover and identify characteristic eggs in feces.

DIAGNOSTIC STAGE

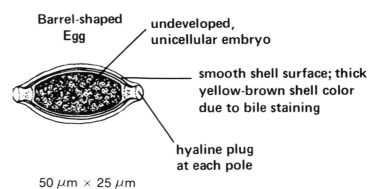

Barrel-shaped
Egg

undeveloped,
unicellular embryo

smooth shell surface; thick
yellow-brown shell color
due to bile staining

hyaline plug
at each pole

50 μm × 25 μm

DISEASE NAMES

• Trichuriasis
• Whipworm infection

MAJOR PATHOLOGY AND SYMPTOMS

1. Persons with slight infection are asymptomatic, with no treatment required.

2. Heavy infection (500 to 5000 worms) simulates ulcerative colitis in children and inflammatory bowel disease in adults. Histology reveals eosinophil infiltrations but no decrease in goblet cells. The surface of the colon may be matted with worms. Patients will have:
   a. Bloody or mucoid diarrhea
   b. Weight loss and weakness
   c. Abdominal pain and tenderness (colitis may be seriously debilitating)
   d. Increased peristalsis and **rectal prolapse,** especially in children
3. Chronic infections in children can stunt growth.
4. Stool is loose with mucus (and obvious blood) in heavy infection.

TREATMENT

Mebendazole

DISTRIBUTION

T. trichiura is prevalent in warm countries and areas of poor sanitation. In the United States, it is prevalent in the warm, humid climate of the South. It is the third most common intestinal helminth in the United States. It is more common among children and mentally handicapped people.

OF NOTE

1. Double infections commonly occur with *Ascaris* because of the similar method of human infection (i.e., ingestion of eggs from fecally contaminated soil). **Pica** is common in children.
2. Drug treatment may cause production of distorted eggs that have bizarre shapes when seen in a fecal specimen.
3. Zoonosis infection can occur with pig or dog species of whipworm.

 FOR REVIEW

1. *Draw the life cycle for whipworm.*
2. *Draw and label a picture of the diagnostic stage for this parasite.*
3. *Why are children more commonly infected than adults?*

_____

4. *Double infections can occur most commonly with* _____.

Ascaris lumbricoides (large intestinal roundworm)

DIAGRAM 2-4

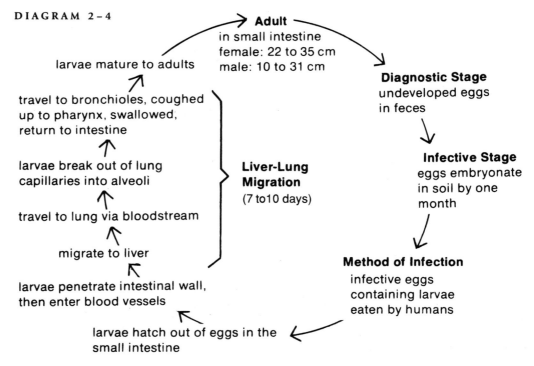

Ascaris lumbricoides (large intestinal roundworm)

METHOD OF DIAGNOSIS

Recover and identify fertile (**corticated** or not) or infertile eggs in feces. Sedimentation concentration test is recommended instead of flotation. Enzyme-linked immunosorbent assay (ELISA) serologic test is available.

DIAGNOSTIC STAGE

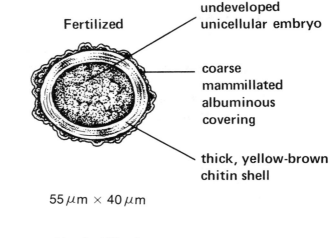

Fertilized

undeveloped
unicellular embryo

coarse
mammillated
albuminous
covering

thick, yellow-brown
chitin shell

55 μm × 40 μm

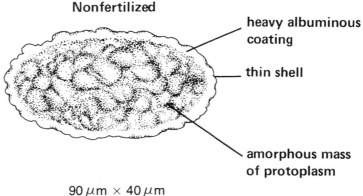

Nonfertilized

heavy albuminous
coating

thin shell

amorphous mass
of protoplasm

90 μm × 40 μm

DISEASE NAMES

- Ascariasis
- Roundworm infection
- Large intestinal roundworm infection

MAJOR PATHOLOGY AND SYMPTOMS

1. Tissue phase: With heavy or repeated infection, pneumonia, cough, low-grade fever, and 30% to 50% eosinophilia (Löffler's syndrome) result from migration of larvae through the lungs (1 to 2 weeks after ingestion of eggs). Allergic asthmatic reaction may occur with reinfection..
2. Intestinal phase: Intestinal or appendix obstruction results from migrating adults in heavy infections.
   a. Vomiting and abdominal pain result from adult migration.
   b. Protein malnutrition can occur in children with heavy infections and poor diets.
   c. Some patients are asymptomatic.
3. Complications from intestinal obstruction are caused by tangling of the large worms or migration of adults to other sites, such as the appendix, bile duct, or liver (detectable by radiograph).
4. Migrating adults (22 to 35 cm long) may exit by the nose, mouth, or anus. They are large, creamy, and white and have a cone-shaped tapered anterior; the male has a curved tail.

TREATMENT

1. Mebendazole or pyrantel pamoate
2. Piperazine citrate
3. Levamisole

4. Corticosteroid treatment (helps symptoms of severe pulmonary phase)
5. Nasogastric suction and drug treatment, or surgery, for intestinal obstruction by adults

DISTRIBUTION

A. lumbricoides is prevalent in warm countries and areas of poor sanitation. It coexists with *T. trichiura* in the United States, which is found predominantly in the Appalachian Mountains and adjacent regions to the east, south, and west. The eggs of these two species require the same soil conditions for development to the infective state, and infection for both is by ingestion of infective eggs.

OF NOTE

1. *Ascaris* is the largest adult intestinal nematode.
2. Adults are active migrators when provoked by fever, certain drugs, and anesthesia, and they may tangle and block the intestine or migrate through the intestine or appendix and come out of the mouth or anus. Mortality mainly results from intestinal complications in heavy infections.
3. *Ascaris* is the second most common intestinal helminth infection in the United States and the most common infection worldwide.
4. The adult female lays up to 250,000 eggs per day.
5. Eggs may remain infective in soil or water for years; they are resistant to chemicals.

 FOR REVIEW

1. *Write the scientific name for the large intestinal roundworm:* _____
2. *Draw and label pictures of the two diagnostic forms of the eggs of this parasite.*
3. *List the route of the migration of the larva after it escapes from the eggshell:*

_____

Necator americanus (New World hookworm) and *Ancylostoma duodenale* (Old World hookworm)

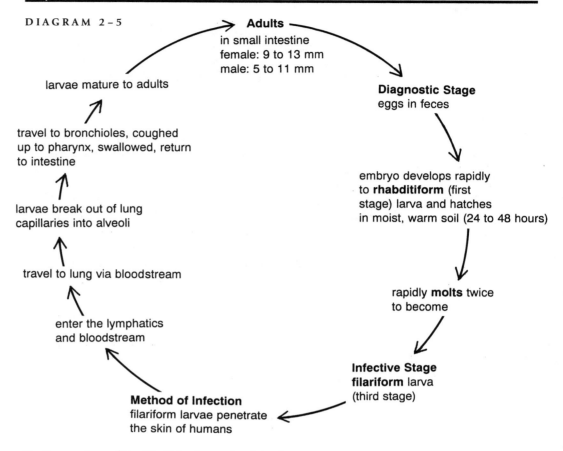

DIAGRAM 2–5

Adults
in small intestine
female: 9 to 13 mm
male: 5 to 11 mm

larvae mature to adults

travel to bronchioles, coughed
up to pharynx, swallowed, return
to intestine

larvae break out of lung
capillaries into alveoli

travel to lung via bloodstream

enter the lymphatics
and bloodstream

Method of Infection
filariform larvae penetrate
the skin of humans

Diagnostic Stage
eggs in feces

embryo develops rapidly
to **rhabditiform** (first
stage) larva and hatches
in moist, warm soil (24 to 48 hours)

rapidly **molts** twice
to become

**Infective Stage
filariform** larva
(third stage)

Necator americanus (New World hookworm) and *Ancylostoma duodenale* (Old World hookworm)

METHOD OF DIAGNOSIS

Recover and identify hookworm eggs in fresh or preserved feces. Species cannot be differentiated by egg appearance.

DIAGNOSTIC STAGE

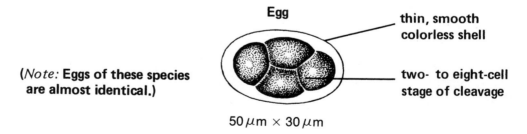

(*Note:* **Eggs of these species are almost identical.**)

Egg

thin, smooth
colorless shell

two- to eight-cell
stage of cleavage

50 μm × 30 μm

DISEASE NAME

Hookworm disease

MAJOR PATHOLOGY AND SYMPTOMS

1. After repeated infection, severe allergic itching develops at site of skin penetration by infective larvae; this condition is known as "ground itch." Penetration stings, and an erythematous papule forms.
2. Larvae migrate through lungs: Intra-alveolar hemorrhage and mild pneumonia with

cough, wheezing, sore throat, bloody sputum, and headache occur in heavy infections. Reaction is more severe in reinfections.

3. Intestinal phase of infection:
   a. Acute (heavy worm burden producing more than 5000 eggs per gram [EPG] of feces): **enteritis,** epigastric distress in 20% to 50%, anorexia, diarrhea, pain, microcytic hypochromic iron deficiency anemia with accompanying weakness, signs of hypoproteinemia, edema, and loss of strength from blood loss caused by adult worms
   b. Chronic (light worm burden showing fewer than 500 EPG): the usual form of this infection; slight anemia, weakness, or weight loss; nonspecific mild gastrointestinal symptoms (may be subclinical)
   c. Symptoms secondary to the iron deficiency anemia caused by blood loss; hyperplasia of bone marrow and spleen
   d. High eosinophilia

TREATMENT

Mebendazole or pyrantel pamoate, iron-replacement therapy, thiabendazole ointment for **cutaneous larval migrans**

DISTRIBUTION

N. americanus is found in North and South America; Asia, including China and India; and Africa. *A. duodenale* is found in Europe; South America; Asia, including China; Africa; and the Caribbean. Other Ancylostoma species are found in the Far East. *A. duodenale* is common in agrarian areas with poor sanitation. Almost one-fourth of the world's population is assumed to be infected with hookworms.

OF NOTE

1. Moist, warm regions and bare-skin contact with sandy soil are optimal conditions for contracting heavy infections in areas of poor sanitation. These parasites are often found in the same soil conditions as *Ascaris* and *Trichuris.*
2. Delayed fecal examination can result in larval development and egg hatching; therefore, *Strongyloides* larvae must be differentiated from hookworm larvae (see Color Plates 21 and 25). Hookworm **rhabditiform larvae** have a long buccal capsule; *Strongyloides* rhabditiform larvae have a short buccal capsule and a bulbous esophagus.
3. Adults are voracious bloodsuckers. Heavy infection can result in 100 mL of blood loss per day; therefore, provide dietary and iron therapy support along with drug treatment, as necessary.
4. Animal species of hookworm larvae can migrate subcutaneously through the human skin after penetration, causing allergic reaction in the migration tracks (cutaneous larval migrans).
5. Differentiate adults by buccal capsule and bursa (see Color Plates 21 and 25).
6. *Ancylostoma* **filariform larvae** can infect orally and possibly by transmammary or transplacental passage.
7. Pica contributes to infection and is a common symptom.

FOR REVIEW

1. *Write the scientific and common names for the two hookworm species:* _____ *and* _____
2. *Why might you find hookworm larvae in a fecal specimen?*

_____

3. *Describe how the two species are differentiated:*

_____

4. *The infective larval form is also called the* _____.

Strongyloides stercoralis (threadworm)

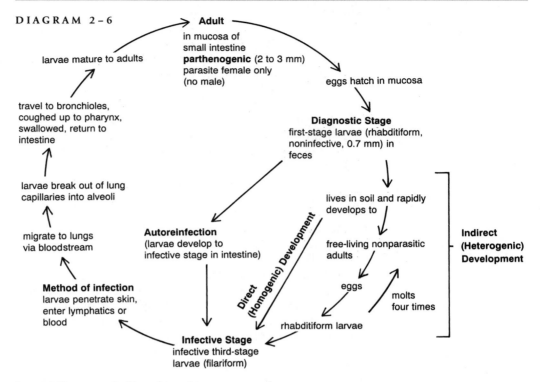

DIAGRAM 2–6

Adult
in mucosa of
small intestine
parthenogenic (2 to 3 mm)
parasite female only
(no male)

larvae mature to adults

travel to bronchioles,
coughed up to pharynx,
swallowed, return to
intestine

eggs hatch in mucosa

Diagnostic Stage
first-stage larvae (rhabditiform,
noninfective, 0.7 mm) in
feces

larvae break out of lung
capillaries into alveoli

migrate to lungs
via bloodstream

lives in soil and rapidly
develops to

Autoreinfection
(larvae develop to
infective stage in intestine)

free-living nonparasitic
adults

**Indirect
(Heterogenic)
Development**

Direct
(Homogenic) Development

Method of infection
larvae penetrate skin,
enter lymphatics or
blood

eggs

molts
four times

rhabditiform larvae

Infective Stage
infective third-stage
larvae (filariform)

Strongyloides stercoralis (threadworm)

METHOD OF DIAGNOSIS

Recover and identify rhabditiform larvae in feces, which are present in low numbers. Also, the presence of hookwormlike eggs or larvae in duodenal drainage fluid or from Entero-Test capsule is diagnostic. (Larvae must be differentiated from hookworm larvae when found in feces; see Color Plates 21 and 25.) Serology is ELISA. Larvae may be in sputum in disseminated strongyloidiasis. In severe cases, intestinal radiograph shows loss of mucosal pattern, rigidity, and tubular narrowing.

DIAGNOSTIC STAGE

Rhabditiform Larva
(*Note:* **Egg resembles hookworm egg.**)

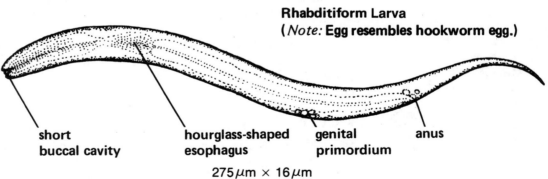

short
buccal cavity

hourglass-shaped
esophagus

genital
primordium

anus

275 μm × 16 μm

DISEASE NAMES

• Strongyloidiasis
• Threadworm infection

MAJOR PATHOLOGY AND SYMPTOMS

1. Major clinical features are abdominal pain, diarrhea, and urticaria, with eosinophilia.
2. Skin shows recurring allergic, raised, itchy, red wheals from larval penetration.

3. Migration of larvae: Primary symptoms are in the lungs; bronchial verminous (from worms) pneumonia.
4. Intestinal symptoms include abdominal pain, diarrhea, constipation, vomiting, weight loss, variable anemia, eosinophilia, and protein-losing enteropathy. Light infections are often asymptomatic; gross lesions are usually absent. The bowel is edematous and congested with heavy infection.
5. *S. stercoralis* has caused sudden deterioration and death in immunocompromised persons because of heavy autoinfection and larval migration throughout body (hyperinfection), with bacterial infection secondary to larval spread and intestinal leakage.

TREATMENT

1. Thiabendazole (not always successful)
2. Albendazole
3. Ivermectin

DISTRIBUTION

Distribution is in warm areas, tropics, and subtropics worldwide (similar to hookworm).

OF NOTE

1. The parasitic female is **parthenogenic;** therefore, multiplication and autoreinfection can develop in the same host.
2. Internal infection can continue for years because of maintenance of autoreinfection.
3. Strongyloidiasis is difficult to treat.
4. Often, T-lymphocyte function is defective.
5. *Strongyloides* larvae are not recovered using the zinc sulfate flotation technique; the sedimentation concentration method is preferred.
6. Heterogonic development with its free-living cycle producing infectious larvae is influenced by environmental conditions.

 FOR REVIEW

1. *Write the scientific name for the threadworm:* _____
2. *How can you recover and identify the diagnostic stage for this parasite?*

_____

3. *List the characteristic(s) that differentiate this parasite's first stage larvae from hookworm larvae:*

_____

4. *Which concentration technique is preferred for this parasite?*

_____

Trichinella spiralis (trichinosis; trichinellosis)

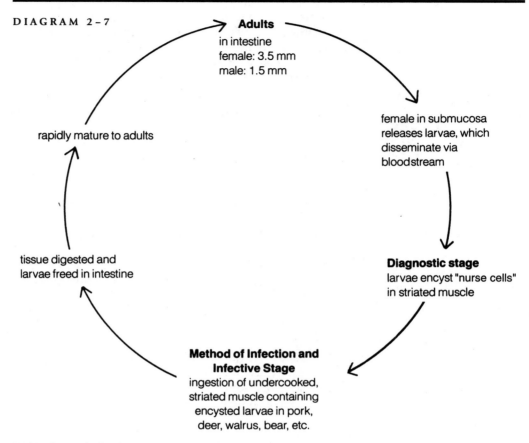

DIAGRAM 2-7

Adults
in intestine
female: 3.5 mm
male: 1.5 mm

female in submucosa
releases larvae, which
disseminate via
bloodstream

rapidly mature to adults

Diagnostic stage
larvae encyst "nurse cells"
in striated muscle

tissue digested and
larvae freed in intestine

**Method of Infection and
Infective Stage**
ingestion of undercooked,
striated muscle containing
encysted larvae in pork,
deer, walrus, bear, etc.

Trichinella spiralis (trichinosis; trichenellosis)

METHOD OF DIAGNOSIS

Identification of encysted larvae in biopsied muscle; serologic testing (ELISA) 3 to 4 weeks after infection. A history of eating undercooked pork or bear, fever, muscle pain, bilateral periorbital **edema,** and rising eosinophilia warrants presumptive diagnosis.

DIAGNOSTIC STAGE

Larva encysted in a muscle cell (called the "nurse cell")

(*Note*: **Granuloma forms around nurse cell and becomes calcified over time.**)

coiled larva

inflammatory infiltrate

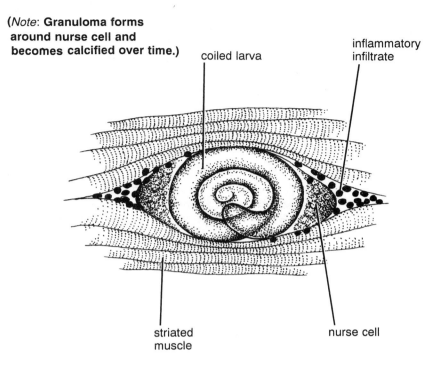

striated muscle

nurse cell

DISEASE NAMES

- Trichinosis
- Trichinellosis

MAJOR PATHOLOGY AND SYMPTOMS

1. Intestinal phase shows small intestine edema and inflammation, nausea, vomiting, abdominal pain, diarrhea, headache, and fever (first week after infection).
2. Migration phase shows high fever (104°F), blurred vision, edema of the face and eyes, cough, pleural pains, and eosinophilia (15% to 40%) lasting 1 month in heavy infection; death can occur during this phase in fourth to eighth week after infection.
3. Muscular phase shows acute local inflammation with edema and pain of the musculature. Other symptoms vary, depending on the location and number of larvae present. Larvae encyst in skeletal muscles of limbs, diaphragm, and face, but they invade other muscles as well. Weakness and fatigue develop.
4. Focal lesions show periorbital edema, splinter hemorrhages of fingernails, retinal hemorrhages, and rash.

TREATMENT

1. Non–life-threatening infection (self-limiting): rest, analgesics, and antipyretics
2. Life-threatening infection: prednisone; thiabendazole (caution—effectiveness not proven; may have side effects)

DISTRIBUTION

Distribution is worldwide among meat-eating populations and rare in the tropics. The prevalence in the United States is about 4% based on autopsy studies; about 100 cases are recognized and reported per year in the United States.

OF NOTE

1. Zoonosis: Carnivorous mammals are the primary hosts. This condition is found in most species.

2. Multiple cases are often related to one source of undercooked infected meat.
3. Cooking meat to 137°F or freezing for 20 days at 5°F will kill larvae.

 FOR REVIEW

1. *Write the scientific name for trichinosis:* _____

2. *Describe the diagnostic stage and method of diagnosis for this parasite:*

   _____

3. *What is the characteristic feature seen in peripheral blood during the migration phase of the life cycle?*

   _____

4. *List three animals that may harbor this parasite:* _____,
   _____, *and* _____

Dracunculus medinensis (Guinea worm)

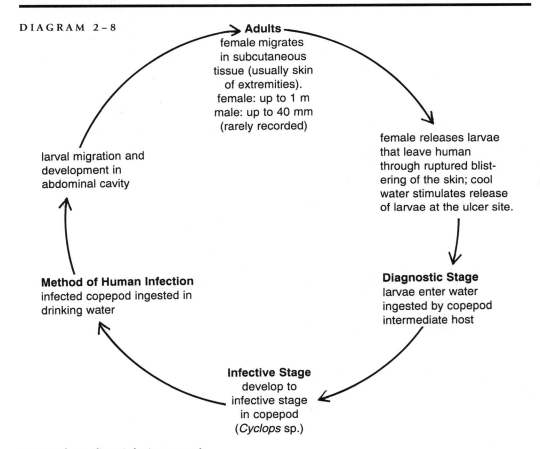

DIAGRAM 2–8

Adults
female migrates
in subcutaneous
tissue (usually skin
of extremities).
female: up to 1 m
male: up to 40 mm
(rarely recorded)

female releases larvae
that leave human
through ruptured blist-
ering of the skin; cool
water stimulates release
of larvae at the ulcer site.

larval migration and
development in
abdominal cavity

Method of Human Infection
infected copepod ingested in
drinking water

Diagnostic Stage
larvae enter water
ingested by copepod
intermediate host

Infective Stage
develop to
infective stage
in copepod
(*Cyclops* sp.)

Dracunculus medinensis (guinea worm)

METHOD OF DIAGNOSIS

Visually observe painful skin blisters or emerging worm; induce release of larvae from skin ulcer when cold water is applied.

DISEASE NAMES

- Dracunculus
- Guinea worm

MAJOR PATHOLOGY AND SYMPTOMS

1. Allergic reaction occurs during migration.
2. The papule develops into a blister, usually on feet or legs, that ruptures.
3. Secondary bacterial infections or reaction to aberrant migration of larvae or adults may cause disability or death.

TREATMENT

1. Removal of adult from skin (slow withdrawal from blister by wrapping it around a revolving small stick over several days; this process may be completed in a few days but usually requires weeks or even months)
2. Surgical removal of adult
3. Aspirin for pain; antihistamines may reduce swelling
4. Prevention of secondary infection

DISTRIBUTION

D. medinensis is found in the Middle East, India, Pakistan, and Africa.

OF NOTE

1. *D. medinensis* is the largest adult nematode parasitic in humans.
2. There is no effective immunity to reinfection.
3. The World Health Organization (WHO) is sponsoring an attempt at global eradication through the promotion of drinking water filtration (T-shirts or gauze can be used) to strain out infected copepods. The WHO also sponsors an education campaign to keep people out of water when adult worms are protruding from the body. Since 1986 the total worldwide caseload has dropped from about 3.5 million to about 100,000 cases in 1996 because of efforts by many organizations.

 FOR REVIEW

1. *Write the scientific name for Guinea worm:* _____
2. *Describe the method of transmission for this parasite:*

_____

> **Review Table 2–2, then proceed to the post-test on intestinal Nematoda if you have mastered the learning objectives.**

Filariae: Tissue Nematodes

Table 2–3 lists the scientific and common names for the members of the superfamily Filarioidea (the tissue roundworms) to be discussed in this section.

General Life Cycle

Adult **filariae** live in various human tissue locations. In general, fertilized adult female filariae living in the tissues produce living embryos **(microfilariae)** that migrate into lymphatics, blood, or skin. These parasites require an arthropod **intermediate host** for transmission of infection. If the arthropod ingests microfilariae while taking a blood meal, the larvae molt twice inside the arthropod intermediate host and become the infective stage filariform larvae. These larvae are released from the insect's proboscis and enter a new human definitive host when the arthropod next feeds on blood. The entering larvae migrate to the appropriate tissue site and develop to become adults. Maturation can take up to 1 year.

In some species, the microfilariae are more prevalent in peripheral blood at specific times of the day or evening (i.e., they exhibit **periodicity**). These times appear to coincide with the usual feeding pattern of the arthropod intermediate host species. Nocturnal or **diurnal** periodicity is noted in Table 2–4.

At least three other species of filariae are common parasites of humans. *Mansonella perstans,* found in Africa and Central and South America, and *Mansonella ozzardi,* found in

TABLE 2–2 □ IMPORTANT INTESTINAL NEMATODE INFECTIONS

Scientific and Common Name	Epidemiology	Disease-Producing Form and Its Location in Host	How Infection Occurs	Major Disease Manifestations, Diagnostic Stage, and Specimen of Choice
Enterobius vermicularis (pinworm)	Worldwide	Adult worms in colon, eggs on perianal region	Infective eggs are discharged by the gravid female on perianal skin eggs are transferred from hand to mouth	Perianal itching caused by local irritation from scratching; diagnosis: eggs found by cellophane test (p. 176)
Trichuris trichiura (whipworm)	Worldwide, especially in moist, warm climates	Adult worms in colon	Ingestion of eggs containing mature larvae from infected soil or food	Light infection—asymptomatic; heavy infection—enteritis, diarrhea, rectal prolapse; diagnosis: eggs in feces
Ascaris lumbricoides (large intestinal roundworm)	Worldwide, especially in moist, warm climate	Larval migration through liver and lungs, adult worms in small intestine	Ingestion of eggs containing mature larvae from infected soil or food	Light infection—asymptomatic; heavy infection—pneumonia from larval migration, diarrhea, and bowel or appendix obstruction; diagnosis: eggs or adults in feces
Trichinella spiralis (trichina worm)	Worldwide	Adults in small intestine, larval migration, larvae encyst in striated muscle	Ingestion of encysted larva in undercooked meat (pork or bear)	Gastric distress, fever, eye edema, acute muscle pain, eosinophilia; diagnosis: encysted larvae in muscle biopsy; serology
Necator americanus (New World hookworm)	United States, West Africa, Asia, and South Pacific	Larval migration, ground itch, adults in small intestine	Eggs shed in feces, mature in soil, larvae hatch and mature, infective (filariform) larvae penetrate host skin, especially feet	Repeated infection results in larval **dermatitis** with later pulmonary symptoms, microcytic hypochromic anemia from chronic blood loss if heavy infection and poor diet; diagnosis: eggs in feces
Ancylostoma duodenale (Old World hookworm)	Europe, Brazil, Mediterranean area, and Asia	As above (for *Necator americanus*)	As above	As above
Strongyloides stercoralis (threadworm)	Worldwide, warm areas	Larval migration, pulmonary signs, adults in small intestine	Immature (rhabditiform) larvae are shed in feces, develop in soil; infective (filariform) larvae penetrate host skin, especially feet; autoreinfection by maturing larvae in intestine; soil-dwelling, nonparasitic adults may produce additional infective-stage larvae	Repeated infection results in larval dermatitis with later pulmonary symptoms, heavy infections—abdominal pain, vomiting, and diarrhea; moderate eosinophilia, immunosuppressed host may suffer severe symptoms or death from heavy worm burdens inasmuch as autoinfection may occur; diagnosis: rhabditiform larvae in feces
Dracunculus medinensis (Guinea worm)	Africa, Asia, South America; no periodicity; *Cyclops* (crustacean)	Adults live in subcutaneous tissues, females migrate (larvae released from skin ulcer)	Ingestion of water containing crustaceans infected with larvae	Systemic allergic symptoms and local ulcer formation; diagnosis: adult in skin ulcer, larvae released into water

TABLE 2–3 □ FILARIAE

Scientific Name	Common Name
Wuchereria bancrofti (wooch-ur-eer'ee-uh/ban-krof'tye)	Bancroft's filaria
Brugia malayi (broog'ee-uh/may-lay eye)	Malayan filaria
Loa loa (lo'uh/lo'uh)	eyeworm
Onchocerca volvulus (onk'o-sur'kuh/vol'vew-lus)	blinding filaria

Central and South America, apparently do not induce pathology but do produce microfilariae in the blood. *Mansonella streptocerca*, found in tropical Africa, produces microfilariae that are found in the skin, as does *Onchocerca volvulus*. Therefore, any microfilariae found in blood or tissue must be differentiated; the diagnostic stages of the species are illustrated to aid in differential diagnosis of filariasis.

Information listed on the following pages is keyed by number according to genus and species. These numbers also will be used in the diagrams: **1** = *Wuchereria bancrofti*; **2** = *Brugia malayi*; **3** = *Loa loa*; **4** = *Onchocerca volvulus*.

TABLE 2–4 □ IMPORTANT FILARIAL INFECTIONS

Scientific and Common Name	Epidemiology, Periodicity, and Intermediate Host	Disease-Producing Form and Its Location in Host	How Infection Occurs	Major Disease Manifestations, Diagnostic Stage, and Specimen of Choice
Wuchereria bancrofti (Bancroft's filaria)	Tropics, nocturnal periodicity; *Culex, Aedes,* and *Anopheles* mosquitoes	Adults live in the lymphatics (microfilariae in blood)	Filariform larvae enter through bite wound into the blood when the mosquito bites a human to take a blood meal	Invades lymphatics and causes granulomatous lesions, chills, fever, eosinophilia, and eventual elephantiasis
Brugia malayi (Malayan filaria)	Far East, nocturnal periodicity, *Anopheles* and *Mansonia* mosquitoes	As above	As above	As above
Loa loa (eyeworm)	Africa, diurnal periodicity, *Chrysops* fly	Adults migrate throughout the subcutaneous tissues (microfilariae in blood)	As above, except the vector is a bloodsucking fly	Chronic and benign disease; diagnosis: microfilariae in blood; serology; Calabar swelling (a transient, subcutaneous swelling)
Onchocerca volvulus (blinding filaria)	Central America and Africa, no periodicity, *Simulium* (blackfly)	Adults live in fibrotic nodules (microfilariae migrate subcutaneously)	As above, except the vector is a bloodsucking fly	Chronic and nonfatal; allergy to microfilariae causes local symptoms—may cause blindness; diagnosis: adults in excised nodules; microfilariae in skin snips of nodule

Filariae

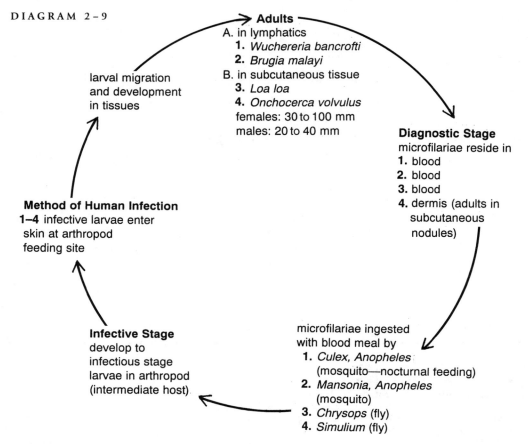

DIAGRAM 2–9

Adults
A. in lymphatics
   1. *Wuchereria bancrofti*
   2. *Brugia malayi*
B. in subcutaneous tissue
   3. *Loa loa*
   4. *Onchocerca volvulus*
   females: 30 to 100 mm
   males: 20 to 40 mm

larval migration
and development
in tissues

Diagnostic Stage
microfilariae reside in
1. blood
2. blood
3. blood
4. dermis (adults in
   subcutaneous
   nodules)

Method of Human Infection
1–4 infective larvae enter
skin at arthropod
feeding site

Infective Stage
develop to
infectious stage
larvae in arthropod
(intermediate host)

microfilariae ingested
with blood meal by
1. *Culex, Anopheles*
   (mosquito—nocturnal feeding)
2. *Mansonia, Anopheles*
   (mosquito)
3. *Chrysops* (fly)
4. *Simulium* (fly)

Filariae

METHOD OF DIAGNOSIS

    A. **1–3.** (Numbers refer to organisms in Diagram 2–9.) Locate microfilariae (200 to 300 μm) in stained blood smear (see p. 177). Also, you can centrifuge blood sample and lyse red blood cells to concentrate microfilariae in the specimen before staining (see p. 180, Knott technique).
       4. Locate microfilariae in skin snips of tissue nodule.
    B. Use serology (lacks specificity).

DIFFERENTIATION OF MICROFILARIAE AS SEEN IN A STAINED BLOOD SMEAR

Examine for the presence or absence of a sheath (a thin, translucent eggshell remnant covering the body of the microfilaria and extending past the head and tail).

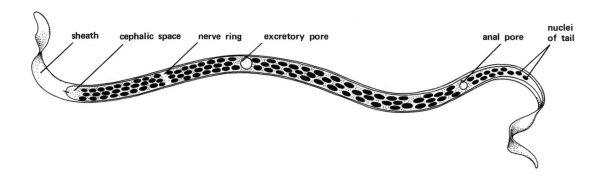

sheath   cephalic space   nerve ring   excretory pore   anal pore   nuclei of tail

Also, examine the tail area of microfilaria for the presence or absence of cells that exhibit a characteristic array of stained nuclei.

A. No nuclei in tailtip

(A1) *Wuchereria bancrofti*
sheath present

(A2) *Mansonella ozzardi* **(nonpathogen)**
no sheath

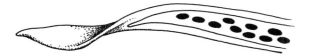
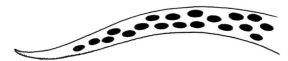

The tail of microfilaria of *Onchocerca volvulus* as seen in a tissue scraping from the nodular mass containing the adult filaria or from a skin snip shows no sheath, nuclei not terminal, and tail straight.

The tail of *Mansonella streptocerca* microfilaria is bent like a fishhook. These microfilariae are also found in skin snips.

(A3) *Onchocerca volvulus*

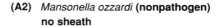

B. Nuclei in tail

(B1) *Loa loa*
continuous row of posterior nuclei;
sheath present

(B2) *Brugia malayi*
nuclei not continuous, two at
tip of tail; sheath present

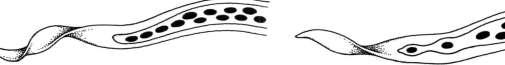
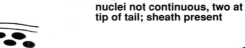

(B3) *Mansonella perstans* **(nonpathogen)**
nuclei in tip of tail; no sheath

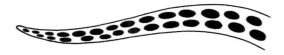

DISEASE NAMES

Filariasis (generic)
1. **Elephantiasis,** Bancroft's filariasis
2. Malayan filariasis
3. Eyeworm
4. Blinding filaria; river blindness

MAJOR PATHOLOGY AND SYMPTOMS

Diagnosis is difficult because symptoms are broad in spectrum. The diagnosis depends on identification of microfilariae.

1–2. In the early acute phase, fever and lymphangitis are seen; after years of repeated exposure, chronic elephantiasis develops because of obstruction of lymphatics, lymph stasis, and lymphedematous changes. Adults in lymphatics sequentially induce dilation, inflammation, and after death of the adult worm, surrounding granulomatous thickening of lymphatic walls. Finally, obstruction and resultant enlargement occur below the blocked area. Malayan filariasis is more often asymptomatic. In endemic areas, "filaria fevers" are seen, with recurrent acute lymphangitis and adenolymphangitis without microfilariae. Also seen is **tropical eosinophilia** or Weingarten's syndrome (which resembles asthma) with high eosinophilia and no microfilariae.

3. Localized subcutaneous edema (Calabar swellings), particularly around the eye, are caused by microfilariae migration and death in capillaries (more serious in visitors to endemic areas). Living adults cause no inflammation; dying adults induce a granulomatous reaction. Proteinuria and endomyocardial fibrosis also occur.

4. Fibrotic nodules on the skin encapsulate adults (onchocercomas). Progressively severe allergic onchodermatitis (pigmented rash) develops; blindness occurs from the presence of microfilariae in all ocular structures (very prevalent in Africa and on Central American coffee plantations).

TREATMENT

1. Diethylcarbamazine; ivermectin kills microfilariae
2. Diethylcarbamazine
3. Diethylcarbamazine (also prophylactic)
4. Ivermectin

DISTRIBUTION

1. Distribution is spotty worldwide; it occurs in tropical and subtropical areas.
2. Filiariae are found in East and Southeast Asia.
3. They are found in the rainforest belt in Africa.
4. They are found in Central America and equatorial Africa.

OF NOTE

1. Mosquito resistance to insecticides and coastal-dwelling human populations are increasing the incidence of exposure to infection.
2. Eosinophilic lung (tropical eosinophilia), an asthmalike syndrome, may be caused by **occult** filariasis or zoonoses.
3. Onchocerciasis is the major cause of blindness in Africa; insect control is difficult because the *Simulium* species (intermediate host) breeds in running water.
4. Filarial infection can induce an **"immunosuppressed** state" in the host that prevents a reaction to the parasite, but immune-mediated inflammatory responses or immunologic hyperreactive immunopathology (elephantiasis response) can still occur.

FOR REVIEW

1. *Write the scientific name for each of the following:*
   a. *Bancroft's filaria:* _____
   b. *blinding filaria:* _____
   c. *eyeworm:* _____
   d. *Malayan filaria:* _____

2. *Define periodicity, and explain why it is important to know the parasite's periodicity:*

   _____

3. *List the general characteristics that must be noted to differentiate the various microfilariae:*

   _____

> **Review Table 2–4 and then proceed to the Filaria post-test.**

● *Zoonoses*

A zoonosis is a biological life-cycle situation—not a class of parasites. Some parasites that normally live only in animals and survive in "the wild" without any life-cycle need for humans can sometimes infect humans. When this happens, the parasite is living in an unnatural host and will cause symptoms in this accidental host. Many types of parasites cause zoonotic infections, but the nematode group has most of the important zoonotic infections seen in humans.

Zoonoses are accidental infections in humans by parasites that usually have other animals as their hosts. Although the animal host and its parasites have evolved together and may tolerate each other well, in an abnormal host, such as a human, the parasite can often cause serious pathology. Table 2–5 lists the scientific names of some nematode zoonotic parasites, their geographic locations and normal animal hosts, and the disease and symptoms produced in humans after accidental infection. Although these parasites do not normally complete full life cycles in humans, it is nevertheless important to study these infections because of the significant pathology they cause in infected individuals.

For example, in the United States, there are large dog and cat pet populations, and these animals commonly have intestinal ascarids (*Toxocara* spp.) and hookworms (*Ancylostoma* spp.). When humans encounter pet feces-contaminated soil, roundworm eggs may be ingested or hookworm larvae may invade exposed skin. Most pet owners do not realize that these dog and cat worms may also infect humans and therefore do not take proper precautions to prevent infections. Small children are particularly at risk because of their play habits (particularly in sandboxes or at public playgrounds) and pica. Various workers (e.g., plumbers, electricians, others who often crawl under raised buildings) and sunbathers sitting on wet beach sand may also be exposed to animal hookworm larvae and are susceptible to larval penetration. Prevention of these infections may be accomplished by monitoring and treating infected pets (especially puppies and kittens) for worms, avoiding potentially contaminated soil, and practicing good hygiene and sanitation.

CASE STUDY 2–1

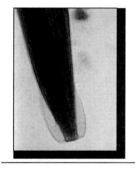

A nurse from a psychiatric facility called the local hospital laboratory to find out how to perform a cellophane tape test ordered for a 40-year-old patient who was exhibiting rectal digging. The technologist on duty explained the procedure, and when the laboratory received it, the technologist noted the parasitic form in the accompanying figure.

1. Was the correct test performed? Why?
2. How is this parasitic infection acquired? How is it maintained within the infected patient?
3. What steps should be taken to ensure that other residents will not become infected with this parasite?

CASE STUDY 2–2

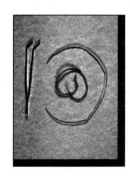

A mother brought the parasite form shown in the accompanying figure to her 5-year-old daughter's pediatrician. She stated that her daughter had been complaining of an upset stomach, had a slight fever, and was having diarrhea "a couple of times" during the last 10 days. Last night, the child vomited this "earthworm" into the toilet.

1. What is the probable identity of this parasite (genus and species)?
2. What other organs are invaded during this parasite's life cycle?
3. What other nematode parasite might commonly be found in patients harboring the worm recovered in this case?
4. What procedure should be performed to rule out other infections?
5. Why did the child vomit out the helminth?

TABLE 2–5 □ IMPORTANT ZOONOTIC INFECTIONS

Scientific and Common Name	Geographic Location	Normal Animal Host	Disease	Symptoms in Humans	Method of Infection of Humans
Ancylostoma braziliense; Ancylostoma caninum (dog hookworms)	Southern United States, Central and South America, Africa, Asia, Northern Hemisphere	Dog and cat; dog	Cutaneous larval migrans; creeping eruption	Allergic response of larvae under the skin; red, itchy tracts, usually on legs	Penetration of the skin by filariform larvae
Angiostrongylus cantonensis (rat lungworm)	China, Hawaii, and tropical islands	Rat	Eosinophilic meningoencephalitis	Eosinophilia and symptoms of meningitis, turbid spinal fluid contains many white blood cells, including increased eosinophils (looks like coconut juice)	Ingestion of infected snail or prawn (intermediate) host)
Angiostrongylus costaricensis	Central America	Rat		Adult worms lay eggs in mesenteric arteries near cecum, cause granulomas and abdominal inflammation	Eating unwashed vegetables contaminated with mucous secretions from infected slug (intermediate host)
Anisakis spp. (roundworm of marine mammals and fish)	Japan, Netherlands	Herring, other fish	Eosinophilic granuloma in stomach or small intestine	Abdominal pain and an eosinophilic granuloma around the migrating larvae of *Anisakis* in the intestinal wall	Ingesting raw fish containing the larval stage
Capillaria philippinensis	Far East	Fish		Malabsorption syndrome, extreme and persistent diarrhea, death from cardiac failure or secondary infection; adults multiply in human intestine and cause blockage	Ingestion of infected raw fish
Dirofilaria spp. (filariae of canines)	Various species worldwide	Dog, raccoon, fox	Tropical eosinophiliae, eosinophilic lung	High eosinophilia, chronic cough, pulmonary infiltrates, high levels of IgE; microfilariae are rarely present in peripheral blood	Bite of mosquito vector carrying infective filaria larvae
Gnathostoma spp.	Far East	Dog, cat		Acute **visceral larval migrans** syndrome, then intermittent chronic subcutaneous swellings; invades nervous system in Southeast Asia	Ingestion of larva from raw, infected fish, or application of infected snake poultice to open lesion; larvae migrate into lesion

Scientific and Common Name	Geographic Location	Normal Animal Host	Disease	Symptoms in Humans	Method of Infection of Humans
Gongylonema pulchrum	Worldwide	Pig		Migrating worm in facial subcutaneous tissue	Accidental ingestion of infected roach or dung beetle
Thelazia spp.	Worldwide	Various mammals		Habitation of conjunctival sac or lacrimal duct by adult, severe irritation of eye	Contract with infected fly or roach
Toxocara canis; T. cati (large intestinal roundworms of dogs or cats)	Worldwide	Dog, cat	Visceral larval migrans (VLM) or systemic toxocariasis; ocular toxocariasis	Eosinophilia, elevated isohemagglutinins, hepatomegaly, pulmonary inflammation with cough and fever, often history of seizures; alternative to VLM is possible encystment of the larvae in the eye (ocular larval migrans), which mimics a malignant tumor (retinoblastoma); all symptoms result from migration of larvae in the tissues of humans	Ingestion of infective-stage larvae in developed eggs from soil; history of pica in children and exposure to puppies

CASE STUDY **2-3**

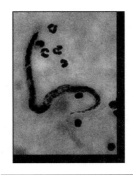

A new internal medicine resident from the Philippines went to the hospital's outpatient drawing area one evening to have his pre-employment blood work done. His laboratory results indicated 1+ proteinuria and rare red blood cells in the urinalysis report. The complete blood count (CBC) indicated mild anemia, and the differential report described the form seen in the accompanying figure.

1. What parasite do you suspect (genus and species)?
2. Would this infection be revealed if the resident had his blood drawn first thing in the morning? Explain your answer.
3. What vector(s) are included in this parasite's life cycle?
4. List other clinical symptoms that may be seen in this disease.

CASE STUDY **2-4**

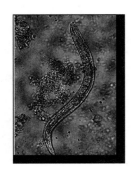

A 50-year-old Vietnam veteran came to the emergency department with severe respiratory symptoms, including fever, wheezing, and a productive cough. Vague gastrointestinal symptoms were also present. The patient had been receiving immunosuppressive therapy since his kidney transplant. He denied exposure to colds or possible intestinal pathogens. The physician ordered a CBC and a sputum culture and Gram stain. Mild eosinophilia was reported in the CBC. The parasite form in the accompanying figure was observed in a wet mount of the patient's sputum following its initial observation in the Gram stain.

1. What nematode parasites have a lung phase in their life cycle?

2. What parasite (genus and species) do you suspect in this case?

3. Describe the life cycle of this parasite, and explain how it can survive for an extended period in the host.

4. List possible complications that may occur if the patient is not successfully treated.

CASE STUDY 2–5   A 25-year-old man went to the doctor complaining of blurred vision and swelling around his eyes. He had been experiencing a low-grade fever and headache for the past 3 days. A CBC was performed, and the differential report revealed eosinophilia of 25%. On further questioning, the patient stated that he was a hunter and had butchered, processed, and eaten a recently killed bear.

1. Based on the patient's symptoms and history, what is the possible parasitic infection (genus and species)?

2. What classic signs are associated with this disease?

3. What other tests should be performed to confirm the diagnosis?

4. What precautions are necessary to prevent infections from this organism?

> You have now completed the chapter covering the Nematoda. After reviewing this material and the related color plates with descriptions, using the learning objectives to direct your studies, proceed to the first post-test. Allow 45 minutes to complete the test. Write your answers on a separate piece of paper. The correct answers are given in the back of the book. If you answer fewer than 80% of the questions correctly, review all the appropriate material and retake the test. Follow this procedure for all chapter post-tests.

Word Puzzles

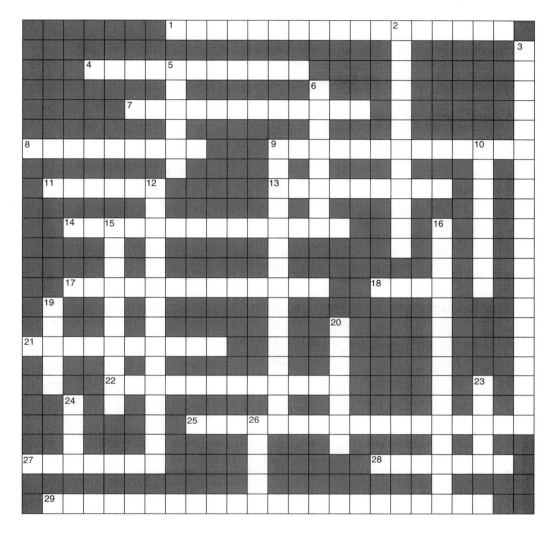

Across

1. Depressed immune response system; can accompany various diseases or can be induced by drugs
4. Recurring at a regular time period
7. The embryo stage of a filaria parasite; usually in the blood or tissue of humans
8. Entrance into a host, growth, development, reproduction, and subsequent transmission of offspring to a new host (2 words)
9. Capable of unisexual reproduction; no fertilization is required
11. Pregnant; female has developing eggs, embryos, or larvae in reproductive organs
13. Inflammation of the intestine
14. Weakening of the rectal musculature resulting in a "falling down" of the rectum (2 words)
17. Indicative of disease; characteristic symptoms suggest the disease
18. Habit of eating dirt or other unusual substances, such as chalk or plaster
21. Inflammation of the skin
22. High levels of circulating eosinophils in the blood
25. Noninfective, feeding, first-stage larva; the larva has an hourglass-shaped esophagus (2 words)
27. The surface of roundworms
28. Occurring during the daytime
29. A disease caused by the migration of larvae of *Ancylostoma* spp. (3 words)

Down

2. The development of a fertilized helminth embryo into a larva
3. A disease syndrome associated with high levels of blood eosinophils and an asthmalike syndrome (2 words)
5. Hidden; not apparent
6. Intense itching; *pruritus ani* refers to anal itching, as in enterobiasis
9. The time elapsing between initial infection with the immature parasite and reproduction by the adult parasite (2 words)
10. A class of the animal phylum Nemathelminthes—the roundworms
12. A developmental stage of a pathogenic organism that can be detected in human body secretions, discharges, feces, blood, or tissue by chemical means or by microscopic observations (2 words)
15. Possessing an outer, mamillated, albuminous coating, as on the eggs of *Ascaris lumbricoides*
16. Infective, nonfeeding, sheathed, third-stage larva; larva has a long, slender esophagus (2 words)
19. Unusual excess fluid in tissue, causing swelling
20. A nematode worm of the order Filariata
23. An immature stage in the development of a worm before becoming a mature adult
24. A process of replacement of the old cuticle with an inner, new one and subsequent shedding of the old, outer cuticle
26. Fan-shaped cartilage expansion at the posterior end of some male nematodes (e.g., hookworms)

```
V  M  R  G  A  R  M  H  O  F  T  L  L  E  G  R  A  V  I  D  E  S  W  C  R
D  A  H  E  Q  V  N  C  L  R  I  L  C  K  T  L  O  M  H  Q  O  A  S  X  A
O  Y  A  N  E  M  R  O  E  A  P  L  N  I  Y  Y  P  R  U  R  I  T  U  S  D
I  C  B  T  P  F  E  A  I  D  U  A  A  U  N  C  S  L  A  N  R  U  I  D  E
R  R  D  E  Q  V  S  F  L  S  E  T  T  R  J  E  E  U  R  R  P  S  K  H  L
E  E  I  R  S  A  P  K  Z  N  S  M  O  H  I  G  G  O  P  A  C  I  P  A  C
P  E  T  I  B  I  A  N  R  P  N  E  A  R  O  F  Z  O  O  D  V  T  N  I  Y
N  P  I  T  A  L  L  O  Y  T  E  O  R  V  E  G  O  A  N  S  R  L  E  R  C
O  I  F  I  W  I  O  I  S  D  D  R  J  P  C  I  N  R  Q  E  H  Q  J  A  E
I  N  O  S  O  H  R  T  A  L  Y  I  I  S  P  O  N  O  M  R  H  O  X  L  F
T  G  R  A  R  P  P  A  I  D  Y  P  A  O  A  U  R  F  M  L  L  T  X  I  I
A  E  M  D  P  O  L  N  R  A  E  T  Y  G  D  E  S  T  E  O  A  G  R  F  L
B  R  L  O  L  N  A  O  A  N  O  R  I  Y  N  I  Z  O  I  C  N  R  D  A  I
U  U  A  T  A  I  T  Y  L  G  U  C  M  D  C  O  C  M  N  C  T  I  V  W  P
C  P  R  A  T  S  C  R  I  F  C  X  C  A  N  N  S  I  E  U  A  I  C  A  S
N  T  V  M  C  O  E  B  F  Q  P  S  K  U  T  U  H  T  T  L  M  T  O  K  A
I  I  A  E  E  R  M  O  G  G  O  Q  R  L  I  C  N  I  Y  C  M  E  N  Z
H  O  D  N  R  V  M  E  R  N  Y  M  O  V  A  T  T  E  L  C  R  I  I  D  L
E  N  S  D  C  Q  H  Q  C  J  L  Y  L  R  O  X  V  I  F  H  S  S  T  E  A
E  L  E  P  H  A  N  T  I  A  S  I  S  Y  E  M  U  E  S  Y  D  T  I  U  G
U  V  M  W  Y  C  X  N  M  E  L  U  S  P  A  C  L  A  C  C  U  B  A  S  C
S  R  D  O  I  R  E  P  T  N  E  T  A  P  E  R  P  U  F  J  M  B  I  G  H
P  S  N  A  R  G  I  M  L  A  V  R  A  L  L  A  R  E  C  S  I  V  R  T  E
P  B  J  A  S  R  U  B  I  N  F  E  C  T  I  V  E  S  T  A  G  E  F  X  O
```

autoreinfection
buccal capsule
bursa
corticated
creeping eruption
cuticle
dermatitis
diagnostic stage
diurnal
edema

elephantiasis
embryonation
eosinophilia
enteritis
fecundity
filaria
filariform larva
gravid
immunosuppression
incubation period

infective stage
larva
life cycle
microfilaria
molt
Nematoda
occult
parthenogenic
pathognomonic
periodicity

pica
prepatent period
pruritus
rectal prolapse
rhabditiform larva
visceral larval migrans

Post-Test

Time: 1 hour

1. Draw the life cycle of *Ascaris lumbricoides* in diagram form. Indicate the diagnostic and infective stages. (**10 points**)

2. The night technician identified the following: (**15 points**)
    a. What is the scientific name of the parasite?
    b. What is the intermediate host?
    c. In what body specimen was this organism identified, and what laboratory technique was helpful in finding the organism?

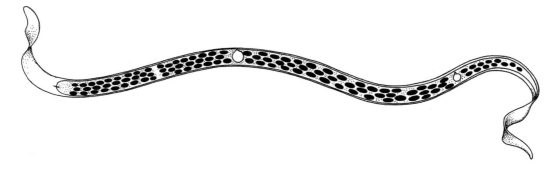

3. Briefly define each of the following: (**25 points**)
    a. Cutaneous larval migrans
    b. Diurnal
    c. Diagnostic stage
    d. Infective stage
    e. Prepatent stage

4. In which of the following sets of nematodes can each organism cause a pneumonia-like syndrome in a person exposed to heavy infection with any of the three parasites? (**5 points**)
    a. *Ascaris lumbricoides, Trichuris trichiura,* or *Onchocerca volvulus*
    b. *Enterobius vermicularis, Dracunculus medinensis,* or *Trichuris trichiura*
    c. *Strongyloides stercoralis, Wuchereria bancrofti,* or *Angiostrongylus costaricensis*
    d. *Necator americanus, Ascaris lumbricoides,* or *Strongyloides stercoralis*

5. A patient presents with vague abdominal pains and a microcytic hypochromic anemia. A possible causative parasite is: (**2 points**)
    a. *Enterobius vermicularis*
    b. *Ancylostoma duodenale*
    c. *Brugia malayi*
    d. *Trichinella spiralis*

6. An immunosuppressed patient is susceptible to autoreinfection with which one of the following nematodes? (**2 points**)
    a. *Strongyloides stercoralis*
    b. *Trichinella spiralis*
    c. *Ascaris lumbricoides*
    d. *Trichuris trichiura*

7. Infection with *Enterobius vermicularis* is best diagnosed by which one of the following? (**2 points**)
    a. Examination of feces for eggs and adults
    b. Serology tests
    c. Perianal itching noted by patient
    d. Examination of a cellophane tape preparation for eggs and adults

8. Human infection with *Loa loa* is best diagnosed by which of the following? (**2 points**)
    a. Examination of an infected *Anopheles* mosquito
    b. Examination of blood smears
    c. Examination of feces
    d. Examination of a skin scraping

9. A child who plays in dirt contaminated with human and pet feces is susceptible to which of the following set of parasites? (**5 points**)
    a. *Ascaris lumbricoides, Trichuris trichiura, Trichinella spiralis, Wuchereria bancrofti*

b. *Loa loa, Capillaria philippinensis, Enterobius vermicularis, Trichinella spiralis*

c. *Strongyloides stercoralis, Toxocara canis, Ascaris lumbricoides, Necator americanus*

d. *Ancylostoma braziliense, Trichuris trichiura, Trichinella spiralis, Necator americanus*

10. All of the following adult parasites live in the intestinal tract **EXCEPT: (2 points)**

a. *Ascaris lumbricoides*
b. *Enterobius vermicularis*
c. *Loa loa*
d. *Trichinella spiralis*

11. The largest adult nematode that is found subcutaneously in infected hosts is: **(2 points)**

a. *Ascaris lumbricoides*
b. *Dracunculus medinensis*
c. *Onchocerca volvulus*
d. *Trichinella spiralis*

12. Each of the following microfilaria have a sheath **EXCEPT: (2 points)**

a. *Brugia malayi*
b. *Loa loa*
c. *Mansonella ozzardi*
d. *Wuchereria bancrofti*

13. For each of the following, match the diagnostic technique(s) associated with the given parasite. **NOTE: Choices may be used more than once or not at all. (10 points)**

a. Blood film examination   _____ *Ascaris lumbricoides*
    _____ *Strongyloides stercoralis*
b. Cellophane tape test
c. Fecal concentration

        _____ *Trichinella spiralis*

method   _____ *Wuchereria bancrofti*

d. Tissue biopsy
e. Serologic test

14. For each of the following, match the insect(s) vector found in each filaria's life cycle: **NOTE: Choices may be used more than once or not at all. (10 points)**

a. *Anopheles* spp. (mosquito)   _____ *Brugia malayi*
    _____ *Loa loa*
b. *Culex* spp. (mosquito)   _____ *Onchocerca volvulus*
c. *Mansonia* spp. (mosquito)   _____ *Wuchereria bancrofti*
d. *Chrysops* (fly)
e. *Simulium* (fly)

15. Visceral larval migrans is caused by: **(3 points)**

a. *Ascaris lumbricoides*
b. *Ancylostoma braziliense*
c. *Dirofilaria* spp.
d. *Toxocara canis*

16. The zoonotic disease known as creeping eruption is caused by: **(3 points)**

a. *Ascaris lumbricoides*
b. *Ancylostoma braziliense*
c. *Dirofilaria* spp.
d. *Toxocara canis*

BIBLIOGRAPHY

Intestinal Nematodes

Anderson, RC: Nematode Parasites of Vertebrates: Their Development and Transmission, ed 2. CABI Publishing, New York, 2000.

Aspock, H, et al: *Trichuris trichiura* eggs in the Neolithic glacier mummy from the Alps. Parasitol Today 12:255–256, 1996.

Banwell, JG, and Schad, GA: Hookworm. Clin Gastroenterol 7: 129–156, 1978.

Behnke, JM: Evasion of immunity by nematode parasites causing chronic infections. Adv Parasitol 26:2–71, 1987.

Booth, M, and Bundy, DAP: Comparative prevalences of *Ascaris lumbricoides, Trichuris trichiura* and hookworm infections and the prospects for combined control. Parasitology 105:151–157, 1992.

Bundy, DAP, and Cooper, ES: *Trichuris* and trichuriasis in humans. Adv Parasitol 28:107–173, 1989.

Centers for Disease Control and Prevention. Trichinosis associated with meat from a grizzly bear—Alaska. Morb Mortal Weekly Rep 30: 115–116, 121, 1981.

Crompton, DW: Hookworm disease: Current status and new directions. Parasitol Today 5:1–2, 1989.

Crompton, DW, et al (eds): Ascariasis and Its Public Health Significance. Taylor and Francis, Philadelphia, 1989.

Cruz, T, et al: Fatal strongyloidiasis in patients receiving corticosteroids. N Engl J Med 275:1093, 1966.

Gillas, HM: Selective primary health care: Strategies for control of disease in the developing world. XVII. Hookworm infection and anemia. Rev Infect Dis 7:111–118, 1985.

Grove, SS, and Elsdon-Dew, R: Internal auto-infection with *Strongyloides stercoralis*. South Afr J Lab Clin Med 4:55, 1958.

Murrell, KD: Beef as a source of trichinellosis. Parasitol Today 10:434, 1994.

Murrell, KD: Trichinosis. In Strickland GT (ed), Hunter's Tropical Medicine, ed 7. WB Saunders, Philadelphia, 1991, pp. 756–761.

Nokes, C, et al: Moderate to heavy infections of *Trichuris trichiura* affect cognitive function in Jamaican school children. Parasitology 104: 539–547, 1992.

O'Brien, W: Intestinal malabsorption in acute infection with *Strongyloides stercoralis*. Trans R Soc Trop Med Hyg 69:69, 1975.

Pawlowski, ZS, et al: Hookworm infection and anatemia: Approaches to prevention and control. World Health Organization, Geneva, 1991.

Pearson, RD, and Guerrant, RL: Intestinal nematodes that migrate through skin and lung. In Strickland GT (ed). Hunter's Tropical Medicine, ed 7. WB Saunders, Philadelphia, 1991, pp. 700–711.

Sato, Y, et al: Efficacy of stool examination for detection of *Strongyloides* infection. Am J Trop Med Hyg 53:248–250, 1995.

Schad, G, and Warren, K (eds): Hookworm Disease: Current Status and New Directions. Taylor and Francis, Philadelphia, 1991.

Siddiqui, AA, et al: *Strongyloides stercoralis:* Identification of antigens in natural human infections from endemic areas of the United States. Parasitol Res 83:655–658, 1997.

Thune, O: Creeping eruption of larval migrans. Int J Dermatol 11:231, 1972.

Filariae

Buck, AA. Filariasis. In Strickland GT (ed), Hunter's Tropical Medicine, ed 7. WB Saunders, Philadelphia, 1991, pp. 713–727.

Chippaux, JP, et al: Severe adverse reaction risks during mass treatment with ivermectin in loiasis-endemic areas. Parasitol Today 12: 448–450, 1996.

Choyce, DP: Epidemiology and natural history of onchocerciasis. Isr J Med Sci 8:1143, 1972.

CIBA Foundation Staff: *Filariasis,* No. 127. Wiley, New York, 1987.

Coolidge, C, et al: Zoonotic Brugia filariasis in New England. Ann Intern Med 90:341, 1979.

Eberhard, ML, et al: A survey of knowledge, attitudes, and perceptions (KAPs) of lymphatic filariasis, elephantiasis and hydrocele among residents in an endemic area in Haiti. Am J Trop Med Hyg 54: 299–303, 1996.

Hougard, MM, et al: Twenty-two years of blackfly control in the Onchocerciasis Control Programme in West Africa. Parasitol Today 13:425–431, 1997.

Kumar, A. Do offspring of filarial infected mothers have a greater risk of becoming microfilaraemic? Acta Tropica 64:219–223, 1997.

Lawrence, RA. Lymphatic filariasis: What mice can tell us. Parasitol Today 12:267–271, 1996.

Michael, E, et al: Re-assessing the global prevalence and distribution of lymphatic filariasis. Parasitology 112:409–428, 1996.

Molyneux, DH: Onchocerciasis control in West Africa: Current status and future of the Onchocerciasis Control Programme. Parasitol Today 11:399–402, 1995.

Nicolas, L. New tools for diagnosis and monitoring of bancroftian filariasis parasitism: The Polynesian experience. Parasitol Today 13: 370–375, 1997.

Olszewski, WL, et al: Bacteriologic studies of skin, tissue, fluid, lymph, and lymph nodes in patients with filarial lymphedema. Am J Trop Med Hyg 57:7–15, 1997.

Ottesen, EA: Filariasis now. Am J Trop Med Hyg 41(suppl 3):9–17, 1989.

Ottesen, EA: Immunological aspects of lymphatic filariasis and onchocerciasis in humans. Trans R Soc Trop Med Hyg 78(suppl):9–18, 1984.

Otteson, RE: Description, mechanisms and control of post-treatment reactions in human filariasis. Ciba Found Symp 127:265–283, 1987.

Pinder, M: *Loa loa*—a neglected filaria. Parasitol Today 4:279–284, 1988.

Price, EW: The mechanism of lymphatic obstruction in endemic elephantiasis of the lower legs. Trans R Soc Trop Med Hyg 69:177, 1975.

Zoonoses

Alicata, JE: The discovery of *Angiostrongylus cantonensis* as a cause of human eosinophilic meningitis. Parasitol Today 7:151–153, 1991.

Alicata, JE, and Jindrak, K: Angiostrongylosis in the Pacific and Southeast Asia. Charles C. Thomas, Springfield, Ill., 1970.

American Heartworm Society. Recommended procedures for the diagnosis and management of heartworm (*Dirofilaria immitis*) infection. American Heartworm Society, Batavia, Ill., 1992.

Beaver, PC, and Orihel, TC: Human infection with the filariae of animals in the United States. Am J Trop Med Hyg 14:1010, 1965.

Centers for Disease Control and Prevention and American Association of Veterinary Parasitologists: How to prevent transmission of intestinal roundworms from pets to people. March 1995 (updated May 1998).

Clayton, DH, and Moore, J (eds): Host-Parasite Evolution. Oxford University Press, New York, 1997.

CRC Handbook Series in Zoonoses, Section C: Parasitic Zoonoses, Vols. 1–3. CRC Press, Boca Raton, Fla., 1982.

Danz, V, et al: Human intestinal capillariasis, 1. Clinical features. Acta Medica Philippina 4:72, 1967.

Freedman, DO (vol ed): Immunopathogenetic aspects of disease induced by Helminth parasites. Karger, New York, 1997.

Glickman, L, et al: Evaluation of serodiagnostic tests for visceral larval migrans. Am J Trop Med Hyg 27:492, 1978.

Hugh-Jones, ME, et al: Zoonoses: recognition, control, and prevention. Iowa State University Press, 2000.

Little, MD, and Most, H: Anisakid larva from the throat of a woman in New York. Am J Trop Med Hyg 22:609, 1973.

Lorõia-Cortez, R, and Lobo-Sanahija, JF: Clinical abdominal angiostrongylosis: A study of 116 children with intestinal eosinophilic granuloma caused by *A. costaricensis.* Am J Trop Med Hyg 29:538, 1980.

Markell, EK: Pseudohookworm infection—Trichostrongyliasis. Treatment with thiabendazole. N Engl J Med 278:831–832, 1968.

Meyers, BJ: The nematodes that cause anasakiasis. J Milk Food Technol 38:774, 1975.

Morera, P, and Cespedes, R: *Angiostrongylus costaricensis* n. sp. (Nematoda: Metastrongyloidea): A new lungworm occurring in man in Costa Rica. Rev Biol Trop 18:173, 1971.

Neafie, RC, and Meyers, WM: Dirofilariasis. In Strickland GT (ed). Hunter's Tropical Medicine, ed 7. WB Saunders, Philadelphia, 1991, pp. 748–749.

Pearson, RD, and Guerrant, RL: Intestinal nematodes that migrate through skin and lung. In Strickland GT (ed). Hunter's Tropical Medicine, ed 7. WB Saunders, Philadelphia, 1991, pp. 700–711.

Polnar, GO, Jr, and Jansson, HB: Diseases of Nematodes (2 vols). CRC Press, Boca Raton, Fla., 1988.

Prociv, P, and Croese, J: Human enteric infections with *Ancylostoma caninum:* Hookworms reappraised in the light of a "new" zoonosis. Acta Tropica 62:23–44, 1996.

Schaad, GA: Hookworms: Pets to humans. Ann Intern Med 120: 434–435, 1994.

Schlotthauer, JC, et al: Dirofilariasis: An emerging zoonosis? Arch Environ Health 19:887, 1969.

Uga, S, and Kataoka: Measures to control *Toxocara* egg contamination by *Toxocara* eggs in public park sandpits. Am J Trop Med Hyg Hyg 52:21–24, 1995.

Uga, S, et al: Defecation habits of cats and dogs and contamination by Toxocara eggs in public park sandpits. Am J Trop Med Hyg 54:122–126, 1996.

World Health Organization: Parasitic Zoonoses. WHO Technical Report No. 637. World Health Organization, Geneva, 1979.

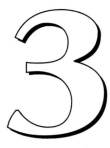

CESTODA

ON COMPLETION OF THIS CHAPTER AND REVIEW OF ITS SUPPLEMENTARY COLOR PLATES AS DESCRIBED, THE STUDENT WILL BE ABLE TO:

1 State the general characteristics of phylum Platyhelminthes.

2 Describe the general morphology of an adult cestode.

3 State the methods of diagnosis used to identify cestode infections.

4 Compare and contrast the phylum Nemathelminthes with Platyhelminthes, using morphologic criteria.

5 Define terminology specifically related to the **Cestoda.**

6 State the scientific and common names of cestodes that parasitize humans.

7 Describe in graphic form the general life cycle of a cestode.

8 Differentiate adult Cestoda using morphologic criteria.

9 Differentiate larval stages of Cestoda using morphologic criteria, the required intermediate host, or both.

10 Differentiate the diagnostic stages of the Cestoda.

11 Discuss the epidemiology and medical importance of cestode zoonoses.

12 Given illustrations or photographs (or actual specimens if you have had laboratory experience), identify diagnostic stages of Cestoda and the body specimen of choice to be used for examination of each.

13 Identify the stage in the life cycle of each cestode (including the zoonoses) that can parasitize humans.

GLOSSARY

anaphylaxis (anaphylactic shock). An exaggerated histamine-release reaction by the host's body to foreign proteins, allergens, or other substances; may be fatal.

anorexia. Loss of appetite.

brood capsule. A structure within the daughter cyst in *Echinococcus granulosus* in which many scolices grow. Each scolex can develop into an adult tapeworm in the definitive host.

Cestoda. A class within the phylum Platyhelminthes

that includes the tapeworms. These helminths have flattened, ribbonlike, segmented bodies.

copepod. A freshwater crustacean; intermediate host in the life cycle of *Diphyllobothrium latum.*

coracidium. A ciliated hexacanth embryo; *D. latum* eggs develop to this stage and then can hatch in fresh water.

cysticercoid. The larval stage of some tapeworms (e.g., *Hymenolepis nana*); a small, bladderlike structure containing little or no fluid in which the scolex is enclosed.

cysticercus. A thin-walled, fluid-filled, bladderlike cyst that encloses a scolex. Also termed a bladder worm. Some larvae develop in this form (e.g., *Taenia* spp.).

embryophore. The shell of *Taenia* spp. eggs and certain other tapeworm eggs as seen in feces.

hermaphroditic. Having both male and female reproductive organs within the same individual. All tapeworms have both sets of reproductive organs in each segment of the adult.

hexacanth embryo. A tapeworm larva having six hooklets (see **onchosphere**).

hydatid cyst. A vesicular structure formed by *E. granulosus* larva in the intermediate host; contains fluid, brood capsules, and daughter cysts in which the scolices of potential tapeworms are formed. Grows slowly and can get quite large.

hydatid sand. Granular material consisting of free scolices, hooklets, daughter cysts, and amorphous material. Found in the fluid of older cysts of *E. granulosus*.

onchosphere. The motile, first-stage larva of certain cestodes; armed with six hooklets (also termed hexacanth embryo).

operculum. The lidlike or caplike cover on certain platyhelminth eggs (e.g., *D. latum*).

parenchyma. Tissue in which the internal organs of Platyhelminthes are embedded.

plerocercoid. The larval stage in the development of *D. latum* that develops after a freshwater fish ingests the procercoid stage. This form has an immature scolex and is infective if eaten by humans.

procercoid. The larval stage that develops from the **coracidium** of *D. latum*. It develops in the body of a freshwater crustacean.

proglottid (proglottis). One of the segments of a tapeworm. Each proglottid contains male and female reproductive organs when mature.

racemose. Clusters with branching, nodular terminations resembling a bunch of grapes. Used in reference to larval cysticercosis caused by the migration and development of *T. solium* larvae in the brain tissue of humans; an aberrant form.

rostellum. The fleshy, anterior protuberance of the scolex of some tapeworms (species specific); may bear a circular row (or rows) of hooks; may be retractable.

scolex (pl. scolices). Anterior end of a tapeworm; attaches to the wall of the intestine of a host by means of suckers and sometimes hooks.

sparganosis. Plerocercoid in human tissue from accidental infection with procercoid of several species of Cestodes.

strobila. Entire body of a tapeworm.

tegument (integument). The body surface of platyhelminths; the Cestode tegument is the site of nutrient and oxygen absorption as well as waste excretion.

transport host. Vector; often a bloodsucking insect.

viscera (sing. viscus). Any of the large organs in the interior of any of the three great body cavities of vertebrates.

● Cestodes

The Platyhelminthes, as a phylum, are known as the flatworms; they are dorsoventrally flattened and have solid bodies with no body cavity. The internal organs are embedded in tissue called the **parenchyma**. There are no respiratory or blood-vascular systems. The life cycles of these organisms are generally indirect; that is, at least one intermediate host is required to support larval development.

The two classes of the phylum Platyhelminthes that contain human parasites are the Cestoda (the tapeworms) and the Digenea (the flukes). The Digenea are covered in Chapter 4. Platyhelminths are all **hermaphroditic** with an important exception: the blood flukes.

The external surface (termed the **tegument**) of both tapeworms and flukes is highly absorptive and even releases digestive enzymes at its surface from microtriches (specialized microvilli). The adult cestodes must absorb all nutrients through the tegument because this class of parasites has no mouth, digestive tract, or vascular system. Waste products are released through the tegument as well.

Members of the class Cestoda are commonly called tapeworms, inasmuch as they are long, ribbonlike, and flattened in cross-section, much like a tape measure. The adult may range from a few millimeters to 20 meters in length, depending on the species.

The adult cestode lives in the intestinal tract of the vertebrate definitive host, whereas the larval stage inhabits tissues of the intermediate host. The anterior end of the adult (termed the **scolex**) is modified for attachment to the intestinal wall of the definitive host. The scolex is usually equipped with four cup-shaped suckers, and some species also have a crown of hooks on the scolex to aid in attachment. A scolex is less than 2 mm long, although the whole tapeworm can be 20 meters in body length. The entire body of an adult tapeworm is termed the **strobila**. The body of the tapeworm consists of segments known as **proglottids**. Segments form by budding from the posterior end of the scolex, an area of germinal tissue for new segment production. Older, mature segments move to the terminal end of the strobila as younger segments are produced.

Each tapeworm is hermaphroditic; that is, every mature proglottid of the body contains both male and female reproductive organs. The reproductive organs in each proglottid mature gradually so that the proglottids toward the terminus of the tapeworm contain fully developed reproductive organs and the uterus is filled with fertilized eggs. The shape of the gravid uterus is distinctive for each species. These posterior segments are termed gravid proglottids and can be found singly or in short chains if they break off from the chain and are expelled in feces. The embryo seen within tapeworm eggs (termed the **onchosphere** or **hexacanth embryo**) bears six tiny hooklets that facilitate entry of the embryo into the intestinal mucosa of the intermediate host. After the embryo hatches from the eggshell in the intestine of the intermediate host, it migrates through the intestinal wall and goes to a specific tissue site.

Table 3–1 lists the scientific names (genus and species) and the common names for the cestodes of medical importance. Use the pronunciation guide and repeat each name out loud several times. The life-cycle diagrams of these tapeworms are shown on the following pages, and Table 3–2, page 55, reviews the pertinent information about tapeworms. Proceed to the post-test when you have learned the vocabulary and the introductory material, have mastered the life cycles and Color Plates 34 to 52, and have reviewed Table 3–2.

TABLE 3–1 □ CESTODA

Order	Scientific Name	Common Name
Cyclophyllidea	*Hymenolepis nana* (high"men-ol'e-pis/nay'nuh	dwarf tapeworm
Cyclophyllidea	*Taenia saginata* (tee'nee-uh/sadj-I-nay'tuh)	beef tapeworm
Cyclophyllidea	*Taenia solium* (tee'nee-uh/so-lee'um)	pork tapeworm
Cyclophyllidea	*Echinococcus granulosus* (eh-kigh"no-kock'us/gran-yoo-lo'sus)	dog tapeworm, hydatid tapeworm
Pseudophyllidea	*Diphyllobothrium latum* (dye-fil"o-both-ree-um/lay'tum)	broadfish tapeworm

Hymenolepis nana (dwarf tapeworm)

DIAGRAM 3–1

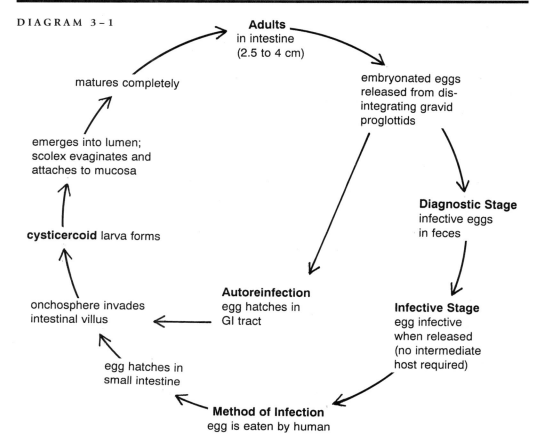

Adults
in intestine
(2.5 to 4 cm)

matures completely

embryonated eggs
released from dis-
integrating gravid
proglottids

emerges into lumen;
scolex evaginates and
attaches to mucosa

Diagnostic Stage
infective eggs
in feces

cysticercoid larva forms

onchosphere invades
intestinal villus

Autoreinfection
egg hatches in
GI tract

Infective Stage
egg infective
when released
(no intermediate
host required)

egg hatches in
small intestine

Method of Infection
egg is eaten by human

Hymenolepis nana (dwarf tapeworm)

METHOD OF DIAGNOSIS

Recover and identify eggs in the feces.

DIAGNOSTIC STAGE

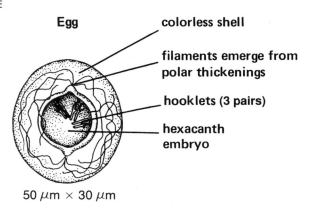

Egg

colorless shell

filaments emerge from
polar thickenings

hooklets (3 pairs)

hexacanth
embryo

50 μm × 30 μm

DISEASE NAME

Dwarf tapeworm infection

MAJOR PATHOLOGY AND SYMPTOMS

1. Light infection is asymptomatic.
2. Heavy infection symptoms include intestinal enteritis, abdominal pain, diarrhea, headache, dizziness, and **anorexia.**
3. Multiple adults are commonly present.

TREATMENT

Praziquantel

DISTRIBUTION

Worldwide, *H. nana* is found in the tropics and subtropics; it most commonly occurs in children and in institutionalized people living in close quarters. It is the most prevalent human tapeworm in the United States, with greater prevalence in the Southeast. Estimated infection rate is 3%.

OF NOTE

1. The dwarf tapeworm requires no intermediate host, but it is common in the house mouse. Fleas and beetles can serve as **transport hosts. Cysticercoid** larvae can develop in the body cavity of these insects and are infective to either humans or rodents if accidentally ingested.
2. Eggs in feces from infected mice and rats are a common source of human infection.

 FOR REVIEW

1. *Write the scientific name for the dwarf tapeworm:* _____
2. *Describe the diagnostic stage of this parasite:*

_____

3. *Explain how autoreinfection with this parasite occurs.*

_____

Taenia saginata (beef tapeworm) and ***Taenia solium*** (pork tapeworm)

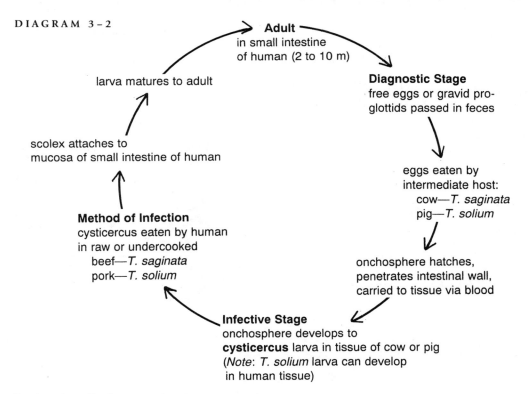

Taenia saginata (beef tapeworm) and *Taenia solium* (pork tapeworm)

METHOD OF DIAGNOSIS

Recover egg or gravid proglottid (or scolex after drug treatment) in feces. Proglottid and scolex identification: *T. saginata* has 15 to 30 lateral uterine branches in each gravid proglottid (can be seen clearly after dye injection into the uterine pore) and a scolex with only four suckers; *T. solium* has a gravid proglottid with 7 to 12 lateral uterine branches, and the scolex has four suckers plus a central crown of hooks. *T. solium* is called the "armed" tapeworm because of the crown of hooks by which the scolex attaches to the intestinal wall (see Color Plate 40). The eggs of these two species are identical. Immunologic methods for cysticercosis are enzyme-linked immunosorbent assay (ELISA) and indirect hemagglutination.

DIAGNOSTIC STAGE

1. Eggs in feces
2. Intact gravid proglottids may be found in feces and must be differentiated (see Color Plates 42 and 43)
3. Radiographic, computed tomography (CT), or magnetic resonance imaging demonstration of *T. solium* **cysticercus** in tissue with accompanying symptoms

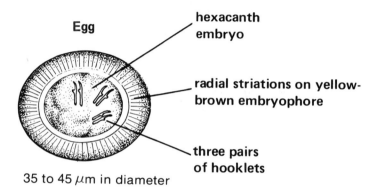

Egg — hexacanth embryo — radial striations on yellow-brown embryophore — three pairs of hooklets

35 to 45 μm in diameter

DISEASE NAMES

- *T. saginata:* taeniasis, beef tapeworm infection
- *T. solium:* taeniasis, pork tapeworm infection, cysticercosis (larval infection in tissue)

MAJOR PATHOLOGY AND SYMPTOMS

1. Most infected people are asymptomatic. Abdominal pain, diarrhea, and weight loss can occur. Eosinophilia is moderate.
2. Humans can serve as accidental intermediate hosts for *T. solium.* If eggs of *T. solium* are accidentally ingested or released from a proglottid in the intestinal tract, the eggs can hatch in the intestine and the larvae will migrate to form cysticercus bladders in any organ or nervous tissue (cysticercosis; neurocysticercosis [NCC], if in the central nervous system). This migration can be fatal if the **racemose** form develops in the brain. Arachnoiditis occurs in 50% of active NCC cases; obstructive hydrocephalus occurs in 25% of active NCC cases. Symptoms include epilepsy, headache, papilledema, and vomiting.

TREATMENT

- For adult tapeworm: praziquantel or niclosamide
- For cysticercosis: albendazole or praziquantel; anticonvulsants for seizures; corticosteroids for NCC symptoms; surgery

DISTRIBUTION

T. saginata: cosmopolitan in countries in which beef is eaten raw or insufficiently cooked. It is found in the southwestern United States.

  T. solium: cosmopolitan when pork is eaten raw or undercooked. It is rare in the United States.

OF NOTE

1. Humans are the only known definitive host for these two *Taenia* spp.
2. The adult worms live for many years, and usually only one worm is present in the intestine.
3. Human cysticercosis is common in Mexico and Central America.
4. Some 60% of patients with cysticercosis have larvae in the brain.

 FOR REVIEW

1. *Write the scientific names for beef and pork tapeworm, respectively:* _____ *and* _____

2. *Draw and label a picture of the diagnostic stage for this parasite.*

3. *State how the two species are differentiated:*

   _____

4. *The species for which humans can serve as an intermediate host is _____. If the stage is found in the brain, it can lead to fatality if the form develops.*

5. *How does a human acquire an adult T. solium infection?*

   _____

6. *How does a human acquire a larval-stage T. solium infection?*

   _____

Diphyllobothrium latum (broadfish tapeworm)

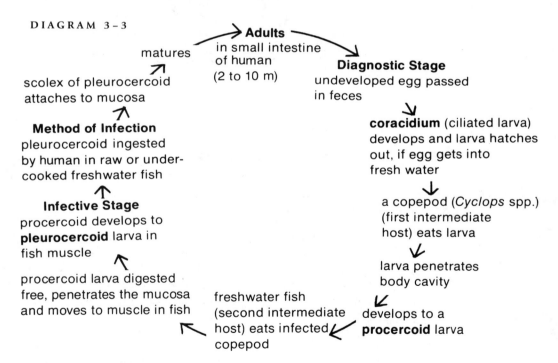

DIAGRAM 3–3

Diphyllobothrium latum (broadfish tapeworm)

METHOD OF DIAGNOSIS

Recover eggs in feces; evacuated proglottids and scolices are also diagnostic in feces but are rarely naturally evacuated intact.

DIAGNOSTIC STAGE

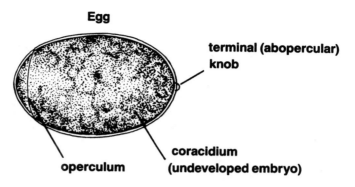

Egg

terminal (abopercular) knob

coracidium (undeveloped embryo)

operculum

75 μm × 45 μm

DISEASE NAMES

- Diphyllobothriasis
- Dibothriocephalus anemia
- Fish tapeworm infection
- Broadfish tapeworm infection

MAJOR PATHOLOGY AND SYMPTOMS

1. Major pathology and symptoms are intestinal obstruction (adult can grow to 20 meters) and abdominal pain. Most infected people exhibit vague digestive symptoms.
2. Weight loss and weakness occur.
3. In about 1% of infected people (usually restricted to people of Scandinavian descent), anemia (macrocytic type) and eventual nervous system disturbances result from a deficiency caused by the tapeworm's utilization of up to 100% dietary B_{12}.

TREATMENT

Niclosamide or praziquantel

DISTRIBUTION

Distribution is in temperate regions where freshwater fish are a common part of the diet or raw fish are eaten (the Great Lakes region of the United States, Alaska, Chile, Argentina, Central Africa, and parts of Asia). In Europe, estimates of infection include 20% of the Finnish people and up to 100% of residents of the Baltic region.

OF NOTE

1. Usually only one adult is present.
2. In addition to humans, a variety of fish-eating mammals can serve as definitive hosts.
3. The **procercoid** may be passed up the food chain in a dormant condition through small to larger game fish (e.g., Northern or walleyed pike).
4. A human can develop a tissue **plerocercoid** if a procercoid in a **copepod** is accidentally ingested. (See **sparganosis** in Table 3–2).

FOR REVIEW

1. *What makes this life cycle different from others you have studied?*

_____

2. *What makes this egg different from others you have studied?*

_____

3. *Humans become infected with taeniasis by eating* _____ *or*

_____.

Echinococcus granulosus (hydatid tapeworm)

DIAGRAM 3–4

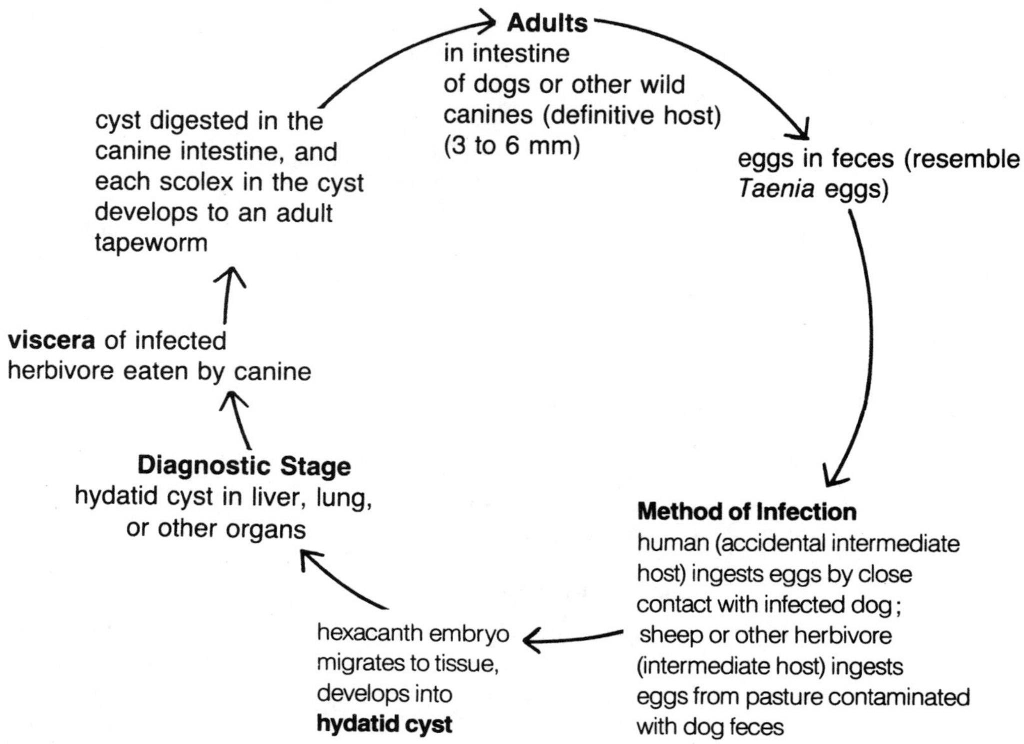

Adults
in intestine
of dogs or other wild
canines (definitive host)
(3 to 6 mm)

eggs in feces (resemble *Taenia* eggs)

cyst digested in the
canine intestine, and
each scolex in the cyst
develops to an adult
tapeworm

viscera of infected
herbivore eaten by canine

Diagnostic Stage
hydatid cyst in liver, lung,
or other organs

hexacanth embryo
migrates to tissue,
develops into
hydatid cyst

Method of Infection
human (accidental intermediate
host) ingests eggs by close
contact with infected dog;
sheep or other herbivore
(intermediate host) ingests
eggs from pasture contaminated
with dog feces

Echinococcus granulosus (hydatid tapeworm)

METHOD OF DIAGNOSIS

1. Serologic tests: indirect hemagglutination, ELISA
2. Presence of scolices, **brood capsules, hydatid sand,** or daughter cysts in the **hydatid cyst** fluid as detected by biopsy (not recommended because leakage of cyst fluid can cause **anaphylaxis**)
3. X-ray examination, ultrasound scan, or CT detection of cyst mass in organ, especially if calcified

DIAGNOSTIC STAGE

Hydatid cyst (partial cross-section)

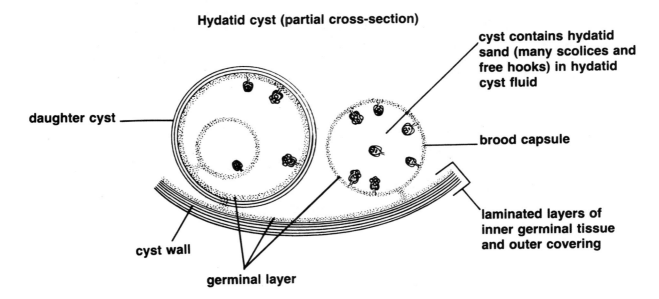

cyst contains hydatid sand (many scolices and free hooks) in hydatid cyst fluid

daughter cyst

brood capsule

laminated layers of inner germinal tissue and outer covering

cyst wall

germinal layer

DISEASE NAMES

- Echinococcosis
- Hydatid cyst
- Hydatid disease
- Hydatidosis

MAJOR PATHOLOGY AND SYMPTOMS

1. Symptoms vary according to location and size of cyst. Expanding cyst causes pressure necrosis of surrounding tissues.
    a. In the liver (most common site), no symptoms develop until the cyst gets large (nearly a year after ingestion of egg); then jaundice or portal hypertension develops.
    b. In the lung, no symptoms appear until cyst becomes large; then coughing, shortness of breath, and chest pain develop.
    c. In other sites, symptoms are related to enlarging cyst pressure.
2. Cyst growth or rupture can result in death.
3. Anaphylactic shock may occur if cyst ruptures (may occur during biopsy procedure).
4. Other findings include eosinophilia, urticaria, and bronchospasm.

TREATMENT

1. Surgery
2. Mebendazole or albendazole

DISTRIBUTION

Distribution is cosmopolitan; human infections occur primarily in sheep-raising areas where domestic dogs are used in herding.

OF NOTE

1. Hydatid disease in the United States is reported mainly in sheep-raising areas of the Southwest (chiefly among the Navaho), Utah, and Alaska; it also is reported in Canada.
2. *Echinococcus* cysts produce daughter cysts and brood capsules, all lined with germinal tissue that buds off many protoscolices, each of which can form the scolex of an adult if ingested by a canine.
3. *E. multilocularis*, which forms alveolar cysts, is rarer in humans, but it is intensely pathogenic and generally fatal without treatment. The disease develops slowly and may not

produce symptoms for several years. Symptoms often mimic those of cirrhosis of the liver or liver cancer. This parasite is found worldwide, mostly in northern latitudes, and is harbored in wild canines (e.g., foxes, coyotes) and in rodents.

4. Hydatid cyst in bone has abnormal, disseminated development in the marrow.
5. A slow-leaking cyst causes allergic sensitization. Cyst rupture (occurring naturally or during surgery) can cause anaphylaxis or spread of germinal tissue to other sites where new cysts can develop.

 FOR REVIEW

1. *Write the scientific name for the hydatid tapeworm:* _____
2. *Explain how hydatid cyst disease is diagnosed in humans.*

_____

3. *The definitive host for this parasite is* _____.
4. *Describe the structure of a growing hydatid cyst:*

_____

TABLE 3–2 □ CESTODA INFECTIONS

HUMAN INFECTIONS WITH CESTODA				
Scientific and Common Name	**Epidemiology**	**Disease-Producing Worm and Its Location in Host**	**How Human Infection Occurs**	**Major Disease Manifestations, Diagnostic Stage, and Specimen of Choice**
Hymenolepis nana (dwarf tapeworm)	Worldwide (common in southeastern United States)	Adults live in small intestine	Egg ingested by human in contaminated food or water or hand to mouth, autoreinfection is common	Light infections are asymptomatic; heavy worm burdens cause abdominal pain, diarrhea, headaches, dizziness; diagnosis: eggs in feces
Taenia saginata (beef tapeworm)	Cosmopolitan in beef-eating countries	Adult lives in small intestine	*Cysticercus bovis* eaten by human in undercooked beef	Most people are asymptomatic, can experience abdominal pain, diarrhea, weight loss; diagnosis: eggs or proglottid in feces
Taenia solium (pork tapeworm)	Worldwide (rare in the United States)	Adult lives in small intestine	*Cysticercus cellulosae* larva eaten by human in undercooked pork	Same as *T. saginata*
Diphyllobothrium latum (broadfish tapeworm)	Temperate areas where freshwater fish is eaten undercooked or raw	Adult lives in small intestine	Plerocercoid larva in freshwater fish ingested by humans	Can cause intestinal obstruction and macrocytic anemia because of B_{12} deficiency, abdominal pain and weight loss; diagnosis: eggs or proglottid in feces
ACCIDENTAL ZOONOTIC HUMAN INFECTIONS WITH CESTODA				
Echinococcus granulosus (dog tapeworm)	Worldwide in sheep-raising areas	Adult lives in the intestine of dogs or other wild canines, larval form in human tissue causes pathology	Human accidentally ingests eggs by close contact with infected dog, usual intermediate host is sheep	Cyst can be found in the liver (most commonly) or lung of humans, lung symptoms include coughing and pain, leakage of hydatid fluid causes allergy and eosinophilia; diagnosis: x-ray, serology
Cysticercosis (*Taenia solium*)	Cosmopolitan	Cysticercoid larva in human tissue, usual host of larva is pig	Human accidentally ingests egg, or eggs, released from proglottid of adult in human intestine	2-cm painless swelling if in skin, pain and other symptoms if in eye, seizures or other neurologic symptoms or death if in brain
Hymenolepis diminuta (rat tapeworm)	Worldwide	Adult lives in the intestine, usual host of adult tapeworm is the rat	Human accidentally ingests cysticercoid larva in infected flea or grain beetle (intermediate host)	Mild symptoms, tapeworms are often lost spontaneously, eggs in feces are diagnostic

Continued on following page

TABLE 3–2 ☐ CESTODA INFECTIONS (Continued)

ACCIDENTAL ZOONOTIC HUMAN INFECTIONS WITH CESTODA				
Scientific and Common Name	Epidemiology	Disease-Producing Worm and Its Location in Host	How Human Infection Occurs	Major Disease Manifestations, Diagnostic Stage, and Specimen of Choice
Dipylidium caninum (dog or cat)	Worldwide	Adult lives in the intestine, usual host of adult tapeworm is the dog or cat	Human accidentally ingests cysticercoid larva in infected dog or cat flea (intermediate host); rare, occurs mainly in children	Mild intestinal disturbances, tapeworms are frequently lost spontaneously, egg packets or proglottids are diagnostic in feces
Sparganosis (*Diphyllobothrium* or *Spirometra* spp. of dog, cat, or other mammals)	Far East freshwater areas	Plerocercoid in tissues	Human accidentally ingests copepod containing a procercoid	Subcutaneous nodules or internal abscesses or cysts

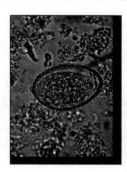

CASE STUDY 3–1

An elderly woman of Mediterranean heritage living in the Great Lakes area went to her doctor. She had been suffering from intermittent diarrhea and abdominal pain for several weeks. After questioning, the patient revealed that she regularly prepared gefilte fish (balls of boneless fish mixed with cracker meal) using freshwater fish purchased from a local grocery store. She said she tasted it often during preparation to make sure the seasonings were correct. Stool cultures and parasitic examinations were ordered. The culture results were negative for enteric pathogens, but the parasitic examination recovered the parasite form shown in the accompanying figure.

1. What parasite (genus and species) do you suspect?
2. How is this parasitic infection acquired? What other parasitic infections could she have gotten by the same means?
3. List other complications that may occur in long-standing infections.
4. What procedure may be performed to ensure that the treatment was successful?

> You have now completed the section on the Cestoda. After reviewing this material and Color Plates 34 to 52 with the aid of your learning objectives, proceed to the post-test.

Word Puzzles

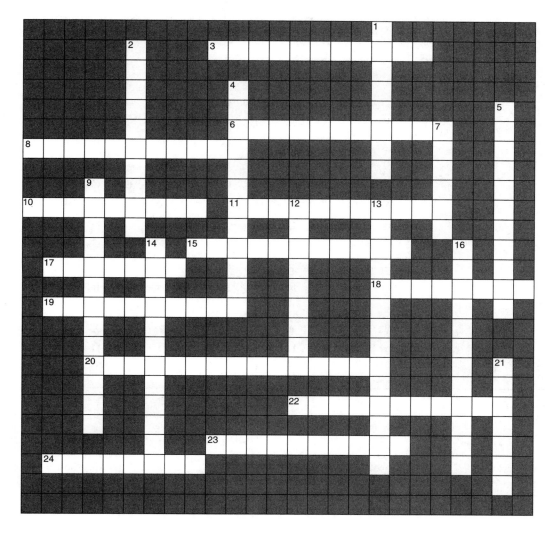

Across

3. Granular material consisting of free scolices, hooklets, daughter cysts, and amorphous material (2 words)
6. Plerocercoid in human tissue from accidental infection with procercoid
8. A vesicular structure formed by *Echinococcus granulosus* larva in the intermediate host (2 words)
10. The lidlike cover on certain platyhelminth eggs
11. The shell of *Taenia* spp. and other tapeworm eggs as seen in feces
15. The motile, first-stage larva of certain cestodes; armed with six hooklets
17. Any large organ in the interior of any of the three great body cavities of vertebrates
18. Loss of appetite
19. A segment of a tapeworm
20. A tapeworm larva having six hooklets (2 words)
22. A thin-walled, fluid-filled bladderlike cyst that encloses a scolex
23. Larval stage that develops from the coracidium of *Diphyllobothrium latum*; develops inside a freshwater crustacean
24. The body surface of platyhelminths; the site of nutrient and oxygen absorption and waste excretion

Down

1. Refers to cysticercosis caused by *T. solium* larvae in the brain tissue of humans
2. A ciliated hexacanth embryo
4. The larval stage of some tapeworms (e.g., *Hymenolepis nana*)
5. An exaggerated histamine-release reaction by the host to foreign protein or allergen
7. Anterior end of a tapeworm; attaches to the host's intestinal wall via suckers and sometimes hooks
9. Vector; often a bloodsucking insect (2 words)
12. The fleshy, anterior protuberance of the scolex of some tapeworms; may bear hooks
13. Having both male and female reproductive organs within the same individual
14. A structure within the daughter cyst in *E. granulosus* (2 words)
16. Larval stage in *D. latum* life cycle; develops after procercoid stage is ingested by freshwater fish
21. A class within the phylum Platyhelminthes that includes the tapeworms

```
V  S  H  I  Y  I  L  P  C  K  V  S  A  T  E  E  E  G  S  V
C  M  T  Z  O  U  U  Y  C  O  I  I  S  E  C  F  A  B  O  V
Y  U  E  R  E  J  A  C  E  X  R  O  S  E  M  I  A  C  J  M
S  L  G  G  X  R  E  R  A  L  H  A  S  C  X  R  E  I  U  P
T  L  U  D  N  C  E  L  O  T  U  C  E  E  X  K  L  X  D
I  E  M  A  J  B  Y  H  R  M  O  S  R  I  E  R  U  J  M  E
C  T  E  K  Q  H  Z  O  P  D  G  O  P  K  D  C  A  L  P  S
E  S  N  B  P  Z  P  N  A  S  N  O  E  A  R  I  I  R  V  O
R  O  T  A  Q  S  G  D  E  A  O  D  F  E  C  B  U  F  N  M
C  R  N  H  N  H  P  K  L  H  T  H  P  I  X  D  W  M  N  E
O  A  H  A  S  N  I  P  U  D  I  O  C  R  E  C  O  R  P  C
I  E  R  O  H  P  O  Y  R  B  M  E  M  N  M  F  F  O  T  A
D  T  X  H  Y  D  A  T  I  D  S  A  N  D  O  D  S  B  R  R
R  D  M  S  S  U  C  R  E  C  I  T  S  Y  C  M  L  I  R  B
O  Z  R  W  D  I  T  T  O  L  G  O  R  P  Z  X  D  M  M  X
Y  C  O  H  E  X  A  C  A  N  T  H  E  M  B  R  Y  O  F  T
S  C  O  L  E  X  B  H  Y  D  A  T  I  D  C  Y  S  T  S  V
L  P  K  A  S  P  A  R  G  A  N  O  S  I  S  X  Y  Y  Z  S
O  S  C  I  T  I  D  O  R  H  P  A  M  R  E  H  H  V  N  V
X  Z  U  H  V  D  I  O  C  R  E  C  O  R  E  L  P  L  D  B
```

anaphylaxis	cysticercus	onchosphere	rostellum
anorexia	embryophore	operculum	scolex
brood capsule	hermaphroditic	plerocercoid	sparganosis
Cestoda	hexcanth embryo	procercoid	tegument
coracidium	hydatid cyst	proglottid	transport host
cysticercoid	hydatid sand	racemose	viscera

Post-Test

1. Define and cite an example of each of the following: **(20 points)**
   a. Hexacanth embryo
   b. Hermaphroditic
   c. "Armed" scolex
   d. Proglottid
   e. Hydatid cyst

2. Matching: Select correct intermediate host(s) for each parasite: **(5 points)**

   a. _____ *Taenia solium*
   b. _____ *Hymenolepis nana*
   c. _____ *Hymenolepis diminuta*
   d. _____ *Diphyllobothrium latum*
   e. _____ *Echinococcus granulosus*

   1. Fish
   2. Copepod
   3. Cow
   4. Human
   5. Pig
   6. Snail
   7. Flea or beetle
   8. Dog
   9. Sheep
   10. None

3. Draw and label the diagnostic stage(s) for each of the following as you would observe them microscopically in human feces: **(40 points)**
   a. Dwarf tapeworm
   b. Broadfish tapeworm
   c. Beef tapeworm
   d. Pork tapeworm

4. Matching: Select one correct match for each parasite: **(7 points)**

   a. _____ *Taenia solium*
   b. _____ *Hymenolepis nana*
   c. _____ *Diphyllobothrium latum*
   d. _____ *Echinococcus granulosus*
   e. _____ *Dipylidium caninum*
   f. _____ Sparganosis
   g. _____ Cysticercosis

   1. Macrocytic anemia, vitamin B_{12} deficiency
   2. Plerocercoid subcutaneously
   3. Neurologic symptoms if in brain
   4. Autoreinfection is common
   5. Proglottid has 7 to 10 lateral uterine branches
   6. Human accidentally ingests infected flea
   7. Cysts found in liver, lungs, or other organs

Questions 5 to 18 are worth **2 points** *each.*

5. A patient from the Great Lakes area presents with vague abdominal symptoms and a macrocytic anemia. Which Cestoda would be the probable cause?
   a. *Diphyllobothrium latum*
   b. *Echinococcus granulosus*
   c. *Taenia saginata*
   d. *Hymenolepis nana*

6. A scolex is recovered in human feces after the patient is treated with medication. The scolex bears four cup-shaped suckers. This parasite is:
   a. *Diphyllobothrium latum*
   b. *Echinococcus granulosus*
   c. *Taenia saginata*
   d. *Hymenolepis nana*

7. The eggs of which two species are infective to humans if ingested, resulting in larval stages and pathology in the host's tissues?
   a. *Taenia solium* and *T. saginata*
   b. *Hymenolepis diminuta* and *Dipylidium caninum*
   c. *Echinococcus granulosus* and *Taenia solium*
   d. *Hymenolepis nana* and *Taenia saginata*

8. The larval stage of which two species are infective to humans if the parasitized insect intermediate host is ingested?
   a. *Taenia solium* and *T. saginata*
   b. *Hymenolepis diminuta* and *Dipylidium caninum*
   c. *Echinococcus granulosus* and *Taenia solium*
   d. *Hymenolepis nana* and *Taenia saginata*

9. Packets of tapeworm eggs encapsulated in a single membrane were recovered in feces. This parasite is:
   a. *Diphyllobothrium latum*
   b. *Dipylidium caninum*
   c. *Hymenolepis nana*
   d. *Taenia saginata*

10. The causative agent of cysticercosis is:
    a. *Echinococcus granulosis*
    b. *Taenia saginata*
    c. *Taenia solium*
    d. *Trichinella spiralis*

11. The examination of human feces is no help in the detection of:
    a. *Ancylostoma duodenale*
    b. *Echinococcus granulosis*
    c. *Hymenolepis nana*
    d. *Strongyloides stercoralis*

12. Mature eggs of an adult tapeworm accumulate in the:

    a. Gravid proglottid
    b. Mature proglottid
    c. Neck region of the strobila
    d. Scolex

13. A type of tapeworm larva with a large bladder, producing daughter cysts, brood capsules, and numerous scolices is:

    a. Cysticercus
    b. Cysticercoid
    c. Hydatid cyst
    d. Plerocercoid
    e. Procercoid

14. Eggs from which tapeworm, when passed, are immediately infective to humans?

    a. *Diphyllobothrium latum*
    b. *Hymenolepis nana*
    c. *Taenia saginata*
    d. *Echinococcus granulosus*

15. In the *Diphyllobothrium latum* life cycle, the infective stage for humans is:

    a. Cysticercus
    b. Cysticercoid
    c. Hydatid cyst
    d. Procercoid
    e. Plerocercoid

16. The human condition resulting from ingestion of the immature larval form of *Diphyllobothrium latum* is called:

    a. Cysticercosis
    b. Hydatid disease
    c. Racemose
    d. Sparganosis

17. The number of uterine branches in the mature proglottid of *Taenia saginata* is:

    a. Less than 14
    b. More than 14

18. The tapeworm scolex without cup-shaped suckers is:

    a. *Diphyllobothrium latum*
    b. *Hymenolepis nana*
    c. *Taenia saginata*
    d. *Taenia solium*
    e. *Echinococcus granulosus*

BIBLIOGRAPHY

Hildreth, MB, et al: *Echinococcus multilocularis:* A zoonosis of increasing concern in the United States. Supplement to the Compendium of Continuing Education for the Practicing Veterinarian 13:727–741, 1991.

Khalil, LF, et al (eds): Keys to the Cestode Parasites of Vertebrates. Oxford University Press, New York, 1997.

Leiby, PD, and Kritsky, DC: *Echinococcus multilocularis:* A possible domestic life cycle in central North America and its public health implications. J Parasitol 58:1213–1215, 1972.

Maurice J: Is something lurking in your liver? New Scientist 19 March:26–31, 1994.

Schmidt, GD: Handbook of Tapeworm Identification. CRC Press, Boca Raton, Fla, 1986.

Schwabe, CW, et al: Hydatid disease is endemic in California. Cal Med 117:13, 1972.

Smyth, JD: The Biology of the Hydatid Organism. In Dawes, B (ed): Advances in Parasitology, Vol. 2. Academic Press, New York, 1964.

Tsang, VCW, and Wilson M: *Taenia solium* cysticercosis. An underrecognized but serious health problem. Parasitol Today 11:124–126, 1995.

Thompson, RCA, and Lymbery, AJ (eds): Echinococcus and Hydatid Disease. Oxford University Press, New York, 1995.

Von Bondsdorff, B: Diphyllobothriasis in Man. Academic Press, New York, 1977.

Von Sinner, WN: Imaging of cystic echinococcosis. Acta Trop 67:67–89, 1997.

World Health Organization: Guidelines for treatment of cystic and alveolar echinococcosis in humans. Bull World Health Organization 74:231–242, 1996.

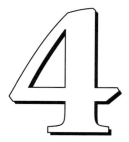

DIGENEA

GLOSSARY

acetabula (sing. **acetabulum**). Muscular suckers found on the ventral surface of the flukes.

cercaria (pl. **cercariae**). The stage of the fluke life cycle that develops from germ cells in a daughter **sporocyst** or **redia**. This is the final development stage in the snail host, consisting of a body with a tail that aids the cercaria in swimming after leaving the snail.

Digenea. A subclass of **Trematoda** in the phylum Platyhelminthes. This subclass includes flukes (trematodes) found in humans and other mammals. These have flattened, leaf-shaped bodies bearing two muscular suckers. Many species are hermaphroditic.

distomiasis. Infection with flukes.

granuloma. A tumor or growth of lymphoid or other cells around a foreign body.

metacercaria (pl. **metacercariae**). The stage of the hermaphroditic fluke life cycle occurring when a cercaria has shed its tail, secreted a protective wall, and encysted as a resting stage on water plants or in a second intermediate host; infective stage for humans.

miracidium (pl. **miracidia**). Ciliated first-stage, free-swimming larva of a Digenea, which emerges from the egg and must penetrate the appropriate species of snail to continue its life cycle.

redia. The second or third larval stage of a trematode that develops within a sporocyst in the snail host. Elongated, saclike organisms with a mouth and a gut. Many rediae develop in one sporocyst. Each redia gives rise to many cercariae.

Schistosoma. A genus of Digenea, commonly called the blood flukes. They have an elongated shape and separate sexes and are found in mating pairs in the blood vessels of their definitive host.

schistosomule. The immature schistosome in human tissues; the stage after the cercaria has lost its tail during penetration of skin.

sporocyst. The larval form of a trematode that develops from a miracidium in the snail intermediate host. A simple saclike structure containing germinal cells that bud off internally and continue the process of larval multiplication, producing many rediae in each sporocyst.

Trematoda. A class of flatworms in the phylum Platyhelminthes. Two subclasses, Digenea and Aspidogastrea, are noted.

● *Digenea*

Digenea (commonly called flukes) belong to the phylum Platyhelminthes, along with the Cestoda. Parasitic species inhabit the intestine or tissue of humans. Flukes in the subclass Digenea are flattened dorsoventrally and are nonsegmented, leaf-shaped helminths. Digenea vary in length from a few millimeters to several centimeters. All adult flukes have two cup-shaped muscular suckers **(acetabula)**: an oral sucker and a ventral sucker. The digestive system is simple: The oral cavity opens in the center of the oral sucker, and the intestinal tract ends blindly in one or two sacs. There is no anal opening, and waste products are regurgitated. The body surface (tegument) of the fluke is metabolically active, as is also true for the Cestoda, and can absorb soluble nutrients and release soluble waste products at the surface microtriches.

There are two types of parasitic flukes that can be present in humans. One type lives in the intestine or in other host organs (e.g., the liver or lungs) and is hermaphroditic, having both male and female sets of complex, highly branched reproductive organs in each adult fluke. These flukes are listed in Table 4–1. The second type includes flukes that live as unisexual adult males and females within the abdominal blood vessels of the definitive host. These are known as the **Schistosoma,** or blood flukes. The body of the male schistosome curves up along the lateral edges and forms a long channel (the gynecophoral canal) that wraps around the larger female worm lying in the channel. They coexist in pairs during their adult life span in the blood vessels. The *Schistosoma* are listed separately in Table 4–2. In both types, sexual reproduction in the adult Digenea occurs within humans, which is followed by asexual multiplication of the larval stages in a specific species of snail.

The life cycles of the flukes are complex (Diagram 4–1). The adult fluke lays eggs that leave the human definitive host via feces, urine, or sputum (depending on the species and host location of the adult fluke). A specific species of freshwater snail is required as an intermediate host for each species of fluke. In general, the life cycle is as follows: The larval stage (a ciliated **miracidium**) emerges from the egg in fresh water and enters the snail host, and the larva undergoes several cycles of asexual multiplication. The final larval stage leaving the snail is known as the **cercaria.** Many hundreds of cercariae result from the asexual multiplication of each miracidium that enters the snail host. Motile cercariae of the *Schistosoma* (blood flukes) then directly penetrate the skin of humans when contact occurs in infected fresh water. However, the cercariae of the hermaphroditic flukes do not penetrate human skin; they either secrete a thick wall and encyst as a **metacercaria** on aquatic vegetation or enter a species-specific second intermediate host (a freshwater fish or crustacean) and encyst. Only a few species of fish or crustaceans may serve as the second intermediate host for each species of hermaphroditic fluke. Human infection by these hermaphroditic flukes occurs when humans eat uncooked water vegetation to which metacercariae are attached or when they eat the undercooked specific species of the second intermediate host containing the encysted metacercaria.

Various studies estimate that at least 30 million people harbor a hermaphroditic fluke infection. Most of these people live in Asia, but some live in the former Union of Soviet Socialist Republics and parts of Europe, Egypt, Cuba, and Peru. The World Health Organization is concerned that infections may increase in other parts of the world via increased international travel and trade of fresh aquatic foods from endemic areas. It is important to carefully wash and thoroughly cook fish and vegetables to prevent infection with these parasites.

DIAGRAM 4-1

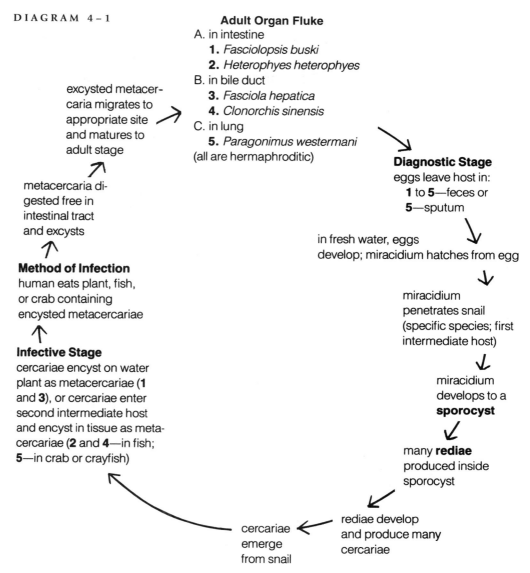

Adult Organ Fluke
A. in intestine
   1. *Fasciolopsis buski*
   2. *Heterophyes heterophyes*
B. in bile duct
   3. *Fasciola hepatica*
   4. *Clonorchis sinensis*
C. in lung
   5. *Paragonimus westermani*
(all are hermaphroditic)

excysted metacer-
caria migrates to
appropriate site
and matures to
adult stage

metacercaria di-
gested free in
intestinal tract
and excysts

Method of Infection
human eats plant, fish,
or crab containing
encysted metacercariae

Infective Stage
cercariae encyst on water
plant as metacercariae (**1**
and **3**), or cercariae enter
second intermediate host
and encyst in tissue as metacercariae (**2** and **4**—in fish;
5—in crab or crayfish)

Diagnostic Stage
eggs leave host in:
   1 to **5**—feces or
   5—sputum

in fresh water, eggs
develop; miracidium hatches from egg

miracidium
penetrates snail
(specific species; first
intermediate host)

miracidium
develops to a
sporocyst

many **rediae**
produced inside
sporocyst

rediae develop
and produce many
cercariae

cercariae
emerge
from snail

General life cycles of Trematoda (organ-dwelling flukes)

Table 4–1 lists the names and pronunciation key for the hermaphroditic flukes. Table 4–2 lists the names and pronunciation key for the blood flukes. Be sure to review the glossary before studying the rest of the chapter.

TABLE 4–1 □ HERMAPHRODITIC FLUKES

Order	Scientific Name	Common Name
Echinostomatiformes	*Fasciolopsis buski* (fa-see'o-lop'sis/bus'kee)	large intestinal fluke
Echinostomata	*Fasciola hepatica* (fa-see'o-luh/he-pat'i-kuh)	sheep liver fluke
Opisthorchiformes	*Clonorchis sinensis* (klo-nor'kis/si-nen'sis)	Chinese liver fluke
Opisthorchiformes	*Heterophyes heterophyes* (het-ur-off'ee-eez/het"ur-off'ee-eez)	heterophid fluke
Opisthorchiformes	*Metagonimus yokogawai* (Met'uh-gon'i-mus/yo-ko-gah-wah'eye)	heterophid fluke
Plagiorchiformes	*Paragonimus westermani* (par"l-gon-'l-mus/wes-tur-man'eye)	Oriental lung fluke

TABLE 4–2 □ BLOOD FLUKES

Order	Scientific Name	Common Name
Strigeiformes	*Schistosoma mansoni* (shis'to-so'muh/man-so'nigh)	Manson's blood fluke
Strigeiformes	*Schistosoma japonicum* (shis'to-so'muh/ja-pon'i-kum)	blood fluke
Strigeiformes	*Schistosoma haematobium* (shis'to-so'muh/hee-muh-toe'bee-um)	bladder fluke

Fasciolopsis buski (large intestinal fluke) and *Fasciola hepatica* (sheep liver fluke)

DIAGRAM 4-2

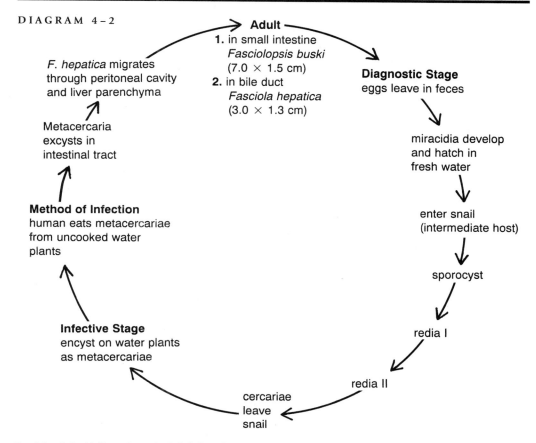

Fasciolopsis buski (large intestinal fluke) and *Fasciola hepatica* (sheep liver fluke)

METHOD OF DIAGNOSIS

Recover eggs in feces. Eggs of these two species are too similar to differentiate. Species diagnosis depends on clinical symptoms, travel history, recovery of adult *Fasciolopsis,* or all these factors.

DIAGNOSTIC STAGE

Egg   (*Note:* Similar for both parasites.)

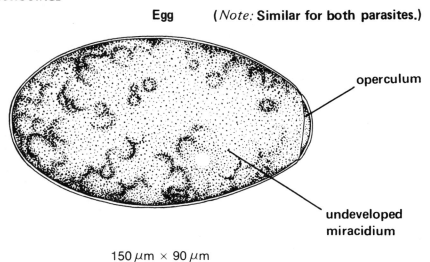

150 μm × 90 μm

DISEASE NAMES

- *F. buski:* fasciolopsiasis
- *F. hepatica:* sheep liver rot

MAJOR PATHOLOGY AND SYMPTOMS

1. *F. buski:* Symptoms include bowel mucosal ulcers and hypersecretion and occasional hemorrhage around worm attachment site. Heavier infections cause pain, nausea, mucoid diarrhea, anemia, intestinal obstruction and malabsorption, generalized edema, and marked eosinophilia. Death can occur with heavy infections.
2. *F. hepatica:* Symptoms are from mechanical irritation, toxic worm metabolites, and mechanical obstruction. Migrating larvae cause local irritation. Fever, hepatomegaly, and eosinophilia in humans from endemic areas suggest clinical diagnosis. Adult flukes in the bile duct induce portal cirrhosis in heavy infections. Jaundice, bile duct obstruction, diarrhea, and anemia may occur in severe infection. Other symptoms may include pruritus, urticaria, and cough.

TREATMENT

- *F. buski:* praziquantel or niclosamide
- *F. hepatica:* bithionol

DISTRIBUTION

- *F. buski* is prevalent in China, Vietnam, Thailand, Indonesia, Malaysia, and the Indian subcontinent.
- *F. hepatica* has cosmopolitan distribution in sheep-raising and cattle-raising countries. It is uncommon in the United States.

OF NOTE

1. The natural definitive host for *F. hepatica* is the sheep; therefore, infection of humans is a zoonotic disease. *F. buski* is common in pigs.
2. *Echinostoma ilocanum* is found in the Philippines as 1-cm adults in the small intestine. The fluke has a spiny collarette around the oval sucker and produces eggs resembling *Fasciolopsis.* Infection results from eating raw snails.

⇨ FOR REVIEW

1. *Write the scientific names for the large intestinal fluke and the sheep liver fluke:*
   _____ *and* _____.
2. *Draw pictures of the diagnostic stages of these parasites.*
3. *Humans become infected with the large intestinal fluke or the sheep liver fluke when*

   _____

4. *The intermediate host for these parasites is* _____.
5. *Why is a human infection with* **F. hepatica** *considered a zoonotic disease?*

   _____

6. *What causes the symptoms of these two diseases?*

   _____

Clonorchis sinensis (Oriental or Chinese liver fluke; *Opisthorchis*)

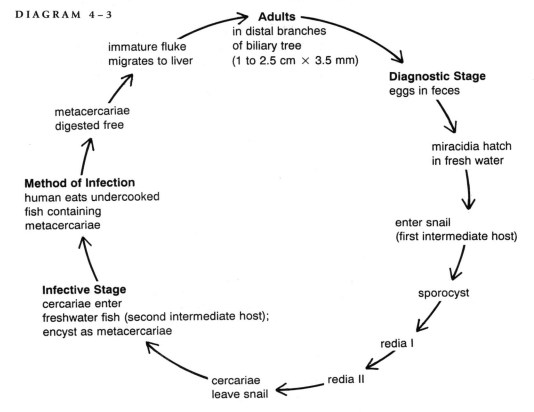

DIAGRAM 4-3

Adults
in distal branches
of biliary tree
(1 to 2.5 cm × 3.5 mm)

immature fluke
migrates to liver

metacercariae
digested free

Method of Infection
human eats undercooked
fish containing
metacercariae

Infective Stage
cercariae enter
freshwater fish (second intermediate host);
encyst as metacercariae

Diagnostic Stage
eggs in feces

miracidia hatch
in fresh water

enter snail
(first intermediate host)

sporocyst

redia I

redia II

cercariae
leave snail

Clonorchis sinensis (Oriental or Chinese liver fluke;
Opisthorchis)

METHOD OF DIAGNOSIS

1. Recover and identify eggs in feces or biliary drainage or from Entero-Test capsule.
2. Perform radiographic studies.

DIAGNOSTIC STAGE

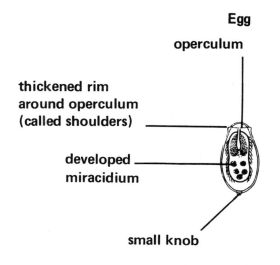

Egg

operculum

thickened rim
around operculum
(called shoulders)

developed
miracidium

small knob

30 μm × 16 μm

DISEASE NAME

Clonorchiasis

MAJOR PATHOLOGY AND SYMPTOMS

1. Light infections are common and may be asymptomatic.
2. Jaundice may develop from bile duct pathology; hyperplastic changes occur.
3. Hepatomegaly may develop, with tenderness in the right upper quadrant.
4. Other symptoms include abdominal pain, diarrhea, and anorexia.
5. Chronic cases with heavy worm burden from repeated infections may induce severe hepatic complications; rarely, pancreatitis, bile duct stones, cholangitis, and cholangiocarcinoma develop.

TREATMENT

Praziquantel or albendazole

DISTRIBUTION

C. sinensis is found in the Far East, especially southern China.

OF NOTE

1. Eggs are passed intermittently; therefore, perform sequential stool examinations.
2. *Clonorchis* and *Opisthorchis* eggs are similar and easily confused with *Heterophyes heterophyes* and *Metagonimus yokogawai*.
3. Dogs and cats are reservoir hosts and may harbor adults.

 FOR REVIEW

1. *The scientific name for the Chinese liver fluke is* _____.
2. *The intermediate host(s) include* _____.
3. *Draw and label a picture of the diagnostic stage for this parasite.*
4. *Humans become infected with this parasite when* _____
   _____.
5. *Eggs of this parasite can be confused with those of* _____.
6. *Reservoir hosts for this parasite include* _____.

Heterophyes heterophyes and *Metagonimus yokogawai* (Heterophyids)

DIAGRAM 4-4

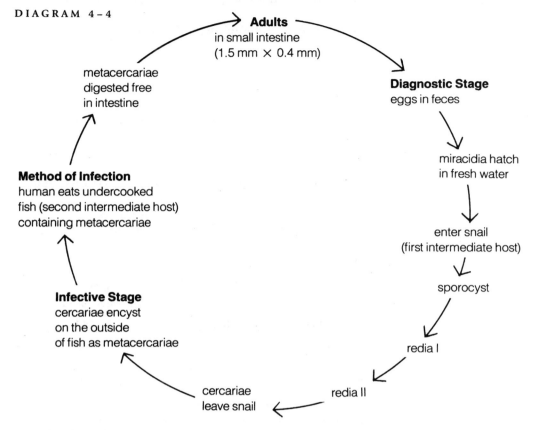

Adults
in small intestine
(1.5 mm × 0.4 mm)

metacercariae
digested free
in intestine

Diagnostic Stage
eggs in feces

Method of Infection
human eats undercooked
fish (second intermediate host)
containing metacercariae

miracidia hatch
in fresh water

enter snail
(first intermediate host)

sporocyst

Infective Stage
cercariae encyst
on the outside
of fish as metacercariae

redia I

redia II

cercariae
leave snail

Heterophyes heterophyes and *Metagonimus yokogawai* (heterophyids)

METHOD OF DIAGNOSIS

Recover and identify eggs in feces or duodenal drainage. Differentiation is difficult (may lack knob at shell end opposite operculum as seen on *C. sinensis* eggs).

DIAGNOSTIC STAGE

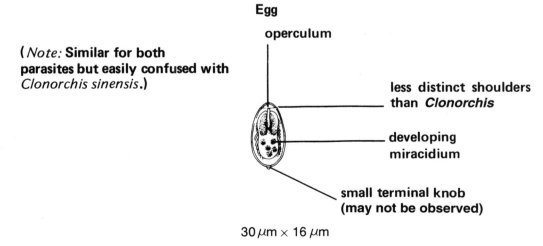

Egg

operculum

(*Note:* **Similar for both
parasites but easily confused with**
Clonorchis sinensis.)

less distinct shoulders
than *Clonorchis*

developing
miracidium

small terminal knob
(may not be observed)

30 μm × 16 μm

DISEASE NAMES

• *Heterophyes heterophyes:* heterophyiasis
• *Metagonimus yokogawai:* metagonimiasis

MAJOR PATHOLOGY AND SYMPTOMS

Infection is asymptomatic unless heavy; heavy infections may induce a chronic mucoid diarrhea and abdominal pain. Worm invasion may produce eggs that travel to the heart or brain, causing symptoms of **granulomas.**

TREATMENT

Praziquantel

DISTRIBUTION

- *H. heterophyes* occurs in the Near East, Far East, and parts of Africa.
- *M. yokogawai* is found in Asia, including Siberia.

OF NOTE

1. Because these are primarily parasites of dogs, cats, and other fish-eating mammals, human infection is a zoonosis.
2. Eggs may travel into tissues, causing granulomas and tissue disorders.
3. *H. heterophyes* adult has a third sucker around the genital opening.

 FOR REVIEW

1. *Write the scientific names for the heterophid flukes:* _____
2. *Draw and label a picture of the diagnostic stage for the heterophid parasites.*
3. *Humans become infected with these parasites when*

_____

4. *The intermediate host(s) include* _____.
5. *Compared with other organ-dwelling flukes, the egg size of these parasites is*

_____.

6. *Other mammals that commonly harbor these parasites include*

_____

Paragonimus westermani (Oriental lung fluke)

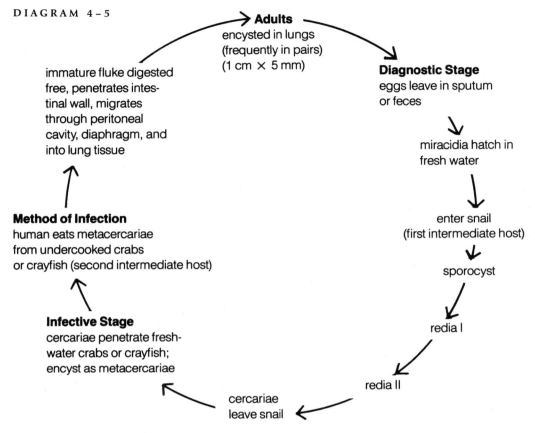

DIAGRAM 4-5

Adults
encysted in lungs
(frequently in pairs)
(1 cm × 5 mm)

immature fluke digested
free, penetrates intes-
tinal wall, migrates
through peritoneal
cavity, diaphragm, and
into lung tissue

Diagnostic Stage
eggs leave in sputum
or feces

miracidia hatch in
fresh water

enter snail
(first intermediate host)

sporocyst

redia I

Method of Infection
human eats metacercariae
from undercooked crabs
or crayfish (second intermediate host)

Infective Stage
cercariae penetrate freshwater crabs or crayfish;
encyst as metacercariae

cercariae
leave snail

redia II

Paragonimus westermani (Oriental lung fluke)

METHOD OF DIAGNOSIS

Recover and identify eggs in bloody sputum (sputum appears to contain rusty iron filings) or in feces (if eggs are swallowed); radiograph of lungs may show patchy infiltrate with modular cystic shadows or calcification.

DIAGNOSTIC STAGE

Egg

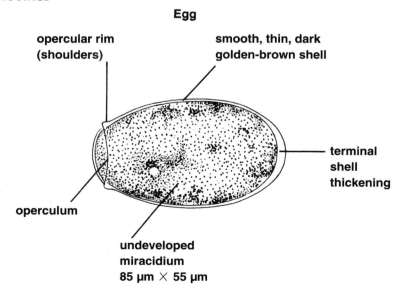

opercular rim
(shoulders)

smooth, thin, dark
golden-brown shell

terminal
shell
thickening

operculum

undeveloped
miracidium
85 μm × 55 μm

DISEASE NAMES

- Paragonimiasis
- Pulmonary **distomiasis**

MAJOR PATHOLOGY AND SYMPTOMS

1. Symptoms include chronic chest pain; cough; blood-tinged sputum (rusty sputum); and lung infiltration, nodules, and abscesses. Adults are present in fibrous cysts; eggs pass through cysts and rupture into bronchioles, causing a cough. Chest radiograph findings and symptoms may resemble those of tuberculosis. Other developments are chronic bronchitis and increasing fibrosis.
2. Cerebral paragonimiasis causes symptoms of a space-occupying lesion. Abdominal paragonimiasis is usually asymptomatic and not rare.

TREATMENT

1. Praziquantel
2. Bithionol

DISTRIBUTION

Infection is most common in the Far East. It also is found in parts of Africa and South America.

OF NOTE

1. At least eight other species of *Paragonimus* are also infectious for humans; *P. mexicanus* is found in Central and South America.
2. Immature flukes may wander aberrantly to other tissues, including the brain (cerebral paragonimiasis), skin, and liver.

 FOR REVIEW

1. *The scientific name for the Oriental lung fluke is* _____.
2. *Draw and label a picture of the diagnostic stage for this parasite.*
3. *Humans become infected with this parasite when*

_____.

4. *The intermediate host(s) include*

_____

5. *Eggs of this parasite can be recovered from what specimen(s):*

_____

Schistosoma spp. (blood flukes)

DIAGRAM 4-6

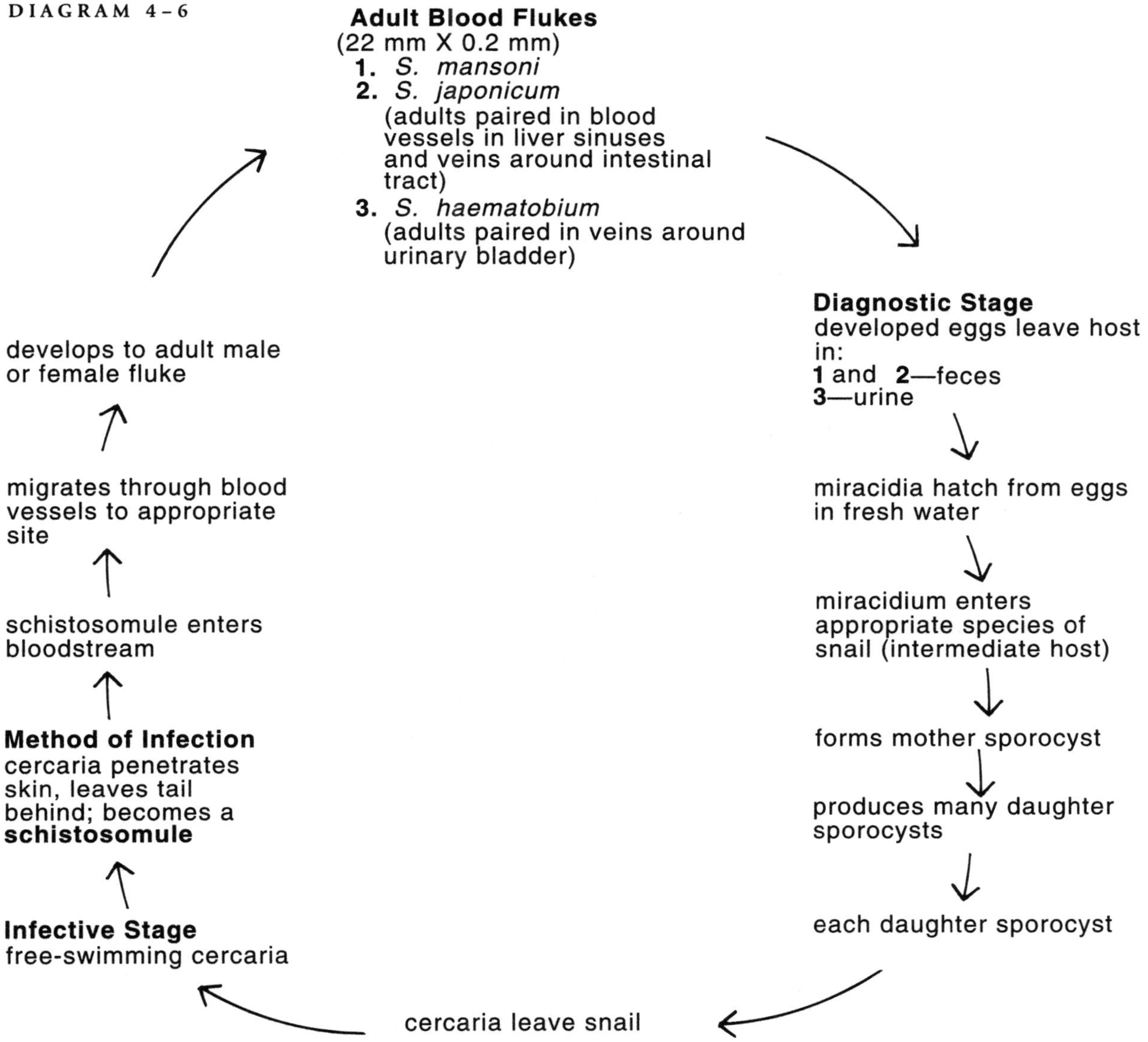

Adult Blood Flukes
(22 mm X 0.2 mm)
1. *S. mansoni*
2. *S. japonicum*
(adults paired in blood vessels in liver sinuses and veins around intestinal tract)
3. *S. haematobium*
(adults paired in veins around urinary bladder)

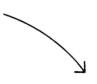

develops to adult male or female fluke

migrates through blood vessels to appropriate site

schistosomule enters bloodstream

Method of Infection
cercaria penetrates skin, leaves tail behind; becomes a **schistosomule**

Infective Stage
free-swimming cercaria

Diagnostic Stage
developed eggs leave host in:
1 and 2—feces
3—urine

miracidia hatch from eggs in fresh water

miracidium enters appropriate species of snail (intermediate host)

forms mother sporocyst

produces many daughter sporocysts

each daughter sporocyst

 cercaria leave snail

Schistosoma mansoni, Schistosoma japonicum, and *Schistosoma haematobium* (blood flukes)

METHOD OF DIAGNOSIS

• *S. mansoni* and *S. japonicum:* Recover eggs in feces or rectal biopsy (may require multiple biopsies for *S. mansoni*).
• *S. haematobium:* Recover eggs in concentrated urine.
• Other diagnostic methods include travel history, clinical symptoms and signs, serology, and enzyme-linked immunosorbent assay.

DIAGNOSTIC STAGES

S. mansoni **egg**

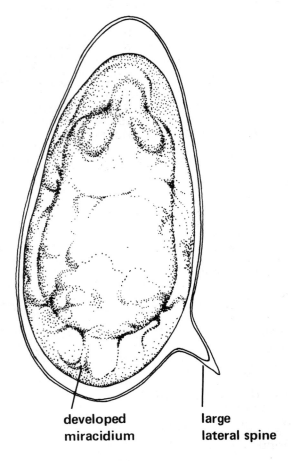

developed
miracidium

large
lateral spine

180 μm × 80 μm

S. japonicum **egg**

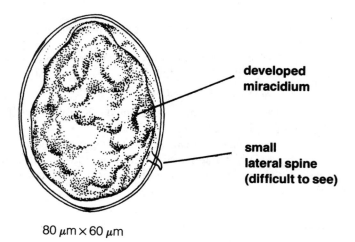

developed
miracidium

small
lateral spine
(difficult to see)

80 μm × 60 μm

S. haematobium **egg**

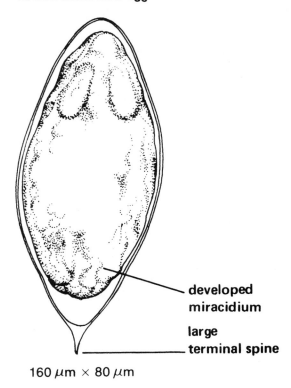

developed
miracidium

large
terminal spine

160 μm × 80 μm

DISEASE NAMES

- Schistosomiasis
- Bilharziasis
- Swamp fever

MAJOR PATHOLOGY AND SYMPTOMS

1. These diseases mainly affect children and adults in endemic areas.
2. The initial reaction may be dermatitis from cercarial penetration.
3. Acute phase of heavy first infection presents with typhoid fever–like symptoms, fever, cough, myalgias, malaise, and hepatosplenomegaly.
4. Cirrhosis of the liver, bloody diarrhea, bowel obstruction, hypertension, and toxic reactions may occur because of granulomas around eggs in liver, urinary bladder, central nervous system, and other tissues.
5. Infected person may develop collateral circulation if hepatic involvement is severe. Eosinophilia is present.
6. Most chronic cases are asymptomatic in endemic areas. Schistosomes feed on red blood cells; brown hematin pigment (identical to malarial pigment) is present in phagocytic cells.
7. Nephrotic syndrome may occur in *S. mansoni* and *S. haematobium*.

TREATMENT

Praziquantel

DISTRIBUTION

- *S. mansoni* is found in Africa and South and Central America. Foci are in the Caribbean, including Puerto Rico and the West Indies.
- *S. haematobium* is found in Africa and the Middle East.
- *S. japonicum* is found in the Far East.

TABLE 4–3 □ DIGENEA

Scientific and Common Name	Epidemiology	Disease-Producing Form and Its Location in Host	How Infection Occurs	Major Disease Manifestations, Diagnostic Stage, and Specimen of Choice
Fasciolopsis buski (large intestinal fluke)	Far East	Adults live in small intestine	Ingestion of encysted metacercariae on raw vegetation	Edema, eosinophilia, diarrhea, malabsorption, and even death in heavy infection; diagnosis: eggs in feces
Fasciola hepatica (sheep liver fluke) (zoonosis)	Worldwide (in sheep-raising and cattle-raising areas), humans (accidental host), sheep (natural host)	Adults live in bile ducts	Ingestion of encysted metacercariae on raw vegetation	Traumatic tissue damage and irritation to the liver and bile ducts, jaundice and eosinophilia can occur; diagnosis: eggs in feces
Clonorchis sinensis (Oriental or Chinese liver fluke)	Far East	Adults live in bile ducts	Ingestion of encysted metacercariae in uncooked fish	Jaundice and eosinophilia in acute phase, long-term heavy infections lead to functional impairment of liver; diagnosis: eggs in feces
Paragonimus westermani (Oriental lung fluke)	Far East, India, and parts of Africa	Adults live encysted in lung	Ingestion of encysted metacercariae in uncooked crab or crayfish	Chronic fibrotic disease resembling tuberculosis (cough with blood-tinged sputum); diagnosis: eggs in sputum or feces
Heterophyes heterophyes; Metagonimus yokogawai (the heterophyids)	Far East	Adults live in small intestine	Ingestion of encysted metacercariae in uncooked fish	No intestinal symptoms unless very heavy infection; diagnosis: eggs in feces
Schistosoma mansoni (Manson's blood fluke, bilharziasis, swamp fever)	Africa, Middle East, and South America	Adult in venules of the colon (eggs trapped in liver and other tissues)	Fork-tailed cercariae burrow into the capillary bed of feet, legs, or arms	Granuloma formation around eggs (i.e., in liver, intestine, and bladder), toxic and allergic reactions: nephrotic syndrome; diagnosis: eggs in feces and rectal biopsy
Schistosoma japonicum (Oriental blood fluke)	Far East	As above (for *Schistosoma mansoni*)	As above	As above, but symptoms are more severe because of greater egg production; diagnosis: eggs in feces and rectal biopsy
Schistosoma haematobium (bladder fluke)	Africa, Middle East, and Portugal	Adults in venules of bladder and rectum, eggs caught in tissues	As above	Bladder colic with blood and pus, nephrotic syndrome, symptomatic symptoms are mild, pulmonary involvement from eggs in lungs, has been associated with cancer of the bladder; diagnosis: eggs in urine
Swimmer's itch (zoonosis)	Worldwide	Cercariae of schistosomes that usually parasitize mammals and birds enter human skin	Fork-tailed cercariae burrow into skin of human in water	Allergic dermal response to repeated penetration, schistosomules *do not* develop to adults

OF NOTE

1. Schistosomiasis ranks second (behind malaria) as a cause of serious worldwide morbidity and mortality, infecting more than 200 million people and killing about 800,000 people per year. Schistosomiasis is spreading and increasing because of new water-control projects that provide increased snail-breeding areas.
2. *S. haematobium* has a clinical correlation with bladder cancer.
3. Repeated infection with avian cercariae may induce allergic dermatitis (swimmer's itch) at freshwater swimming resorts. This occurs in North America.
4. Persistent *Salmonella* infection may be associated with *S. mansoni* and *S. japonicum*.
5. *S. intercalatum* in Africa and *S. mekongi* in the Mekong Basin infect humans.
6. *S. japonicum* infects many mammals.
7. Niclosamide lotion on the skin helps prevent cercarial penetration.
8. Pipestem fibrosis and collateral blood circulation may occur if liver involvement is severe.

FOR REVIEW

1. *Write the scientific names and location of adults for each of the blood flukes:*

_____

2. *Draw and label pictures of the diagnostic stage for each of these parasites.*
3. *Humans become infected with these parasites when*

_____

4. *The intermediate host(s) include* _____.
5. *Compare and contrast the morphology of organ-fluke eggs and blood-fluke eggs:*

_____

CASE STUDY 4–1

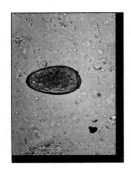

A 17-year-old American foreign exchange student returned home to the United States after finishing his school year in Japan. He complained to his mother that he had been coughing a lot and that his sputum was reddish. His mother noted a fever and took him to the doctor. The physician ordered cultures for routine bacteriology and tuberculosis. When the report indicated "normal flora" and no acid-fast bacteria were noted, the doctor questioned the young man further and found out that he had enjoyed eating unusual Japanese foods. His favorite was crayfish because they "tasted like shrimp" and weren't "weird like sushi." The physician then ordered a new examination of his sputum for eggs and parasites. The laboratory found the parasite form shown in the accompanying figure.

1. What parasite (genus and species) do you suspect?
2. Why did the physician order a parasitic examination of the patient's sputum?
3. What intermediate hosts are included in this parasite's life cycle?
4. What other specimen could be used to diagnose this disease? What parasitic form would be noted?

> **You have now completed the chapter on Digenea. After reviewing this material and Color Plates 53 to 71, with the aid of your learning objectives, proceed to the post-test.**

Word Puzzles

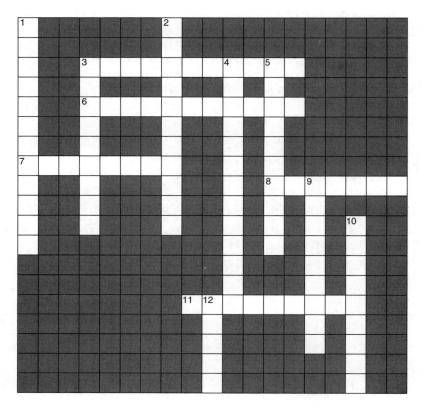

Across

3. A genus of Digenea, commonly called the blood flukes
6. The motile, first-stage larva of certain cestodes; armed with six hooklets
7. The stage of the fluke life cycle that develops from germ cells in a daughter sporocyst or redia
8. A subclass of Trematoda in the phylum Platyhelminthes
11. A class of flatworms in the phylum Platyhelminthes

Down

1. The stage of the fluke life cycle occurring when a cercaria has shed its tail, secreted a protective wall, and encysted as a resting stage
2. Infection with flukes
3. The larval form of a trematode that develops from a miracidium in the snail host
4. The immature schistosome in human tissues
5. Ciliated first-stage, free-swimming larva of a Digenea
9. A tumor or growth of lymphoid or other cells around a foreign body
10. Muscular suckers found on the ventral surface of the flukes
12. The second or third larval stage of a trematode that develops within a sporocyst in the snail host

T	Q	Z	Y	J	B	G	J	H	N	W	W	H	I	M	Y	P	E	L	C
F	O	T	S	Y	C	O	R	O	P	S	S	N	D	B	B	A	D	V	S
M	V	K	Y	Q	Z	A	C	Y	K	Z	O	G	E	Y	I	E	Z	G	L
C	E	C	W	P	S	D	J	Q	H	Q	J	L	Y	S	Q	N	X	V	G
R	E	T	H	F	L	S	C	H	I	S	T	O	S	O	M	U	L	E	M
U	E	F	A	K	P	M	B	J	S	T	R	E	M	A	T	O	D	A	C
M	J	E	T	C	Y	Y	G	X	A	S	P	S	I	O	O	W	Y	Z	V
H	P	L	D	U	E	V	G	R	U	A	I	R	A	C	R	E	C	W	D
I	T	Z	T	M	A	R	L	K	A	Y	P	Y	R	T	G	T	Z	W	F
D	P	A	M	I	G	M	C	U	C	N	M	G	L	X	U	J	K	A	A
K	N	R	M	C	G	G	F	A	I	U	U	X	B	Q	W	W	E	E	G
Q	M	Y	G	C	U	L	M	W	R	L	N	L	U	S	J	Q	D	N	D
R	V	B	P	Z	P	B	K	X	K	I	P	M	O	W	N	Y	Q	E	W
S	I	S	A	I	M	O	T	S	I	D	A	Z	X	M	D	L	S	G	W
X	C	O	L	A	M	O	S	O	T	S	I	H	C	S	A	A	B	I	R
U	E	I	C	S	Q	Q	P	S	K	A	I	D	E	R	O	R	A	D	N
M	U	P	R	M	Z	N	D	C	T	N	X	S	O	V	A	R	R	L	L
Y	D	J	X	H	M	I	R	A	C	I	D	I	U	M	X	J	S	Y	S
Q	N	W	V	G	Y	E	A	L	U	B	A	T	E	C	A	H	F	K	T
T	E	F	K	V	M	B	I	Z	C	M	Q	K	A	Y	Y	X	A	S	P

acetabula	distomiasis	miracidium	schistosomule
cercaria	granuloma	redia	sporocyst
Digenea	metacercaria	Schistosoma	Trematoda

Post-Test

1. Number these terms from 1 to 7 to describe the chronologic sequence of the life cycle of an intestinal trematode. **(10 points)**

   ___Egg   ___Adult

   ___Metacercaria   ___Sporocyst

   ___Miracidium   ___Cercaria

   ___Redia

2. You have decided to move to the Great Lakes area of the Unites States to become a sheepherder. You will be a hermit, enjoying a completely self-sustained life by the edge of a lake with your sheepdog and sheep. Which of the following sets of Platyhelminthes are you most likely to contract? Why did you reject each of the other answer sets? **(16 points)**

   a. *Fasciola hepatica, Paragonimus westermani, Taenia solium*
   b. *Schistosoma mansoni, Echinococcus granulosus, Clonorchis sinensis*
   c. *Fasciolopsis buski, Diphyllobothrium latum, Schistosoma japonicum*
   d. *Fasciola hepatica, Echinococcus granulosus, Diphyllobothrium latum*
   e. *Heterophyes heterophyes, Hymenolepis nana, Dipylidium caninum*

3. **(24 points)**
   a. Give the scientific and common name for each parasite represented in the following illustration of the diagnostic stage.
   b. State the method of human infection by each of the parasites represented.

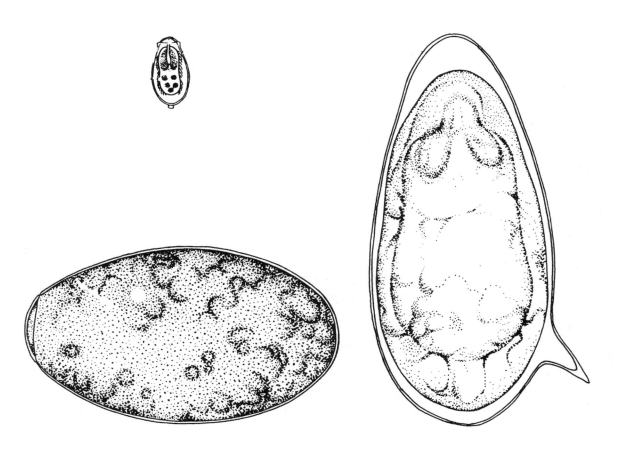

4. Why are methods of infection and control for the blood flukes different from those for the intestinal flukes? **(6 points)**

*Questions 5 to 15 are worth **4 points** each.*

5. Humans can be infected with the larval stage of all except one of the following parasites. Which of these Digenea cannot develop as a viable larva in the tissues of humans?

   a. Hydatid tapeworm
   b. Bird schistosomes
   c. Manson's blood fluke
   d. Sheep liver fluke

6. Which of the Platyhelminthes infects humans by skin penetration and has an association with bladder cancer?

   a. *Schistosoma mansoni*
   b. *Schistosoma haematobium*
   c. *Clonorchis sinensis*
   d. *Schistosoma japonicum*

7. Eggs of all of the following flukes are undeveloped when passed in feces **EXCEPT:**

   a. *Fasciola hepatica*
   b. *Paragonimus westermani*
   c. *Schistosoma japonicum*
   d. *Clonorchis sinensis*

8. The preferred specimen for the diagnosis of paragonimiasis is:

   a. Bile drainage
   b. Duodenal aspirate
   c. Rectal biopsy
   d. Sputum

9. The three species of human blood flukes have as intermediate host:

   a. A cyclops
   b. An aquatic snail
   c. An insect
   d. A freshwater fish

10. The fluke acquired by eating contaminated vegetation is:

    a. *Clonorchis sinensis*
    b. *Fasciolopsis buski*
    c. *Heterophyes heterophyes*
    d. *Paragonimus westermani*
    e. *Schistosoma mansoni*

11. Fish carrying metacercariae may transmit:

    a. *Clonorchis sinensis*
    b. *Fasciolopsis buski*
    c. *Paragonimus westermani*
    d. *Schistosoma haematobium*
    e. None of these

12. *Paragonimus westermani* infection is acquired by:

    a. Drinking contaminated water
    b. Eating infected crustacea
    c. Eating infected fish
    d. Eating infected water chestnuts

13. *Schistosoma cercariae* enter the human body:

    a. In flesh of infected fish
    b. By skin penetration
    c. In contaminated drinking water
    d. On contaminated vegetation
    e. Either b or c

14. The Digenea infection for which bloody urine is often a symptom is:

    a. *Schistosoma haematobium*
    b. *Schistosoma japonicum*
    c. *Schistosoma mansoni*
    d. b or c only
    e. None of these

15. The fluke most commonly found in the United States is:

    a. *Fasciola hepatica*
    b. *Fasciolopsis buski*
    c. *Heterophyes heterophyes*
    d. *Schistosoma mansoni*
    e. None of these

BIBLIOGRAPHY

Contis, G, and David, AR: The epidemiology of bilharziasis in ancient Egypt: 5000 years of schistosomiasis. Parasitol Today 12:253–255, 1996.

Farid, Z: Schistosomes with terminal-spined eggs: Pathological and clinical aspects. In Jordan P, et al (eds): Human Schistosomiasis. CAB International, Wallingford, 159–193, 1993.

Gibson, DI, and Bray, RA: The evolutionary expansion and host-parasite relationships of the Digenea. Int J Parasitol 24:1213–1226, 1994.

Healy, GR: Trematodes transmitted to man by fish, frogs, and crustacea. J Wildl Dis 6:255, 1970.

Hillyer, GV, and Apt W: Food-borne trematode infections in the Americas. Parasitol Today 13:87–88, 1997.

How, PC: The relationship between primary carcinoma of the liver and infestation with *Clonorchis sinensis*. J Pathol Bacteriol 72:239, 1965.

Jordan, P, et al (eds): Human Schistosomiasis. CAB International, Wallingford, 1993.

Price, TA, et al: Fascioliasis: Case reports and review. Clin Infect Dis 17:426–430, 1993.

Viranuvatti, V, and Stitnimankarn, T: Liver fluke infection and infestation in Southeast Asia. Prog Liver Dis 4:537–547, 1972.

Yokogawa, J: *Paragonimus* and paragonimiasis. In Dawes, B (ed): Advances in Parasitology. Academic Press, New York, 1969.

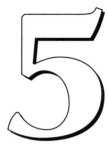

PROTOZOA

LEARNING OBJECTIVES

ON COMPLETION OF THIS CHAPTER AND REVIEW OF ITS SUPPLEMENTARY COLOR PLATES AS DESCRIBED, THE STUDENT WILL BE ABLE TO:

1 State the general characteristics of each class of Protozoa.

2 Define terminology specific for protozoa.

3 State the recommended methods of diagnosis of protozoal infections.

4 State any vector or intermediate host involved in the transmission of protozoal diseases.

5 Describe in graphic form the general life cycles for the protozoa in each class.

6 State the type of pathology caused by infection with protozoa.

7 State and correctly spell the scientific and common names of protozoa that parasitize humans.

8 Identify accidental protozoal infections of humans that are of medical importance.

9 Identify the type of specimen that would most likely contain the diagnostic stages of each pathogenic protozoon.

10 Discriminate between cyst and trophozoite stages of protozoa on the basis of both the morphologic criteria and the infectivity of various genera.

11 Discriminate between pathogenic and nonpathogenic amoebae on the basis of morphologic criteria.

12 Differentiate species of *Plasmodium* and *Trypanosoma* by morphology, symptomatic criteria, or both.

13 Discuss the medical importance of accurate identification of protozoa in humans.

14 Discuss the importance of protozoal zoonoses.

15 Discuss how the development of genetic resistance to chemicals affects protozoal diseases, such as malaria.

16 Given an illustration or photograph (or an actual specimen, given sufficient laboratory experience), identify diagnostic stages of protozoa.

17 Differentiate the diagnosis of protozoa and helminth infections.

18 Compare and contrast life cycles of protozoa and helminths.

19 Predict the effects of immunosuppression on patients harboring various protozoal or helminth parasites.

GLOSSARY

accolé. On the outer edge.

amastigote. A small, ovoid, nonflagellated form of the order *Kinetoplastid flagellata.* Notable structures

include a mitochondrial kinetoplast and a large nucleus. Also called L.D. (Leishman-Donovan) body or leishmanial form.

Apicomplexa. A phylum containing protozoa whose life cycle includes feeding stages (trophozoites), asexual multiplication (schizogony), and sexual multiplication (gametogony and sporogony).

arthropod. An organism having a hard segmented exoskeleton and paired, jointed legs (see Chap. 6).

atria(sing. **atrium**). An opening; in a human, refers to the mouth, vagina, and urethra.

axoneme. The intracellular portion of a flagellum.

axostyle. The axial rod functioning as a support in flagellates.

blepharoplast. The basal body origin of the flagella that supports the undulating membrane in kinetoplastid flagellates.

bradyzoites. Slowly multiplying intracellular trophozoites of *Toxoplasma gondii*; intracellular tissue cysts in immune hosts contain bradyzoites that continue dividing within the cyst. Bradyzoites are also found in sarcocysts.

chromatin. Basophilic nuclear DNA.

chromatoid bar (or body). A rod-shaped structure of condensed RNA material within the cytoplasm of some amoeba cysts.

cilia. Multiple hairlike processes attached to a surface of a cell; functions for motility through fluids at the surface of a protozoa.

Ciliophora. A phylum containing protozoa that move by means of cilia; have two dissimilar nuclei.

costa. A thin, firm, rodlike structure running along the base of the undulating membrane on certain flagellates.

cryptozoite. The stage of *Plasmodium* spp. that develops in liver cells from the inoculated sporozoites. Also called the exoerythrocytic stage or tissue stage.

cutaneous. Pertaining to the skin.

cyst. The immotile stage protected by a resistant cyst wall formed by the parasite. In this stage, the protozoan is readily transmitted to a new host.

cytostome. The rudimentary mouth.

dysentery. A disorder marked by bloody diarrhea and/or mucus in feces.

ectoplasm. The gelatinous cytoplasmic material beneath the cell membrane.

endoplasm. The fluid inner cytoplasmic material in a cell.

endosome. The small mass of chromatin within the nucleus, comparable to a nucleolus of metazoan cells (also termed karyosome).

epimastigote. A flattened, spindle-shaped, flagellated form seen primarily in the gut (e.g., in the reduviid bug) or salivary glands (e.g., in the tsetse fly) of the insect vectors in the life cycle of trypanosomes; it has an undulating membrane that extends from the flagellum (attached along the anterior half of the organism) to the small kinetoplast located just anteriorly to the larger nucleus located at the midpoint of the organism.

excystation. Transformation from a cyst to a trophozoite after the cystic form has been swallowed by the host.

exflagellation. The process whereby a sporozoan microgametocyte releases haploid flagellated microgametes that can fertilize a macrogamete and thus form a diploid zygote (ookinete).

flagellum (pl. flagella). An extension of ectoplasm that provides locomotion; resembles a tail that moves with a whiplike motion.

fomites. Objects that can absorb and harbor organisms and cause human infection through direct contact (e.g., doorknob, pencil, towel).

gamete. A mature sex cell.

gametocyte. A sex cell that can produce gametes.

gametogony. The phase of the development cycle of the malarial and coccidial parasite in the human in which male and female gametocytes are formed.

hypnozoite. A long-surviving modified liver schizont of *P. vivax* that is the source of relapsing infections in this species.

karyosome. *See* **Endosome.**

kinetoplast. An accessory body found in many protozoa, especially in the family Trypanosomatidae, consisting of a large mitochondrion next to the basal granule (blepharoplast) of the anterior or undulating membrane flagellum; contains mitochondrial DNA.

L.D. body (Leishman-Donovan body). Each of the small ovoid amastigote forms found in tissue macrophages of the liver and spleen in patients with *Leishmania donovani* infection.

Mastigophora. A subphylum containing organisms that move by means of one or more flagella.

merogony. Asexual multiplication in coccidian life cycle. Usually occurs in intestinal epithelium.

merozoite. Each of the many trophozoites released from human red blood cells or liver cells at maturation of the asexual cycle of malaria.

nosocomial. An infection that originates in and is acquired from a medical facility. Infections present or incubating inside patients when they are admitted to the facility are *not* included in this definition.

oocyst. The encysted form of the ookinete that occurs on the stomach wall of *Anopheles* spp. mosquitoes infected with malaria.

ookinete. The motile zygote of *Plasmodium* spp.; formed by microgamete (male sex cell) fertilization of a macrogamete (female sex cell). The ookinete encysts (*see* **oocyst**).

paroxysm. The fever-chills syndrome in malaria. Spiking fever corresponds to the release of merozoites and toxic materials from the rupturing parasitized red blood cells, and shaking chills occur during subsequent schizont development. Occurs in malaria cyclically every 36 to 72 hours, depending on the species.

patent. Apparent or evident.

promastigote. A flagellate form of trypanosoma in which the kinetoplast is located at the anterior end of the organism; has no undulating membrane. This form is seen in the midgut and pharynx of vectors in the life cycle of the leishmania parasites and is the form that develops in culture media in vitro.

Protozoa. A subkingdom consisting of unicellular eukaryotic animals.

pseudopod. A protoplasmic extension of the trophozoites of amoebae that allows them to move and engulf food.

pseudocyst. A cyst with a membrane covering formed by the host following an acute infection with *Toxoplasma gondii.* The cyst is filled with bradyzoites in immunocompetent hosts; may occur in brain or other tissues. Latent source of infection that may become active if immunosuppression occurs.

recrudescence. A condition that may be seen in any malarial infection; infected red blood cells and accompanying symptoms reappear after a period of apparent "cure." This situation reflects an inadequate immune response by the host or an inadequate response to treatment.

relapse (malaria). A condition seen subsequent to apparent elimination of the parasite from red blood cells; caused by a reactivation of sequestered liver merozoites that begin a new cycle in red blood cells. True relapses occur only in *Plasmodium vivax* and *P. ovale* infections.

Sarcodina. A subphylum containing amoebae that move by means of pseudopodia.

sarcocyst. Infective cyst containing banana-shaped bradyzoites.

schizogony (merogony). Asexual multiplication of *Apicomplexa;* multiple intracellular nuclear divisions precede cytoplasmic division.

schizont. The developed stage of asexual division of the *Sporozoa* (e.g., *Plasmodium* spp. in a human red blood cell; *Isospora belli* in the intestinal wall).

sporocyst. The fertilized oocyst in which the sporozoites of *Plasmodium* have developed.

sporogony. Sexual reproduction of *Apicomplexa.* Production of spores and sporozoites.

sporozoite. The form of *Plasmodium* that develops inside the sporocyst, invades the salivary glands of the mosquito, and is transmitted to humans.

subpatent. Not evident, subclinical.

tachyzoites. Rapidly growing intracellular trophozoites of *Toxoplasma gondii.*

trophozoite (pl. trophozoites). The motile stage of protozoon that feeds, multiplies, and maintains the colony within the host.

trypomastigote. A flagellate form with the kinetoplast located at the posterior end of the organism and the undulating membrane extending along the entire body from the flagellum (anterior end) to the posterior end at the blepharoplast. This form is seen in the blood of humans with trypanosomiasis and is the infective stage transmitted by the insect vectors.

undulating membrane. A protoplasmic membrane with a flagellar rim extending out like a fin along the outer edge of the body of certain protozoa; it moves in a wavelike pattern.

xenodiagnosis. Infections with *Trypanosoma cruzi* may be diagnosed by allowing an uninfected Triatoma bug to feed on the patient (the bite is painless); the insect's feces are later examined for parasites (trypomastigote forms).

zygote. The fertilized cell resulting from the union of male and female gametes.

● *Introduction*

The subkingdom Protozoa includes eukaryotic unicellular animals. The various life functions are carried out by specialized intracellular structures known as organelles. Each group of protozoa exhibits morphologic differentiation by which it can be identified. Most protozoa multiply by binary fission. However, certain groups have more specialized modes of reproduction, which are individually discussed.

Each species of parasitic protozoa is frequently confined to one or a few host species. At least 30 species of protozoa parasitize humans, and many of these parasitic species are widely distributed throughout the world. Many species of vertebrates and invertebrates harbor protozoan parasites, often without clinical signs. Parasites (including the parasitic protozoa) that have had a long coevolution with their host species have evolved adaptations, such as antigenic variations of their surface proteins, that permit evasion of the host's immune recognition and response mechanisms. Effective, affordable vaccines for humans generally have not been developed to date.

There are two major methods of transmission of protozoal infection: through ingestion of the infective stage of the protozoa or via an **arthropod** vector. A few are transmitted by sexual contact. The mode of transmission is specific for each species.

The following groups of protozoa are considered:

1. Amoebae that move by means of **pseudopodia**
2. Protozoa that possess one to several flagella
3. Protozoa that move by means of many **cilia** on the cell surface
4. Protozoa that do not exhibit an obvious mode of mobility, but can glide nonetheless (This same group uses sexual reproduction during the life cycle.)

Each group is listed in separate tables preceding the general discussion of each class of organisms. You should review the glossary before studying the rest of the chapter.

Amoebae in the order Amoebida (Table 5–1), which include parasites of humans, can be found worldwide. The motile, reproducing, feeding stage (the **trophozoite**) lives most commonly in the lower gastrointestinal tract. Many of these amoebae can form a nonfeeding, nonmotile **cyst** stage, which is the stage that is infective for humans. Transmission of amoebae is generally by ingestion of cysts in fecally contaminated food or water. When cysts are swallowed and pass to the lower intestine, they **excyst** and begin to multiply as feeding trophozoites.

The structure of the nucleus is quite different for each genus of amoeba, and identification of stained nuclear structure aids in diagnosis. Cysts of amoebae may have varying numbers of nuclei, depending on their stage of development; therefore, it is critical to look at nuclear structure as well as numbers for correct identification. A permanent stain—such as the trichrome stain used on a thin, fixed fecal smear—is particularly helpful in allowing identification of nuclear and other intracellular structures and is highly recommended as a routine procedure in a diagnostic laboratory.

Other diagnostic features of the motile amoeba include size, cytoplasmic inclusions, and type of motility exhibited by the pseudopodia formed by trophozoites in a wet-mount preparation. In the cyst stage, diagnostic features include nuclear structure, the size and shape of the cyst, the number of nuclei, and other inclusion bodies present.

Entamoeba histolytica is the major pathogen in this group and the cause of amebic dysentery in humans. It can occur in other primates, dogs, cats, and rats. All other amoebae seen in feces are considered nonpathogenic commensals. It is important, however, that

● *Class Lobosea*

TABLE 5–1 □ AMOEBAE

Order	Scientific Name	Common Name
Amoebida	*Entamoeba histolytica* (en'tuh-mee'buh/his-toe-lit'i-kuh)	amebic dysentery
Amoebida	*Entamoeba dispar* (en'tuh-mee'buh/dis'par)	commensal
Amoebida	*Entamoeba hartmanni* (en'tuh-mee'buh/hart-man'nee)	commensal (formerly "small race of *E. histolytica*)
Amoebida	*Entamoeba coli* (en'tuh-mee'buh/ko'lye)	*E. coli,* commensal
Amoebida	*Entamoeba polecki* (en'tuh-mee'buh/po-lek'ee)	commensal
Amoebida	*Entamoeba gingivalis* (en'tuh-mee'buh/gin-gi-val'is)	commensal
Amoebida	*Blastocystis hominis* (blast'o-sis-tis/hom-in'is)	*Blastocystis,* commensal
Amoebida	*Endolimax nana* (en'doe-lye'macks/nay'nuh)	*E. nana* commensal
Amoebida	*Iodamoeba bütschlii* (eye-o'duh-mee'buh/bootch'leee-eye)	*I. bütschlii* commensal
Amoebida	*Acanthamoeba* spp. (ay-kanth'uh-mee'buh)	none
Schizopyrenida	*Naegleria fowleri* (nay'gleer-ee'uh/fow-ler'i)	primary amebic meningoencephalitis

each species be correctly identified to ensure proper therapy, if needed, and to avoid unnecessary or inappropriate treatment because of misdiagnosis.

The nucleus of *E. histolytica* has a small central **karyosome (endosome)** and uniform peripheral chromatin granules lining the nuclear membrane. Spokelike chromatin may also radiate outward from the karyosome to the nuclear membrane. *E. histolytica* invades the intestinal wall and multiplies in the mucosal tissue. In the cytoplasm of the trophozoite, one often can see ingested red blood cells (RBCs); the trophozoite voraciously feeds on RBCs when it is invasive in tissue. The RBCs can appear either whole or partially digested. These blood cells are not seen in the trophozoite of any other amoeba, and their presence is required for differential diagnosis. The trophozoite of *E. histolytica* extends thin, pointed pseudopodia and exhibits active, progressive motility in a saline wet mount.

The cyst of *E. histolytica* contains one, two, or four nuclei because nuclear divisions accompany cyst maturation. The nuclear structure in stained cysts and in trophozoites is the same. The cyst of the pathogenic *E. histolytica* is round and is 10 to 20 μm. It may also contain cigar-shaped **chromatoid bars.** *E. hartmanni* is nonpathogenic and may be confused with *E. histolytica.* Formerly known as the "small race" of *E. histolytica, E. hartmanni* forms cysts of less than 10 μm, and trophozoites are less than 12 μm in size. A calibrated ocular micrometer (see p. 167) is required to measure cyst diameters to differentiate these species.

Another nonpathogenic species is *Entamoeba dispar.* Cysts and trophozoites are morphologically identical to *E. histolytica,* except that *E. dispar* is noninvasive and never ingests RBCs. Because patients harboring *E. dispar* are asymptomatic and may not require treatment, when no trophozoites with ingested RBCs are found in submitted specimens, the laboratory report should say "*Entamoeba histolytica/E. dispar*—unable to differentiate unless trophozoites are seen containing ingested RBCs." If trophozoites with ingested RBCs are noted or an immunoassay specific for *E. histolytica* is performed, the report can confirm the presence of this parasite.

Pathology caused by *E. histolytica* includes flask-shaped ulcerations of the intestinal wall and bloody dysentery. If amoebae penetrate the intestinal wall and spread via blood, ulceration may occur in the liver, lungs, brain, or other tissues. Liver abscesses are most common, and lung invasion usually results from erosion of the liver abscess. Any of these extraintestinal infections can be fatal.

Prevalence is very high in the subtropics and tropics (more than 50%), and focal epidemics can occur anywhere. The infection can be transmitted sexually by gay men and is one cause of the disease known as "gay bowel syndrome." Up to 30% of some populations of this at-risk group can harbor *E. histolytica/E. dispar.* Prevalence in the general population in the United States and Europe is approximately 5% and includes many asymptomatic carriers. Although many people worldwide are infected with *E. histolytica/E. dispar,* only a small number of people harboring the parasite ever develop symptoms. The fact that so many carriers do not exhibit symptoms may be explained by the misdiagnosis of the nonpathogenic *E. dispar* infections. More realistic estimates of true *E. histolytica* infections are probably only 10% of the totals reported before *E. dispar* was correctly characterized.

Entamoeba coli (a nonpathogenic commensal) is most commonly confused with *E. histolytica.* The nucleus of *E. coli* differs from *E. histolytica;* it has a large eccentric karyosome and irregular peripheral chromatin clumping along the nuclear membrane. The trophozoite exhibits granular cytoplasm and ingested bacteria but not RBCs. Motility is sluggish, and the pseudopods are blunt. The cyst stage often has up to eight nuclei of characteristic structure rather than a maximum of four as in *E. histolytica.* Chromatoid bars, if present, have splintered or pointed ends rather than rounded ends. Mature *E. coli* cysts become more impermeable to fixatives; therefore, it is sometimes possible to observe cysts better in the concentrated sediment than in permanently stained smears. The pale or distorted appearance of cysts on stained smears may lead to confusion.

Entamoeba polecki, found primarily in pigs and monkeys, is occasionally found in humans. It closely resembles both *E. histolytica* and *E. coli* morphologically. Great care is needed when identifying this organism because it is not pathogenic and unnecessary treatment results if it is incorrectly differentiated as *E. histolytica.* This organism is identified by noting the usual one nucleus in mature cysts. Rarely, there may be two or four nuclei. A large glycogen "inclusion mass" may also be present. Chromatoid bodies are abundant and are pointed rather than rounded as in *E. histolytica.*

Entamoeba gingivalis, found in the mouth in soft tartar between teeth or in tonsillar crypts, is considered nonpathogenic, but occasionally it can be found in sputum and must be differentiated from *E. histolytica.* Two important features help in this regard: *E. gingivalis* has no cyst stage, and it is the only species known to ingest white blood cells. Nuclear fragments of white cells can be seen in the trophozoite's large food vacuoles when permanently stained smears are examined.

Two common nonpathogenic species also found in the intestinal tract include *Endolimax nana* and *Iodamoeba butschlii.* These organisms must be differentiated from pathogens to avoid misdiagnosis and mistreatment. Diagnostic features of these protozoa are found on pages 93–95.

Blastocystis hominis is a strictly anaerobic intestinal protozoan that has been variously classified since its discovery in 1912. It multiplies by binary fission or sporulation. Fecal-oral transmission through contaminated food or water is probably the route of infection. This parasite generally does not seem to cause clinical disease in humans, but it must be considered when found in large numbers in patients with abdominal symptoms who have no other apparent etiologic agent. Metronidazole is the drug of choice when treatment is needed.

When present, *B. hominis* protozoa are easily recovered and are identified using the trichrome stain. The organism is round and varies greatly in size from 6 to 40 μm in diameter. The central area of the cell resembles a large vacuole surrounded by several small, dark-staining nuclei. These organisms may be confused with yeast cells. When fecal samples are being processed, only saline should be used to wash the specimen because water destroys *B. hominis,* causing a false-negative report.

Several species of free-living amoebae may become opportunistic parasites of humans. These organisms are found in fresh or salt water, moist soil, and decaying vegetation. In most instances, no disease is produced by these organisms. In a few cases, however, severe consequences result. The notable potential pathogens are *Naegleria fowleri* and, less commonly, *Acanthamoeba* spp. *Naegleria* is an ameboflagellate because in the free-living state it alternates from an ameboid phase to a form possessing two flagella. Only the ameboid phase is found in host tissues.

The disease caused by *N. fowleri* occurs most often during the summer months (Diagram 5–1). The parasite gains entry through the nasal mucosa when the host is diving and swimming in ponds or small lakes that are inhabited by the parasite. It then migrates along the olfactory nerves and, within several days, invades the brain. This parasite is highly thermophilic and survives at water temperatures up to 45°C. It also tolerates chlorinated water and has even been found in an indoor swimming pool. Furthermore, infections have been acquired by drinking unfiltered, chlorinated tap water. Upon infection, the clinical symptoms are dramatic, and the disease runs a rapid and usually fatal course. Symptoms of primary amebic meningoencephalitis (PAM) begin with headache, fever, nausea, and vomiting within 1 or 2 days. Typical symptoms of meningoencephalitis follow, leading to irrational behavior, coma, and death. The clinical course rarely lasts more than 6 days.

Diagnosis is often made on autopsy; however, a purulent spinal fluid containing high numbers of neutrophils (200 to 20,000/μL) without bacteria should add amebic meningoencephalitis to the differential diagnosis. Motile amoebae may be noted in unstained preparations. A drop of unrefrigerated spinal fluid sediment should be examined on a clean glass slide for parasite motility because the organism resembles a leukocyte when observed on a counting chamber. Warming the prepared slide to 35°C will promote amebic movement. Phase microscopy is preferred, but the motile trophozoite may be observed using a bright-field microscope with reduced light. Giemsa or trichrome stain is helpful to differentiate the organism. Trophozoites may also be seen in Wright-stained cytospin preparations. Its ameboid form is elongated with a tapered posterior and ranges from 7 to 20 μm. The rounded form is 15 μm with a large central nuclear karyosome and granular, vacuolated cytoplasm. Treatment is usually unsuccessful; however, when given promptly, amphotericin B and sulfadiazine have been effective in a very few cases.

DIAGRAM 5-1

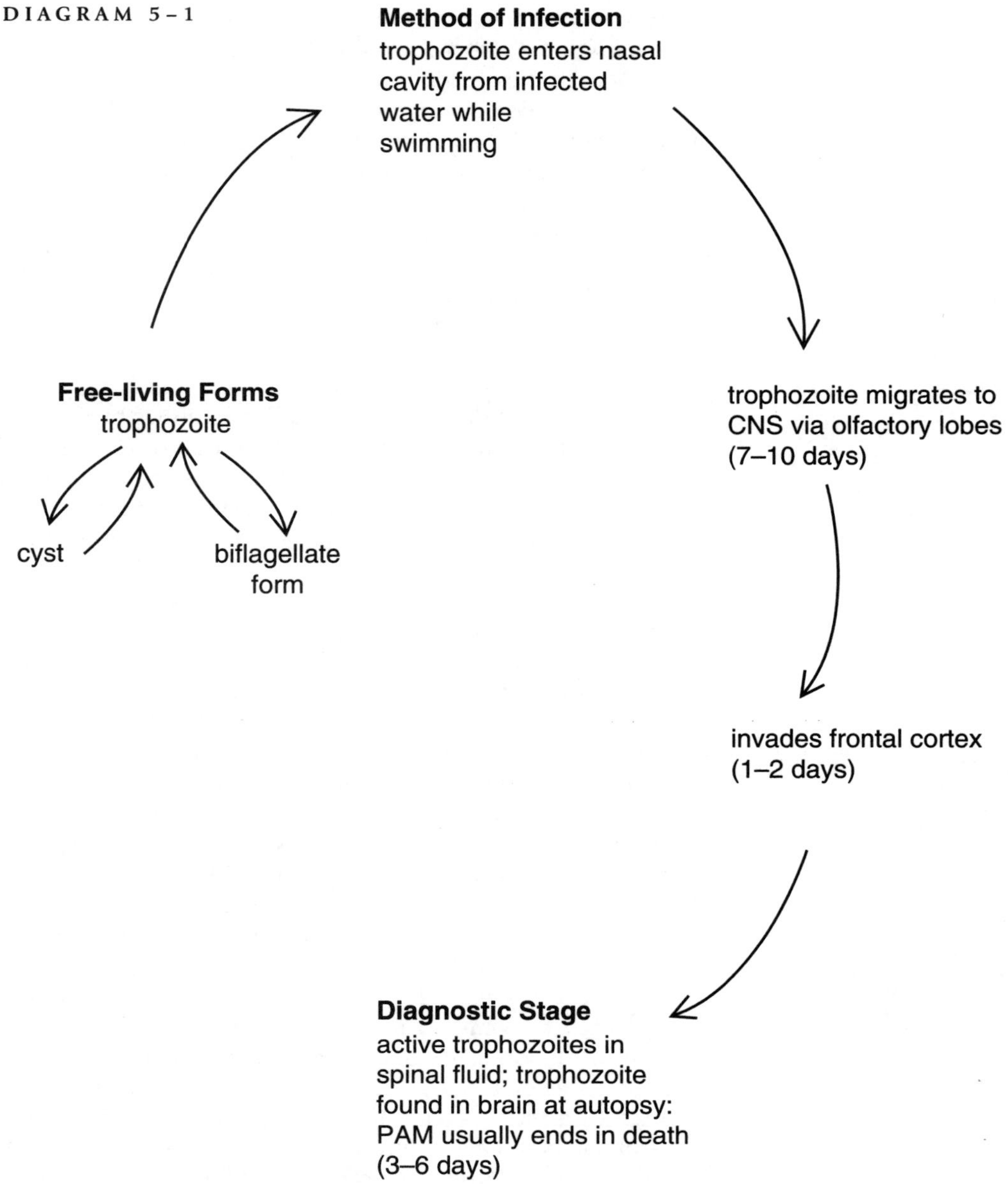

Method of Infection
trophozoite enters nasal
cavity from infected
water while
swimming

Free-living Forms
trophozoite

cyst   biflagellate
                        form

trophozoite migrates to
CNS via olfactory lobes
(7–10 days)

invades frontal cortex
(1–2 days)

Diagnostic Stage
active trophozoites in
spinal fluid; trophozoite
found in brain at autopsy:
PAM usually ends in death
(3–6 days)

Life cycle of *Naegleria fowleri*

At least six species of *Acanthamoeba* are known to cause granulomatous amebic encephalitis (GAE), a more chronic form of meningoencephalitis (Diagram 5-2). Infected patients often have compromised immunologic systems. Onset of symptoms is slow—usually
weeks to months or even years. Chronic granulomatous lesions in brain tissue may contain
both trophozoites and cysts. *Acanthamoeba* have been isolated from the upper respiratory
tract of healthy individuals and seem to grow best in the upper airways of susceptible patients. Apparently, infections occur through either inhalation of contaminated dust or
aerosols or through invasion of broken skin or mucous membranes. These parasites have
been found in the lungs, nasal and sinus passages, eyes, ears, skin lesions, and vagina.

There have also been several hundred cases of *Acanthamoeba keratitis* related to poor
contact lens care. Direct examination of a patient's cornea using a confocal microscope can
aid in diagnosing *A. keratitis*. Direct examination and culture of corneal scraping can also
lead to a correct diagnosis. Using contaminated saline cleaning solutions and wearing
lenses while swimming in contaminated water are the usual causes of these infections.

A related amoeba, *Balamuthia mandrillaris*, has been reported as another causative agent
of GAE. It is rare, however. It **has** also been found in immunocompetent children. This

DIAGRAM 5–2

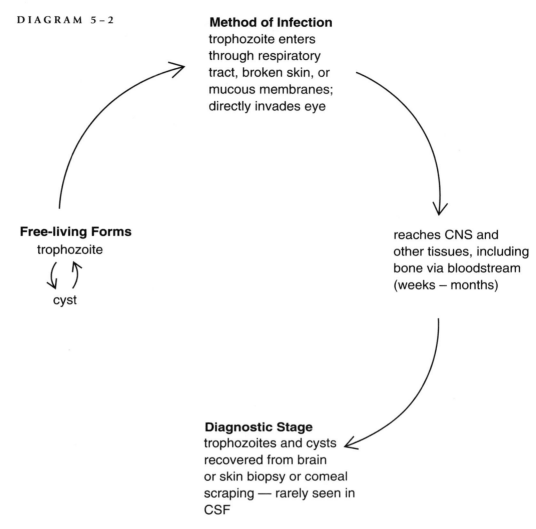

Method of Infection
trophozoite enters
through respiratory
tract, broken skin, or
mucous membranes;
directly invades eye

Free-living Forms
trophozoite

cyst

reaches CNS and
other tissues, including
bone via bloodstream
(weeks – months)

Diagnostic Stage
trophozoites and cysts
recovered from brain
or skin biopsy or comeal
scraping — rarely seen in
CSF

Life cycle of *Acanthamoeba* ssp.

parasite has been found in many primates (e.g., gorillas, gibbons, monkeys) and sheep and horses. One-third of the few cases reported in the United States were in patients with AIDS.

Cysts of *Acanthamoeba* spp., like *Naegleria* spp., are also resistant to chlorination and drying. *Acanthamoeba* spp. trophozoites have spinelike pseudopodia but are rarely seen motile. They average 30 μm and have a large central karyosome in the nucleus. The 10- to 25-μm cyst is round with a single nucleus and has a double wall; the outer cyst wall may be slightly wrinkled with a polyhedral inner wall. *Acanthamoeba* spp. vary in sensitivity to antimicrobial agents. Treatment of *Acanthamoeba keratitis* is often successful, but only rare cases of central nervous system (CNS) infections have responded to therapy. In vitro studies suggest that *B. mandrillaris* is susceptible to pentamidine isothiocyanate.

Entamoeba histolytica (amoeba)

DIAGRAM 5-3

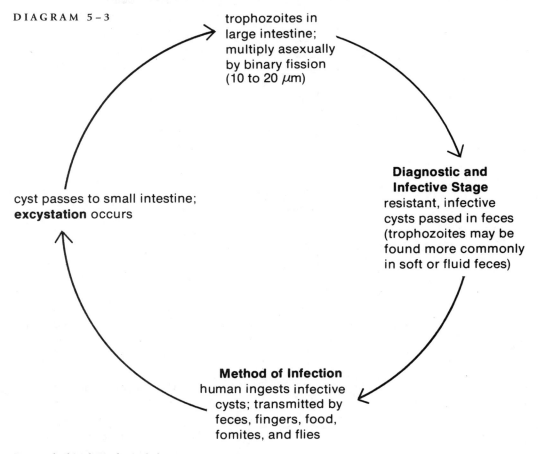

trophozoites in
large intestine;
multiply asexually
by binary fission
(10 to 20 μm)

**Diagnostic and
Infective Stage**
resistant, infective
cysts passed in feces
(trophozoites may be
found more commonly
in soft or fluid feces)

cyst passes to small intestine;
excystation occurs

Method of Infection
human ingests infective
cysts; transmitted by
feces, fingers, food,
fomites, and flies

Entamoeba histolytica (amoeba)

METHOD OF DIAGNOSIS

Recover and identify trophozoites or cysts in feces or intestinal mucosa.

SPECIMEN REQUIREMENTS

1. At least three fresh stool specimens should be examined for the presence of parasites. A permanently stained smear and a concentration procedure must be performed on each specimen submitted for examination. A saline mount may be performed on fresh liquid or soft stool to observe trophozoite motility.
2. Six permanent smears from different sites should be prepared while a sigmoidoscopy is being performed.
3. Serologic methods are most useful in extraintestinal diseases.

DIAGNOSTIC STAGE

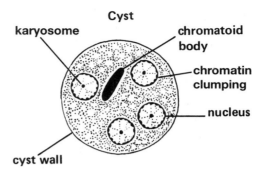

Cyst

karyosome — chromatoid body — chromatin clumping — nucleus — cyst wall

10 to 20 μm

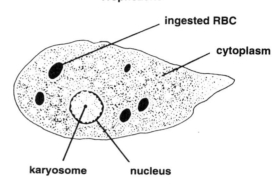

Trophozoite

ingested RBC — cytoplasm — karyosome — nucleus

10 to 20 μm

Note: Even pattern
of nuclear chromatin on the nuclear rim
with spokelike pattern from the karysome.

DISEASE NAMES

- Amebiasis
- Amebic dysentery
- Amebic hepatitis (if liver is involved)

MAJOR PATHOLOGY AND SYMPTOMS

Patient may be asymptomatic or exhibit vague abdominal discomfort, malaise, diarrhea alternating with constipation, or bloody dysentery and fever (in cases of acute illness). The pathogen invades the intestinal submucosa via lytic enzymes in 2% to 8% of infections; lateral extension leads to typical flask-shaped lesions. In amebic hepatitis, there is an enlarged liver, fever, chills, and leukocytosis.

TREATMENT

Depending on the location of infection, iodoquinol, paromomycin, metronidazole, dehydroemetine, and combinations (see *Medical Letter* items in Bibliography on p. 211). All positive cases should be treated.

DISTRIBUTION

Distribution is worldwide.

OF NOTE

1. Chronic infection may last for years.
2. Although the pathogenic *E. histolytica* and the nonpathogenic species, *E. dispar*, can be

differentiated definitively only by using DNA probes, it is acceptable to use the finding of ingested RBCs as a means of identifying *E. histolytica*.

3. Onset of invasive disease may be gradual or sudden and is characterized by blood-tinged mucous dysentery with up to 10 stools **per day**. Severe, sudden-onset cases may mimic appendicitis.

4. It must be differentiated from ulcerative colitis, **carcinoma**, other intestinal parasites, and diverticulitis. Also, the hepatic form must be differentiated from hepatitis, hydatid cyst, various gallbladder problems, cancer, and lung disease.

5. Amoebae can invade the lungs, brain, skin, and other tissues. Amebic hepatitis is the most common and gravest complication. Usually, only a single abscess develops in the right lobe of the liver. Any of the various imaging techniques reveals the abscess.

6. This parasite has been added to the list of sexually transmitted diseases.

COMPARATIVE MORPHOLOGY OF INTESTINAL AMOEBAE AND OTHERS

TABLE 5–2 □ DIAGNOSTIC CHARACTERISTICS OF AMOEBA CYSTS AND TROPHOZOITES

Parasite	Size of Cyst and Troph (μm)	Number of Nuclei	Nuclear Appearance	Cytoplasmic Inclusions	Cyst	Trophozoite
Entamoeba histolytica (pathogen)	10–20	**Cyst** = 1, 2, or 4 **Troph** = 1	Small central karyosome with even chromatin	**Cyst** = cigar-shaped chromatoid body **Troph** = red blood cells		
Entamoeba hartmanni (commensal)	<10	**Cyst** = 1, 2, or 4 **Troph** = 1	Small central karyosome with even chromatin	**Cyst** = cigar-shaped chromatoid body **Troph** = none		

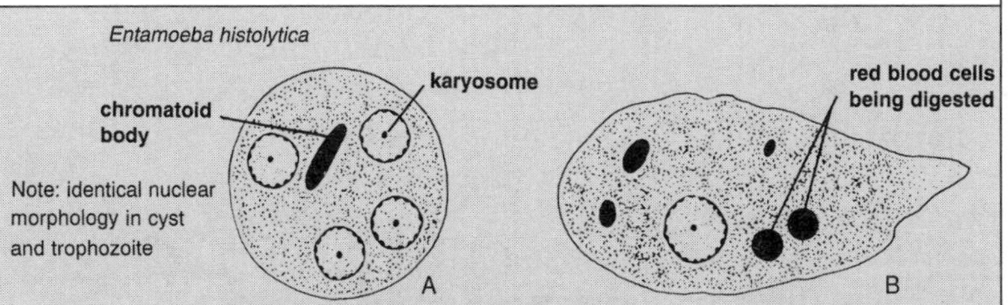

Entamoeba histolytica

karyosome

chromatoid body

A

red blood cells being digested

B

Note: identical nuclear morphology in cyst and trophozoite

diameter over 10 μm, up to 4 nuclei in cyst, central karyosome, even nuclear chromatin at edges, and spokelike rays of chromatin from karyosome outward; chromatoid body has blunt, rounded ends that are noted more frequently than those seen in *E. coli* cysts; precysts may have a glycogen vacuole that stains reddish brown

Entamoeba hartmanni (small race of *E. histolytica*; nonpathogenic)

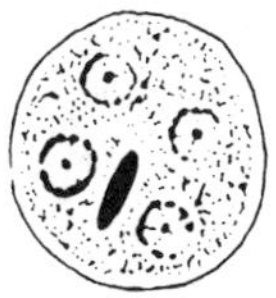

diameter less than 10 μm

A

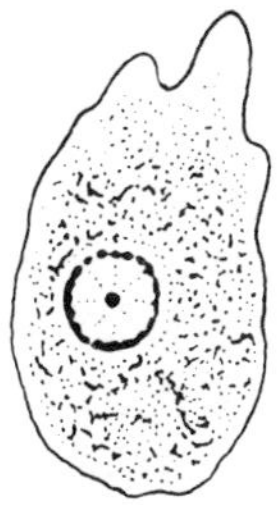

B

Continued on following page

TABLE 5-2 □ DIAGNOSTIC CHARACTERISTICS OF AMOEBA CYSTS AND TROPHOZOITES (Continued)

Parasite	Size of Cyst and Troph (μm)	Number of Nuclei	Nuclear Appearance	Cytoplasmic Inclusions	Cyst	Trophozoite
Entamoeba coli (commensal)	>10	Cyst = 1–8 Troph = 1	Eccentric karyosome with irregular chromatin	Cyst = splinter-shaped, rough-pointed, rough-edged chromatin body Troph = ingested bacteria	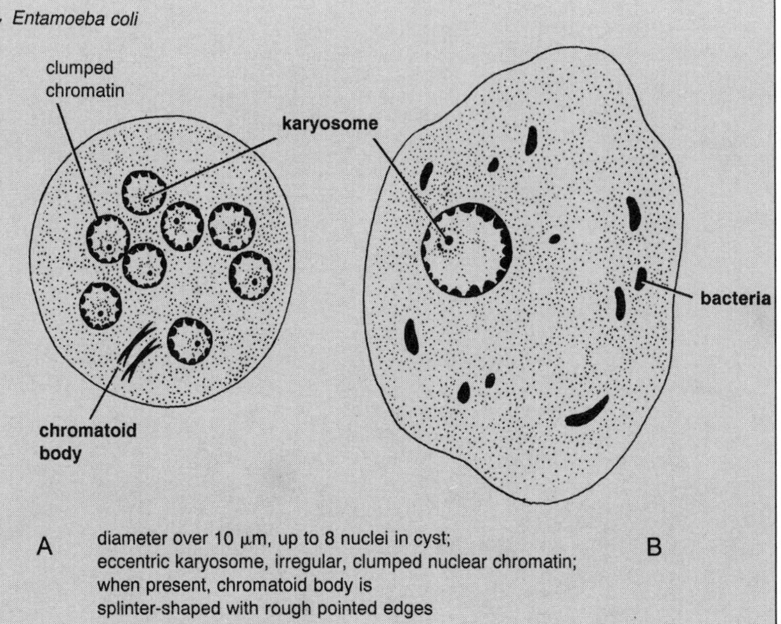	
Endolimax nana (commensal)	6–12	Cyst = 1–4 Troph = 1	Irregular clumped karyosome with no peripheral chromatin	Cyst = none Troph = none	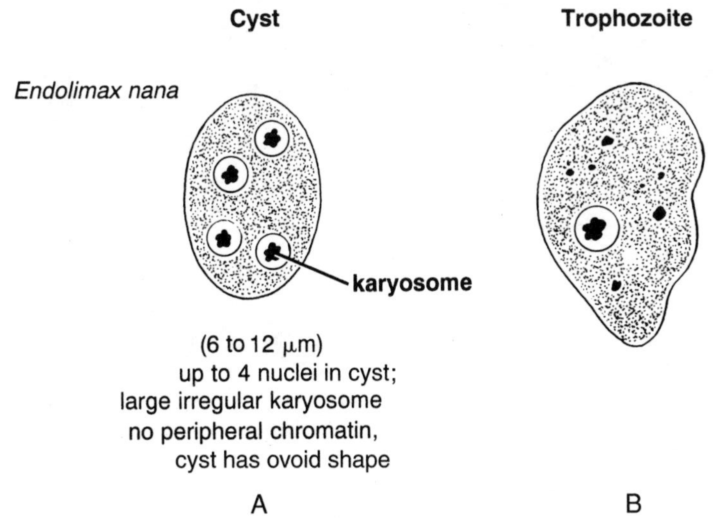	

Entamoeba coli diagram labels:
- bacteria
- karyosome
- clumped chromatin
- chromatoid body

A — diameter over 10 μm, up to 8 nuclei in cyst; eccentric karyosome, irregular, clumped nuclear chromatin; when present, chromatoid body is splinter-shaped with rough pointed edges

B — Trophozoite

Endolimax nana diagram labels:
- Trophozoite
- Cyst
- karyosome

A — (6 to 12 μm) up to 4 nuclei in cyst; large irregular karyosome no peripheral chromatin, cyst has ovoid shape

B

Endolimax nana

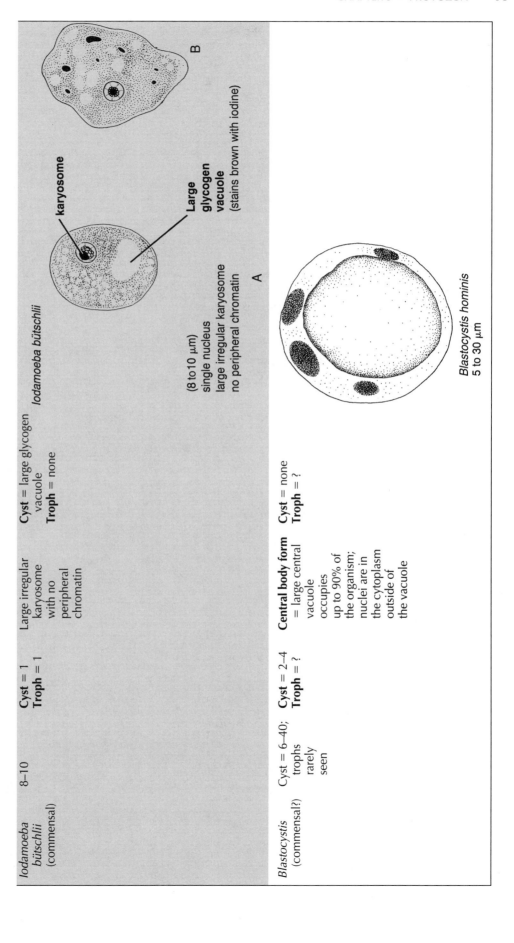

Iodamoeba bütschlii
(commensal)

8–10

Cyst = 1
Troph = 1

Large irregular
karyosome
with no
peripheral
chromatin

Cyst = large glycogen
vacuole
Troph = none   *Iodamoeba bütschlii*

karyosome

**Large
glycogen
vacuole**
(stains brown with iodine)

B

A

(8 to 10 µm)
single nucleus
large irregular karyosome
no peripheral chromatin

Blastocystis
(commensal?)

Cyst = 6–40;
trophs
rarely
seen

Cyst = 2–4
Troph = ?

Central body form
= large central
vacuole
occupies
up to 90% of
the organism;
nuclei are in
the cytoplasm
outside of
the vacuole

Cyst = none
Troph = ?

Blastocystis hominis
5 to 30 µm

TABLE 5–3 ☐ COMPARATIVE MORPHOLOGY OF OPPORTUNISTIC AMEBIC PATHOGENS OF THE CENTRAL NERVOUS SYSTEM

Parasite	Size of Cyst and Troph (μm)	Number of Nuclei	Nuclear Appearance	Cytoplasmic Inclusions	Cyst	Trophozoite
Acanthamoeba spp.	Cyst = 15–20 Troph = 10–45	Cyst = 1 Troph = 1	Both cyst and troph = distinct nucleus with smooth-staining cytoplasm when viewed in tissue no chromatin	Cyst = double-walled wrinkled appearance in tissue Troph = none		
Naegleria fowleri	Cyst = none in humans Troph = 7–20	Troph = 1	Troph = large, centrally located karyosome	Cyst = none Troph = numerous WBCs and no bacteria are present when motile trophs are seen in CSF	Naegleria fowleri no cyst present in tissue	

FOR REVIEW

1. Describe the nuclear structure for E. histolytica.

2. State the microscopic characteristics used to differentiate E. histolytica from E. dispar.

3. How is E. hartmanni differentiated from E. histolytica?

4. List and describe the characteristics used to differentiate cysts of E. histolytica from E. coli.

5. The most prominent diagnostic feature seen in the cyst of Iodamoeba butschlii is

_____.

6. Describe the microscopic appearance of B. hominis.

7. Compare and contrast the cause and diagnostic features of PAM and GAE.

● *Superclass Mastigophora*

Flagellates in the class Zoomastigophorea include the pathogenic protozoa that inhabit the gastrointestinal tract, **atria,** bloodstream, or tissues of humans. The pathogenic gastrointestinal flagellates include two species: *Giardia lamblia* and *Dientamoeba fragilis.* Two common nonpathogenic species also found in the intestinal tract are *Chilomastix mesnili* and *Trichomonas hominis.* These organisms must be differentiated from the pathogens to avoid misdiagnosis and mistreatment. *T. vaginalis* is the only pathogenic atrial protozoan that inhabits the vagina and urethra.

    G. lamblia is the most common intestinal protozoa in the United States. Of the intestinal flagellates, it is important to differentiate *G. lamblia* from the several nonpathogenic flagellates that can be found in the intestinal tract. The trophozoite and the cyst are illustrated

TABLE 5–4 □ FLAGELLATES

Order	Scientific Name	Common Name
Diplomonadida	*Giardia lamblia* (gee′are-dee′uh/lamb-blee′uh)	traveler's diarrhea
Trichomonadida	*Dientamoeba fragilis* (dye-en′tuh-mee′buh/fradj″i-lis)	*Dientamoeba*
Trichomonadida	*Trichomonas vaginalis* (trick″o-mo′nas/vadj-I-nay′lis)	trich
Kinetoplastida	*Trypanosoma brucei rhodesiense* (trip-an″o-so″muh/brew′see″I/ro-dee″zee-en′see)	East African sleeping sickness
Kinetoplastida	*Trypanosoma brucei gambiense* (trip-an″o-so′muh/brew′see″I/gam-bee-en′see)	West African sleeping sickness
Kinetoplastida	*Trypanosoma cruzi* (trip-an″o-so′muh/kroo′zye)	Chagas' disease
Kinetoplastida	*Leishmania tropica* complex (leesh-may′nee-uh/trop′i-kuh)	Oriental boil
Kinetoplastida	*Leishmania mexicana* complex (leesh-may′nee-uh/mex-I-can′uh)	New World leishmaniasis, diffuse cutaneous leishmaniasis
Kinetoplastida	*Leishmania braziliensis* complex (leesh-may′nee-uh/bra-zil″I-en′sis)	New World leishmaniasis
Kinetoplastida	*Leishmania donovani* complex (leesh-may′nee-uh/don″o-vay′nigh)	kala-azar

on page 100. The trophozoite of *G. lamblia* (10 to 20 μm × 5 to 15 μm) is bilaterally symmetric and has two anterior nuclei and eight **flagella.** A sucking disk concavity on the ventral side is the means of attachment to the intestinal mucosa. The cysts are oval, with two or four nuclei located at one end. The clustered nuclei and the central **axoneme** give the cyst the appearance of a little old lady wearing glasses. The cytoplasm of the cyst stage is often retracted from the cyst wall, leaving a clear space under the wall. This parasite has often been associated with traveler's diarrhea, and both trophozoites and cysts can be found in the diarrheic feces along with unusual amounts of mucus. These are not tissue invaders; however, prolonged heavy infection may result in malabsorption by the intestinal mucosa. Transmission is by ingestion of the cyst stage in fecally contaminated water or food.

D. fragilis also has been associated with cases of diarrhea. It lives in the cecum and colon and does not form cysts; the method of transmission is uncertain. The trophozoite has two nuclei connected by a division spindle filament. It has no observable flagella but is classified in the flagellate order Trichomonadida. It moves by means of pseudopodia when seen in feces. The trophozoite is 6 to 20 μm and exhibits sluggish nondirectional motility. *D. fragilis* may occasionally have more or fewer than two nuclei in the trophozoite stage; therefore, it could be confused with developing cysts of *Endolimax nana* or other amoeba.

T. vaginalis multiplies in the genitourinary atrium of both men and women. Usually, only women exhibit symptoms, whereas men serve as asymptomatic carriers. Transmission of *T. vaginalis* is direct and generally by sexual intercourse. Trichomonad species do not form cysts. Motile trophozoites may be identified in fresh urine or in a saline preparation of urethral or vaginal discharge by its characteristic structure, jerky motility, and the "rippling" motion of its undulating membrane. It has a large anterior nucleus, four anterior flagella, an **axostyle,** and an **undulating membrane.** Men are usually asymptomatic; thus, all sex partners should be treated to prevent reinfection.

Giardia lamblia (flagellate)

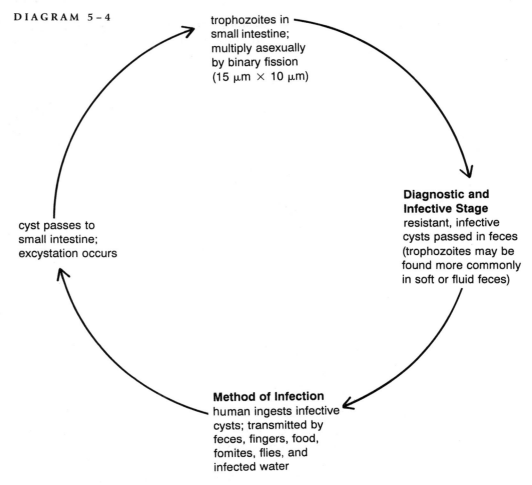

DIAGRAM 5-4

trophozoites in small intestine; multiply asexually by binary fission (15 μm × 10 μm)

Diagnostic and Infective Stage resistant, infective cysts passed in feces (trophozoites may be found more commonly in soft or fluid feces)

cyst passes to small intestine; excystation occurs

Method of Infection human ingests infective cysts; transmitted by feces, fingers, food, fomites, flies, and infected water

Giardia lamblia (flagellate)

METHOD OF DIAGNOSIS

Recover and identify trophozoites or cysts in feces or duodenal contents.*

SPECIMEN REQUIREMENTS

1. At least three stool specimens should be examined for possible parasites. Because trophozoites adhere to the duodenal intestinal mucosa via their sucking disk, there may be intermittent shedding of organisms; therefore, more than three specimens may be required to diagnose this infection.
2. A permanently stained smear for each specimen should be prepared and examined.
3. Be sure to examine areas of mucus in feces for the possible presence of parasites.
4. The string test (Entero-Test; see p. 178) may be helpful if fecal examinations are negative.

---

*A commercially available, orally retrievable string device swallowed in a gelatin capsule—Entero-Test (available from "Hedeco," Health Development Corp., East Palo Alto, CA)—can be examined for the presence of trophozoites in duodenal mucus adherent on the string, which is pulled up after the capsule has been swallowed. The device is also useful for recovering *Strongyloides stercoralis* eggs and/or larvae.

DIAGNOSTIC STAGE

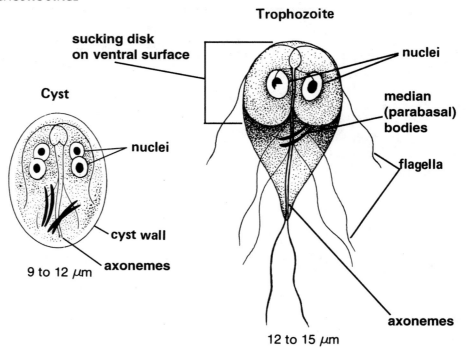

DISEASE NAMES

- Giardiasis
- Traveler's diarrhea

MAJOR PATHOLOGY AND SYMPTOMS

Symptoms include abdominal pain, foul-smelling diarrhea, foul-smelling gas (known as the "purple burps" and smells like rotten eggs), and mechanical irritation of intestinal mucosa with shortening of villi and inflammatory foci. Malabsorption syndrome may occur in heavy infections. People with an IgA deficiency may be more susceptible. Unlike bacillary dysentery, stool does not contain red or white blood cells.

TREATMENT

1. Quinacrine
2. Metronidazole or furazolidone

DISTRIBUTION

Distribution is worldwide.

OF NOTE

1. Outbreaks have been related to cross-contamination of water and sewage systems and contamination of streams by wild animals, such as beavers, that serve as reservoir hosts.
2. Travelers to endemic areas (e.g., St. Petersburg, Russia; some areas of the United States) experience severe diarrhea on infection, but permanent residents of the endemic areas generally do not exhibit symptoms.
3. Increased numbers of gay men harbor this infection.

Dientamoeba fragilis (intestinal flagellate)

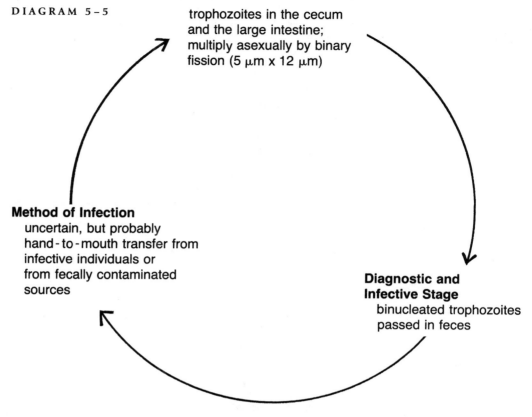

DIAGRAM 5–5

trophozoites in the cecum and the large intestine; multiply asexually by binary fission (5 μm x 12 μm)

Method of Infection
uncertain, but probably hand-to-mouth transfer from infective individuals or from fecally contaminated sources

Diagnostic and Infective Stage
binucleated trophozoites passed in feces

Dientamoeba fragilis (intestinal flagellate)

METHOD OF DIAGNOSIS

Identify trophozoites in feces (no cyst stage known).

SPECIMEN REQUIREMENTS

1. At least three stool specimens should be examined for parasites.
2. A permanently stained smear for each specimen should be prepared and examined for trophozoites.
3. Trophozoites can be found in formed stools.

DIAGNOSTIC STAGE

Dientamoeba fragilis

No cyst stage known

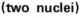

(two nuclei)

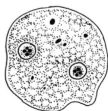

MAJOR PATHOLOGY AND SYMPTOMS

Disease is usually asymptomatic, but it may be associated with diarrhea, anorexia, and abdominal pain.

TREATMENT

Iodoquinol, tetracycline, or paromomycin

DISTRIBUTION

Distribution is worldwide.

OF NOTE

1. A fairly high association between *Enterobius vermicularis* and *D. fragilis* infections has been noted. These findings suggest that *D. fragilis* may also be transmitted via pinworm eggs.
2. No cyst stage is known for this parasite.
3. Most organisms have two nuclei.

Trichomonas vaginalis (Atrial Flagellate)

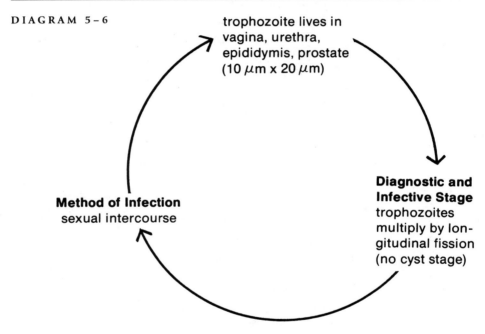

DIAGRAM 5-6

trophozoite lives in vagina, urethra, epididymis, prostate (10 μm x 20 μm)

Diagnostic and Infective Stage
trophozoites multiply by longitudinal fission (no cyst stage)

Method of Infection
sexual intercourse

Trichomonas vaginalis (atrial flagellate)

METHOD OF DIAGNOSIS

Recover and identify motile trophozoites in fresh urethral discharge, vaginal smear, or urine. *T. vaginalis* can be recognized in a Papanicolaou-stained cervical smear.

SPECIMEN REQUIREMENTS

1. Fresh vaginal or urethral discharges or prostatic secretions are examined as a wet mount diluted with a drop of saline. Note jerky, "rippling" pattern of motility.
2. Several specimens may be needed before diagnosis is confirmed.

DIAGNOSTIC STAGE

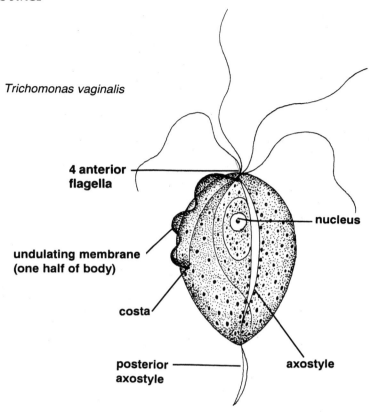

Trichomonas vaginalis

4 anterior
flagella

undulating membrane
(one half of body)

costa

posterior
axostyle

nucleus

axostyle

Trophozoite (no cyst stage form)
15 μm

DISEASE NAMES
- Trichomonad vaginitis
- Urethritis
- Trich

MAJOR PATHOLOGY AND SYMPTOMS
1. In women, the following symptoms are common:
   a. Persistent vaginal inflammation
   b. Yellowish, frothy, foul-smelling vaginal discharge
   c. Burning on urination
   d. Itching and irritation in the vaginal area
2. In men, the disease is generally asymptomatic.

TREATMENT
Metronidazole

DISTRIBUTION
Distribution is worldwide.

 FOR REVIEW

1. *Write the scientific names for two flagellates that do not form cysts.* _____
   and _____
2. *For G. lamblia, C. mesnili, D. fragilis, T. vaginalis, and T. hominis, write the respective body locations where these parasites are found.*

3. *Compare and contrast the diagnostic features of G. lamblia, C. mesnili, D. fragilis, T. vaginalis, and T. hominis.*

4. *Compare and contrast the clinical symptoms for diseases caused by G. lamblia, D. fragilis, and T. vaginalis.*

● *Nonpathogenic Intestinal Flagellates*

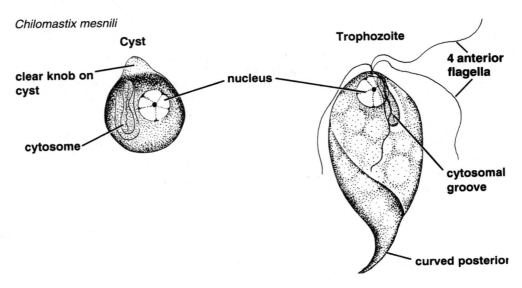

Chilomastix mesnili

Cyst

clear knob on cyst

cytosome

nucleus

Trophozoite

4 anterior flagella

cytosomal groove

curved posterior

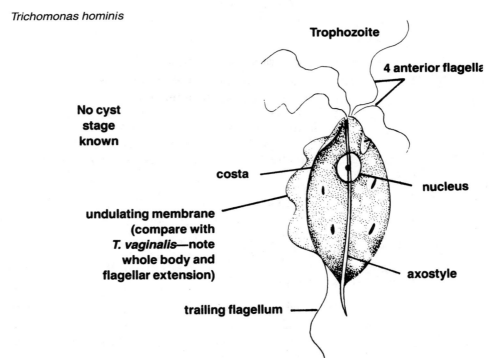

Trichomonas hominis

No cyst stage known

Trophozoite

4 anterior flagella

costa

nucleus

undulating membrane (compare with *T. vaginalis*—note whole body and flagellar extension)

axostyle

trailing flagellum

● *Kineto-plastida*

In the order Kinetoplastida, the pathogenic *Trypanosoma* and *Leishmania* flagellates are found multiplying in the blood (hemoflagellates) or tissue of humans. All species require an arthropod intermediate host. These hemoflagellates exhibit varying morphology in specific locations in both humans and arthropods.

In the genus *Trypanosoma*, two subspecies—*T. brucei rhodesiense* and *T. brucei gambiense*—cause East and West African sleeping sickness, respectively. These diseases are transmitted by the tsetse fly intermediate host (*Glossina* spp.). Organisms are injected when the infected fly takes a blood meal. The **trypomastigote** form can be found extracellularly in a human blood smear in the plasma, or in tissues such as lymph-node biopsies, or in the CNS late in the disease.

The species *T. cruzi*, primarily found in Central and South America, causes a debilitating condition known as Chagas' disease. *T. cruzi* is transmitted by the *Triatoma* bug intermediate host. When the *Triatoma* takes a blood meal, infective organisms are deposited on the skin in the feces of the bug and are rubbed into the wound when the itching bite site is scratched. *T. cruzi* organisms multiply in macrophages of the reticuloendothelial system and are found multiplying as the **amastigote** form in tissues such as the heart. However, trypomastigote forms may be found in the bloodstream early during the infection. Chagas' disease can result in an enlarged heart, esophagus, and colon. Eventually, death may occur if the disease is untreated. In children, an acute fatal disease course is not uncommon.

In the genus *Leishmania*, there are four pathogenic "species complexes" with subspecies in each complex: *L. tropica* (Old World), *L. mexicana* (New World), *L. braziliensis*, and *L. donovani*. Speciation has traditionally been based on clinical symptomology, geographic location, and case history. All *Leishmania* species are transmitted by the sandfly intermediate host, *Phlebotomus* spp. The bite of an infected sandfly initially results in a self-healing skin lesion at the bite site; the lesion may last up to 1 year and may be a wet or dry ulcer, depending on the species. Amastigote forms can be found multiplying intracellularly in local macrophages of the lesion. *L. tropica* and *L. mexicana* cause cutaneous, spontaneously healing ulcers, although some subspecies of *L. mexicana* spread to cause disfiguring from diffuse cutaneous leishmaniasis (DCL). *L. braziliensis* affects the mucosa of the nasopharynx and mouth. In addition, *L. braziliensis* can become **subpatent** and flare up years later, resulting in subsequent erosion of cartilage in the nose and ears.

Unlike the others, *L. donovani* does not stay localized in the skin lesion; the organisms spread to the viscera, multiplying in macrophages of all internal organs and eventually causing death if the patient is untreated. In tissue sections (e.g., liver, spleen), *L. donovani* can be seen as intracellular multiplying amastigote forms (**L.D. bodies**). All species of *Leishmania* that infect humans are zoonotic; the usual host is a vertebrate, such as a dog, fox, or rodent.

Trypanosoma brucei rhodesiense (East African sleeping sickness) and *Trypanosoma brucei gambiense* (West African sleeping sickness)

DIAGRAM 5–7

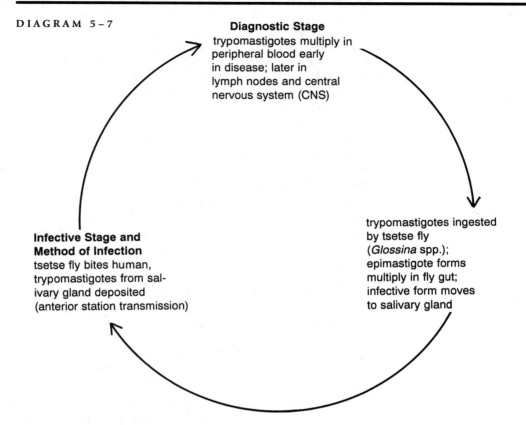

Diagnostic Stage
trypomastigotes multiply in
peripheral blood early
in disease; later in
lymph nodes and central
nervous system (CNS)

trypomastigotes ingested
by tsetse fly
(*Glossina* spp.);
epimastigote forms
multiply in fly gut;
infective form moves
to salivary gland

**Infective Stage and
Method of Infection**
tsetse fly bites human,
trypomastigotes from sal-
ivary gland deposited
(anterior station transmission)

Trypanosoma brucei rhodesiense (East African sleeping sickness) and
Trypanosoma brucei gambiense (West African sleeping sickness)

METHOD OF DIAGNOSIS

Examine fluid from bite site chancre or buffy coat of blood for trypomastigotes during febrile period. Thick blood smears (see pp. 177 and 179) increase the chance of diagnosis. Multiple whole-blood specimens may be needed. Thick and thin blood smears are stained with Giemsa or Wright's stain. Late in infection, trypomastigotes are best found in lymph nodes or cerebrospinal fluid (CSF). Concentrating CSF by centrifugation may increase the chance of recovering parasites. Animal inoculation (mice or young rats) may be helpful; trypomastigotes in patient's blood multiply in the animal and then may be detected more easily.

DIAGNOSTIC STAGE

Trypomastigote form in plasma

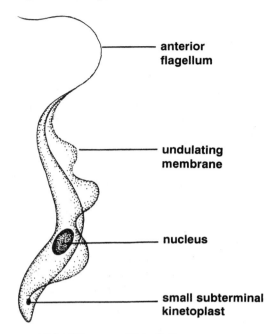

anterior
flagellum

undulating
membrane

nucleus

small subterminal
kinetoplast

15 to 30 μm x 15 to 3.5 μm

Note: Trypomastigote form
may be seen dividing
in peripheral blood.

MAJOR PATHOLOGY AND SYMPTOMS

Pathology and symptoms for both parasites include the following:

1. Lesion at bite site (chancre), usually seen in non-Africans
2. Enlarged lymph nodes, especially posterior cervical chain (Winterbottom's sign)
3. Fever, headache, night sweats
4. Joint and muscle pain
5. CNS impairment in 6 months to 1 year with *T. b. gambiense* or in 1 month with *T. b. rhodesiense*
6. Lethargy and motor changes
7. Coma and death; death from cardiac failure may precede CNS symptoms in *T. b. rhodesiense*

TREATMENT

Treatment depends on the phase of the disease:

1. Early: suramin or pentamidine
2. Late: melarsoprol or tryparsamide, when CNS involvement has occurred

DISTRIBUTION

Distribution is primarily East or West Africa, as noted.

OF NOTE

1. RBC autoagglutination is commonly observed in vitro.
2. High levels of both IgM and spinal fluid proteins are characteristic.
3. IgM in spinal fluid is diagnostic.
4. Enzyme-linked immunosorbent assay (ELISA) method to detect antigen in serum and CSF is useful for clinical staging of the disease and evaluating therapy.

⇨ **FOR REVIEW**

1. *East and West African sleeping sickness is caused by* _____ *and* _____ , *respectively.*
2. *Only the* _____ *form is found in humans and transferred to a new host by the* _____ .
3. *Trypomastigote forms are seen in* _____ .

Trypanosoma cruzi (Chagas' disease)

DIAGRAM 5–8

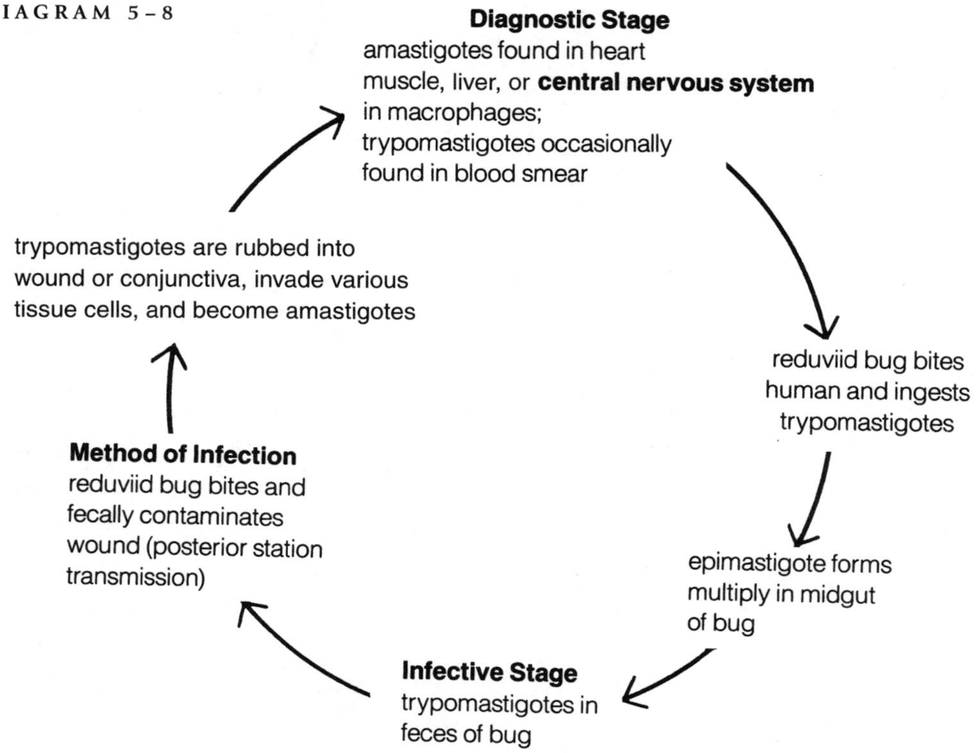

Diagnostic Stage
amastigotes found in heart
muscle, liver, or **central nervous system**
in macrophages;
trypomastigotes occasionally
found in blood smear

trypomastigotes are rubbed into
wound or conjunctiva, invade various
tissue cells, and become amastigotes

reduviid bug bites
human and ingests
trypomastigotes

Method of Infection
reduviid bug bites and
fecally contaminates
wound (posterior station
transmission)

epimastigote forms
multiply in midgut
of bug

Infective Stage
trypomastigotes in
feces of bug

Trypanosoma cruzi (Chagas' disease)

METHOD OF DIAGNOSIS

1. Find amastigotes in stained tissue scraping of skin lesion (chagoma) at bite site.
2. Identify C-shaped trypomastigotes in blood smear during acute exacerbation of symptoms.
3. Allow uninfected bugs to feed on patient, then later examine bug feces for parasite (xenodiagnosis).
4. Perform Machado complement fixation test, intradermal test, or indirect hemagglutination test (serology); endocardial, vascular, and interstitial (EVI) antibodies present; chemiluminescence, ELISA.
5. L.D. bodies (amastigotes) appear in heart muscle postmortem.
6. Culture for epimastigotes in diphasic Novy-MacNeal-Nicolle (NNN) medium (see p. 191).
7. Polymerase chain reaction using *T. cruzi* DNA is being used to detect the presence of the parasite in chronic cases.

DIAGNOSTIC STAGE

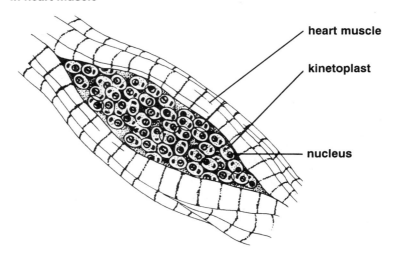

**Pseudocyst containing amastigote stages
in heart muscle**

heart muscle

kinetoplast

nucleus

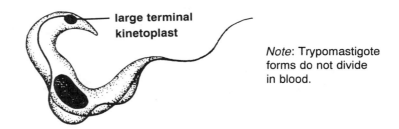

**C- or S-shaped trypomastigote
form in blood**

large terminal
kinetoplast

Note: Trypomastigote
forms do not divide
in blood.

DISEASE NAMES

- Chagas' disease
- American trypanosomiasis

MAJOR PATHOLOGY AND SYMPTOMS

1. In chronic cases, usually in adults, there may be no history of acute illness, but an enlarged, weakened heart may cause sudden death.
2. Symptoms may include fever; weakness; and enlarged spleen, liver, and lymph nodes.
3. Acute infection (most common in children) results in initial chagoma reaction at bite site with periorbital edema if bitten near the eye (Romaña's sign), cardiac ganglia destruction, megacolon, and often rapid death.

TREATMENT

Nifurtimox

DISTRIBUTION

Distribution is primarily in Mexico, Central America, and South America; seropositivity rates range from 60% to 70% in Brazil and Bolivia. It may be the cause of 30% of adult deaths in Brazil and Bolivia. A few cases have been reported in Texas and California.

OF NOTE

1. Many animals serve as reservoir hosts in the warmer southwestern states of North America.
2. Reduviid bugs feed at night on warm-blooded hosts, frequently on the conjunctiva of the eye.
3. *T. cruzi* can cross the placenta and cause the disease prenatally.
4. Autoimmune reaction by antibodies that cross-react with EVI antibodies may play a role in heart, colon, and esophagus dilation and atony.
5. Nonpathogenic *T. rangeli* trypomastigotes may be present in humans in Central and South America and may confuse diagnosis.

 FOR REVIEW

1. *Write the scientific names for the organisms that cause Chagas' disease and East and West African sleeping sickness:* _____ *and* _____

2. *Compare and contrast the life cycles of Chagas' disease and the African sleeping sicknesses. Be sure to include the vectors, the names of morphologic forms, and where they are found in the host.*

_____

3. *Identify the major disease symptoms from trypanosomal infections:*

_____

***Leishmania tropica, L. mexicana, L. braziliensis,* and *L. donovani* species complexes (Leishmaniasis)**

DIAGRAM 5–9

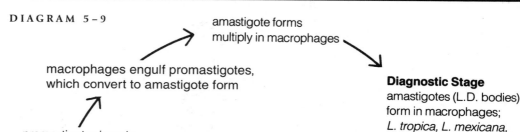
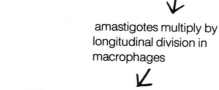

amastigote forms multiply in macrophages

macrophages engulf promastigotes, which convert to amastigote form

promastigotes invade tissue at wound site

Method of Infection
vector bites human and regurgitates promastigotes (anterior station transmission)

Diagnostic Stage
amastigotes (L.D. bodies) form in macrophages; *L. tropica, L. mexicana,* and *L. braziliensis* invade skin-lesion macrophages only; *L. donovani* also invades bone marrow, liver, and spleen macrophages

amastigotes multiply by longitudinal division in macrophages

Infective Stage
promastigote form multiplies in gut of *Phlebotomus* spp.

biting sandfly (*Phlebotomus* spp. intermediate host) ingests infected macrophages containing amastigotes

***Leishmania tropica, L. mexicana, L. braziliensis,* and *L. donovani* species complexes (leishmaniasis)**

METHOD OF DIAGNOSIS

- *L. tropica* and *L. mexicana:* Identify amastigotes in macrophages of skin lesion.
- *L. braziliensis:* Identify amastigotes at the periphery of the lesion.
- *L. donovani:* Identify amastigotes in early skin lesion and L.D. bodies later in reticuloendothelial system, spleen, lymph nodes, bone marrow, and liver. They are also present in feces, urine, and nasal discharges. The clinical symptoms of a person in an endemic area are presumptive; bone marrow smears are helpful. A striking increase in gamma globulin should be noted; serology, skin testing, culture, and animal inoculations are helpful.

SPECIMEN REQUIREMENTS

1. Fine-needle aspiration from the base of the lesion using the aseptic technique is recommended. Several slides should be made and stained with Giemsa stain.
2. Cultures should be attempted for a complete diagnosis, using aspirated material and a suitable medium, such as NNN.

DIAGNOSTIC STAGE

Amastigotes multiplying in tissue macrophages

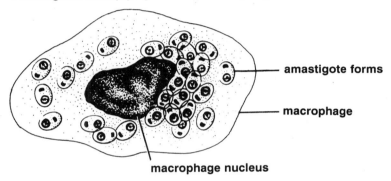

amastigote forms

macrophage

macrophage nucleus

DISEASE NAMES

- *L. tropica:* cutaneous or Old World leishmaniasis, Oriental boil, Baghdad or Delhi boil
- *L. braziliensis:* mucocutaneous or New World leishmaniasis, uta, espundia
- *L. donovani:* visceral leishmaniasis, kala-azar, Dumdum fever

MAJOR PATHOLOGY AND SYMPTOMS

The type of illness results from immunopathology in specific tissue sites.

1. *L. tropica* complex: Incubation period is several months (*L. tropica*) or as short as 2 weeks (*L. major*). One or more ulcerated, pus-filled lesions appear on the body (indurated with macrophages) and are self-healing. Lesions often are moist and short-term in rural areas (infection by *L. major* lasting 3 to 6 months) or dry and long-lasting in urban areas (infection by *L. tropica* lasting 12 to 18 months).
2. *L. mexicana:* Symptoms are similar to *L. tropica.* Two subspecies may cause DCL.
3. *L. braziliensis:* Symptoms include a red, itchy, indurated ulcer; lesions may metastasize along lymphatics and sequester; lesion is self-healing. Disfigurement of nose and ears may occur years later from chronic mucosal ulceration. DCL, seen mainly in Brazil, has an absence of cell-mediated immune reactivity. *Note:* The cause may be *L. pifanoi.*
4. *L. donovani:* The incubation period is long. With the initial lesion, short-term, small papules are at the bite site. Malarialike spiking chills and fever ensue (however, double fever spikes occur), along with sweating, diarrhea, dysentery, and weight loss. Splenomegaly and hepatomegaly develop after leishmania disseminate and multiply in visceral reticuloendothelium. Hyperplasia of tissue and organs occurs, along with progressive anemia. Death often occurs within 2 years if untreated (75% to 95% mortality).

TREATMENT

1. *L. tropica* complex: (1) antimony (as sodium stibogluconate [Pentostam]), (2) local heat (three 30-second treatments of 50°C at weekly intervals on chancre)
2. *L. mexicana:* (1) pentostam, (2) amphotericin B
3. *L. braziliensis:* (1) pentostam, (2) amphotericin B
4. *L. donovani:* (1) pentostam, (2) pentamidine isethionate

DISTRIBUTION

- *L. tropica* complex is found in the Mediterranean area, southwestern Asia, central and northwest Africa, Central America and South America; recent cases have been seen in Texas (may be L. *mexicana*).
- *L. braziliensis* occurs in Central America and South America; the highest concentration is in Brazil and the Andes. The disease is rural.
- *L. donovani* occurs primarily in young children in North Africa and East Africa, Asia, the Mediterranean area, and South America. In India and Bangladesh, disease is found primarily in adults.

OF NOTE

1. Cutaneous lesions may appear as ulcers, cauliflower-like masses, or nodules.
2. Host's genetic, nutritional, and immunologic status plays a large role in pathology.
3. Various animals serve as reservoir hosts (e.g., gerbils and other rodents, monkeys, and in the New World, dogs).
4. Vaccination against *L. tropica* is common in the former Soviet Union.
5. Leishmanin (Montenegro) skin test becomes positive in DCL and kala-azar only after cured; positive reactions are usually found in cutaneous and mucocutaneous leishmaniasis.
6. Elevated globulin levels are present in visceral leishmaniasis.
7. *L. tropica* is generally transmitted from humans; other parasites in the complex are primarily zoonoses.

 FOR REVIEW

1. *For each of the following parasites, name the morphologic form found in humans, state where this form is found in the infected host, and describe the pathology that the organism produces:*
   a. L. tropica:

   _____

   b. L. braziliensis:

   _____

   c. L. donovani:

   _____

2. *Name the insect vector in the Leishmania spp. life cycle, and describe the morphologic form found in the vector:*

   _____

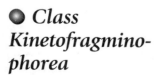
Class Kinetofragmino-phorea

Organisms in the Kinetofragminophorea class are characterized by ectoplasmic cilia covering the surface, two different kinds of nuclei (a large kidney-shaped macronucleus and a small micronucleus), and other well-developed organelles, such as an oral **cytostome.** Ciliates multiply asexually by binary fission and also sexually reproduce by conjugation, with exchange of micronuclei.

Balantidium coli is the largest parasitic protozoon (60 μm × 40 μm) and is the only ciliate that is pathogenic for humans. B. coli causes dysentery in severe intestinal infections and can be found in feces in either the trophozoite or cyst state. It is probable that human infections are directly acquired through ingestion of cysts in fecally contaminated food or water.

This parasite is a tissue invader and produces intestinal lesions along the submucosa. There are also reports of vaginal infections with this organism, probably acquired by fecal contamination of the vaginal atrium.

Balantidium coli (ciliate)

DIAGRAM 5-10

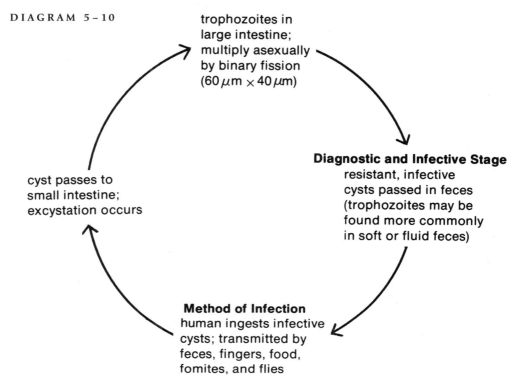

Balantidium coli (ciliate)

METHOD OF DIAGNOSIS

Identify trophozoites or cysts in feces or intestinal mucosa.

SPECIMEN REQUIREMENTS

1. One to three stool specimens are usually sufficient. The large organisms can be noted easily under low power (100×).
2. Wet mounts of fresh or concentrated specimens are best. The organisms stain very darkly in permanently stained preparations.

DIAGNOSTIC STAGE

Cyst

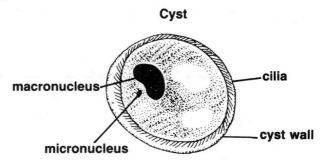

40 to 50 μm

Trophozoite

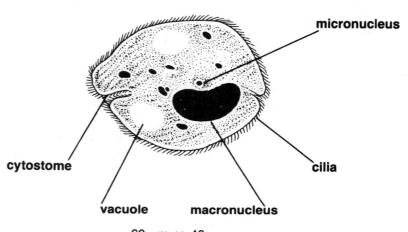

60 μm × 40 μm

DISEASE NAMES

• Balantidiasis
• Balantidial dysentery

MAJOR PATHOLOGY AND SYMPTOMS

Disease may be asymptomatic. When symptoms occur, they are usually abdominal discomfort with mild to moderate chronic recurrent diarrhea or acute dysentery. A healthy person is less likely to develop illness.

TREATMENT

1. Tetracycline
2. Iodoquinol or metronidazole

DISTRIBUTION

Distribution is worldwide, especially in the tropics, but the disease is rare in the United States.

OF NOTE

1. Pig feces are regarded as a potential source of infection because pigs can harbor this parasite.
2. *B. coli* may invade the intestinal mucosa, spreading horizontal lesions and causing

hyperemia and hemorrhage of the bowel surface. However, the organism does not spread via the bloodstream.

3. This is the largest protozoa and the only ciliated protozoa to infect humans.

 FOR REVIEW

1. *Write the scientific name for the only ciliate pathogenic in humans:* _____

2. *Describe the nuclear features of this parasite and its mode of reproduction:*

_____

3. *Differentiate the disease symptoms associated with B. coli and E. histolytica:*

_____

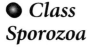 ## ● *Class Sporozoa*

Sporozoan parasites are obligate endoparasitic protozoa with no apparent organelles of locomotion. This class includes some of the most important and widespread parasites of humans, including those that cause malaria and toxoplasmosis (Table 5–5). Most species produce a spore form that is infective for the definitive host after it is ingested or injected by a biting arthropod vector. All genera have a life cycle that includes both sexual (**gametocyte** production and **sporogony**) and asexual (**schizogony**) phases of reproduction. Most have a two-host life cycle.

The genus *Plasmodium* includes the sporozoon that causes human malaria. The asexual cycle (schizogony) begins when the infected female *Anopheles* mosquito (the definitive host) bites a human and injects infective **sporozoites**, which then enter cutaneous blood vessels. The sporozoites travel via blood and invade liver cells. Each becomes a **cryptozoite**, reproducing intracellularly by asexual division and forming many **merozoites.** This is the exoerythrocytic cycle and is completed in 1 to 2 weeks.

The merozoites escape from the liver cells and invade circulating RBCs. Merozoites entering RBCs become trophozoites (also known as ring forms), which then mature through the **schizont** stage in 36 to 72 hours. Each schizont produces 6 to 24 new merozoites. The timing to maturation of the schizont and the number of new merozoites produced differentiate the species of *Plasmodium*. When the schizont is mature, the RBC ruptures, releasing the merozoites, which invade new RBCs. The cycle of RBC invasion, schizogony, and cell

TABLE 5–5 □ SPOROZOANS

Order	Scientific Name	Common Name
Eucoccidiida	*Plasmodium vivax* (plaz-mo'dee-um/vye'vacks)	benign tertian malaria
Eucoccidiida	*Plasmodium falciparum* (plaz-mo'dee-um/fal-sip'uh-rum)	malignant tertian malaria
Eucoccidiida	*Plasmodium malariae* (plaz-mo'dee-um/ma-lair'ee-ee)	quartan malaria
Eucoccidiida	*Plasmodium ovale* (plaz-mo'dee-um/ova'lee)	ovale malaria
Piroplasmida	*Babesia* spp. (bab-ee"zee'-uh)	none
Eucoccidiida	*Toxoplasma gondii* (tock"so-plaz'muh/gon'dee-eye)	toxoplasma
Eucoccidiida	*Sarcocystis* spp. (sahr"ko-sis-tis)	(*Isospora hominis* reclassified)
Eucoccidiida	*Isospora belli* (eye"sos'puh-ruh/bell-eye)	none
Eucoccidiida	*Cryptosporidium parvum* (krip"toe-spor-i'dee-um/par'vum)	none
Eucoccidiida	*Cyclospora cayetanensis* (sye'klo-spor-a/kay'e-tan'en-sis)	none

rupture continually repeats itself, producing symptoms. This is the erythrocytic cycle: merozoite enters RBC → trophozoite → schizont production → RBC rupture → merozoites released to penetrate new RBCs. Each cycle induces a **paroxysm** when toxic materials are released from the many ruptured RBCs. The paroxysm begins suddenly and is characterized by a 10- to 15-minute (or longer) period of shaking chills, followed by a high fever lasting from 2 to 6 hours or longer. The patient begins sweating profusely as the temperature returns to normal. The paroxysm is in part an allergic response to released parasitic antigens.

Later in the infection, some merozoites develop into microgametocytes (male sex cells) and macrogametocytes (female sex cells). The sexual cycle (sporogony) begins when a female *Anopheles* mosquito (definitive host) ingests gametocytes as she takes a blood meal from an infected person. The **gametes** unite in the stomach of the mosquito, forming a motile **zygote** (the **ookinete**), which then moves through and encysts on the mosquito's stomach wall. After further maturation to an **oocyst** containing many infective sporozoites, the sporozoites are released from the oocyst and migrate to the mosquito's salivary glands. The mosquito bite is now infective to the next human victim. Infective sporozoites enter the bite site via the saliva of the mosquito and travel to the liver; the life cycle begins again. Malaria can also be transmitted via blood transfusion and from contaminated needles of intravenous drug users.

Drug-resistant strains of *Plasmodium* species and insecticide-resistant strains of mosquitoes have recently and rapidly evolved, posing major problems in controlling the spread of this disease worldwide. Control measures have essentially eliminated the disease from some countries, including the United States, but it is still a major problem in Africa, Asia, Central and South America, and areas of Europe, and it could be reintroduced into controlled areas.

Of the four species included in the life-cycle diagram, *P. falciparum* is the most deadly; these parasites promote physiologic changes of the red cell (which develops a "knobby" surface), which causes agglutination and lysis. Schizogony takes place in the capillaries and blood sinuses of the brain, visceral organs, and placenta, with infected cells tending to adhere to one another and to the surrounding vessel walls. Vessels become blocked, causing local infarction damage to the regional tissue. Symptoms vary according to the degree of tissue anoxia and rupture of blocked capillaries. Many uninfected red cells also lyse during a paroxysm. Host responses to red-cell remnants and other parasitic debris lead to more RBC lysis and enlargement of the spleen and liver. Another complication is renal failure caused by renal anoxia. The sudden massive intravascular lysis of RBCs, followed by hemoglobin passage in urine (blackwater fever, or hemoglobinuria) is related to treatment with quinine in susceptible individuals. The most severe complication—cerebral malaria—occurs when blood vessels in the brain become affected. Coma and death may follow.

Pathology caused by the other *Plasmodium* species is less severe, primarily because these parasites are unable to invade both young and old red cells, as are *P. falciparum* parasites. In addition, the other species do not cause changes to the red-cell membrane such as those seen with *P. falciparum*. Merozoites of *P. malariae* can invade only older cells; those of *P. vivax* and *P. ovale* infect primarily reticulocytes (immature RBCs). Inasmuch as these young red-cell populations are small at any given time, the infection is limited.

P. vivax is the most widely disseminated and most prevalent parasite causing malaria. There is repeated exoerythrocytic development in the liver; therefore, *P. vivax* can cause relapses, with erythrocytic cycles starting again years after the initial infection sequence. This is thought to result from sequestered hypnozoites in the liver.

Plasmodium species (malaria)

DIAGRAM 5-11

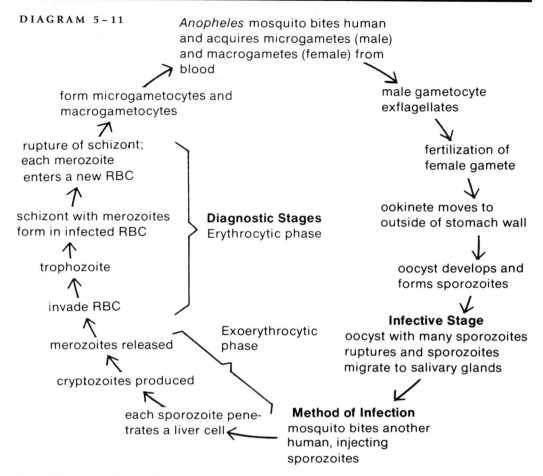

Anopheles mosquito bites human and acquires microgametes (male) and macrogametes (female) from blood

form microgametocytes and macrogametocytes

rupture of schizont; each merozoite enters a new RBC

schizont with merozoites form in infected RBC

trophozoite

invade RBC

merozoites released

cryptozoites produced

each sporozoite penetrates a liver cell

Diagnostic Stages
Erythrocytic phase

Exoerythrocytic phase

male gametocyte exflagellates

fertilization of female gamete

ookinete moves to outside of stomach wall

oocyst develops and forms sporozoites

Infective Stage
oocyst with many sporozoites ruptures and sporozoites migrate to salivary glands

Method of Infection
mosquito bites another human, injecting sporozoites

Plasmodium species (malaria)

METHOD OF DIAGNOSIS

Demonstrate and identify trophozoites, schizonts, or gametocytes in peripheral blood. Ideally, blood should be drawn between paroxysms because the greatest number of parasites is likely to be present in the specimen at this time. Blood should be drawn immediately when the patient arrives at the hospital, however, even though the infection is not yet synchronized. The initial test must be considered a STAT request, and subsequent specimens should be drawn at 6- to 12-hour intervals. Both thick and thin smears should be examined. Negative morning and afternoon thick-stained smears for 3 consecutive days during symptoms indicate absence of infection. Serology is helpful but is not readily available in the United States. See Disease Names (p. 119) for the timing of the cycle of paroxysms for each species.

SPECIMEN REQUIREMENTS

Ethylenediaminotetraacetic acid–preserved whole blood is preferred if anticoagulants are used for collection, but smears should be made within 1 hour because true stippling of immature RBCs may not be retained (e.g., *P. vivax*). Giemsa stain is preferred, but parasites are visible when stained with Wright's stain.

DIAGNOSTIC STAGES

P. falciparum

Trophozoites

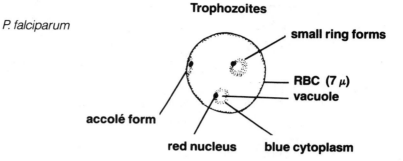

small ring forms

RBC (7 μ)

vacuole

accolé form

red nucleus   **blue cytoplasm**

**Gametocyte
(crescent-shaped)**

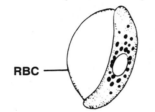

RBC

Note: Advanced trophozoites
and schizonts
generally not seen in
peripheral blood.

P. malariae

**Trophozoite
(single ring)**

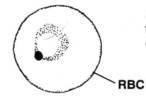

Note: Trophozoite
forms band across RBC
during early schizogony.

RBC

**Schizont
(6 to 12 merozoites)**

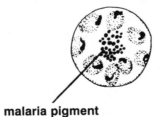

malaria pigment

**Gametocyte
(ovoid)**

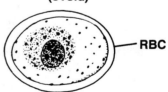

RBC

P. vivax

**Trophozoite
(single ring)**

**Reticulocyte
(immature RBC 7 to 10 μ)** —

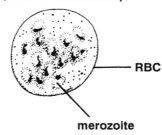

Schüffner's dots

Note: Single ring,
one-third diameter of
an RBC; invades only
immature RBCs so that
large bluish-staining cells are
parasitized.
RBC shows red-stained
Schüffner's dots, which
become visible between
15 and 20 hours following
invasion of the cell.
Note: Trophozoite is very
ameboid and assumes bizarre
shapes during early schizogony.

**Schizont
(12 to 24 merozoites)**

RBC

merozoite

**Gametocyte
(round)**

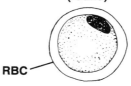

RBC

P. ovale
(rare)

Note: Single ring, one-third diameter of
RBC. RBC is oval, shows Schüffner's dots.

DISEASE NAMES

Scientific Name	Common Name	Cyclic Paroxysms	Relapses
P. falciparum	Malignant malaria	Every 36 to 48 hours	No
P. vivax	Tertian malaria	Every 48 hours	Yes
P. malariae	Quartan malaria	Every 72 hours	No
P. ovale	Ovale malaria	Every 48 hours	Yes

MAJOR PATHOLOGY AND SYMPTOMS

All cause splenic enlargement, fever and chill paroxysms, pain in the joints, and anemia from red-cell destruction. Nausea, vomiting, and diarrhea often are among the initial symptoms seen on admission to the hospital. Malaria pigment is deposited in tissues. *P. falciparum* infection can cause high fever, bloody urine, massive hemolysis, brain damage from clumping of RBCs, resultant blocking of capillaries, and subsequent rapid death. *P. falciparum* infection also can result in severe blackwater fever and renal failure. A sudden life-threatening respiratory distress syndrome may also occur with *P. falciparum*. High IgM and IgG levels suggest current or recurrent malaria infection; elevated IgG alone indicates past infection. Quartan malaria nephropathy is immunopathologic from immune complex deposition in kidneys.

Suspicion must be high and response must be rapid for the diagnosis of malaria when a patient who has visited or lived in a malarious area shows symptoms of this disease. Death can occur quickly if treatment is delayed.

TREATMENT

Chloroquine, quinine, pyrimethamine, sulfadiazine, and tetracycline

DISTRIBUTION

- *P. falciparum* and *P. malariae* are found in the tropics.
- *P. vivax* is found in the tropics, subtropics, and some temperate regions; it is the most prevalent malaria species.
- *P. ovale* is found in West Africa.
- *P. vivax* and *P. falciparum* account for more than 95% of infections.

OF NOTE

1. *P. vivax* and *P. ovale* may cause relapses years later because of secondary exoerythrocytic cycles (hypnozoites in liver); primaquine is used to kill the liver-phase organisms of malaria.
2. *P. vivax* invades reticulocytes preferentially; therefore, counterstaining blood for reticulocytes can aid identification.
3. As many as 70% of African Americans and West Africans are negative for the Duffy blood group, which may be related to resistance to *P. vivax* infection in the indigenous people. Inherited glucose-6-phosphate dehydrogenase deficiency and hemoglobin gene alterations (e.g., sickle cell inheritance) may play an evolutionary role in survival of humans in endemic areas, inasmuch as these genetic variants are incompatible with parasite survival.
4. Presence of *P. falciparum* schizonts in peripheral blood indicates very grave prognosis.
5. *P. malariae* infections may cause a recrudescence or series of recrudescences for many years because of low-grade parasitemia.
6. Malaria is primarily a rural disease; its incidence is significantly increasing because of drug-resistant malaria strains, insecticide-resistant mosquitoes, and inadequate resources to prevent infection from spreading.

 FOR REVIEW

1. *Blackwater fever is caused by* _____, *and the diagnostic features are* _____.

2. *The most prevalent malaria parasite is* _____, *and the diagnostic features are* _____.

3. *Relapses may be found in P.* _____*infections, and recrudescences may be found in P.* _____ *infections.*

4. *"Band" form trophozoites are noted in P.* _____ *infections.*

5. *Reticulocyte infections are seen in P.* _____ *infections.*

6. *For each of the following, list two diagnostic morphologic features seen in peripheral blood films:*
   a. *P. malariae:* _____ *and* _____
   b. *P. vivax:* _____ *and* _____
   c. *P. ovale:* _____ *and* _____
   d. *P. falciparum:* _____ *and* _____

7. *Why are P. falciparum infections more severe than infections caused by the other Plasmodium spp.?*

_____

Babesia species

Ticks are the definitive hosts for the sporozoa of the *Babesia* species (subclass Piroplasmia). Occasional tick-transmitted human infections have been reported. In the human intermediate host, the organisms multiply in RBCs. Trophozoites are generally pear-shaped (2 to 4 μm), lying in pairs or tetrads. Unlike malarias, extracellular trophozoites may occasionally be observed. Clinical signs follow the bite of an infected tick in about 2 to 3 weeks and resemble symptoms of malaria, including nonsynchronous fever, chills, sweats, anorexia, and myalgia. There may also be hemolytic anemia and mild spleen and liver disease. Although most infections are subclinical, more severe cases may exhibit renal failure, disseminated intravascular coagulation, and respiratory syndrome.

Studies comparing disease symptoms found in patients in the northeastern United States with those found in patients in California indicate that more than one species of *Babesia* causes disease in humans. Cases in the Northeast are more acute, and several patients have died, whereas the infections in California tend to be subclinical except in splenectomized or immunocompromised patients. *Babesia* spp. infections have been transmitted through blood transfusions.

METHOD OF DIAGNOSIS

The diagnosis is made by examination of multiple thin and thick blood smears. Parasites in RBCs usually lie in pairs at an acute angle or as a tetrad in a Maltese cross formation, although they are rarely observed. As many as four or five ring forms per erythrocyte may be seen in babesiosis. Care must be taken not to confuse *Babesia* spp. with malarial ring forms of *Plasmodium*, especially *P. falciparum*, which often has multiple small ring forms in RBCs. When absolute species identification is impossible, it is advisable to add the statement that "*Plasmodium falciparum* cannot be excluded" to the laboratory report. Paired sera tested against infected hamster RBCs using an indirect fluorescent antibody method can be helpful in diagnosing chronic infections.

DIAGNOSTIC STAGE

Babesia microti

Trophozoites

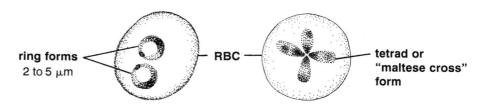

ring forms
2 to 5 μm — RBC — tetrad or "maltese cross" form

SPECIMEN REQUIREMENTS

- Whole blood or capillary blood may be used.
- Giemsa stain is preferred, but parasites are visible when stained with Wright's stain.

TREATMENT

1. Clindamycin and quinine
2. Chloroquine phosphate, which provides symptomatic relief but does not reduce the parasitemia

DISTRIBUTION

Distribution is worldwide.

OF NOTE

Automated differential counting instruments can lead to diagnostic problems because these machines are not designed to detect bloodborne parasites such as *Malaria* or *Babesia*. Therefore, infections may be missed, especially if the affected individual is asymptomatic.

FOR REVIEW

1. *The definitive host for Babesia spp. is a(n)* _____.
2. *The diagnostic forms seen in RBCs appear and may be confused with* _____.

● *Subclass Coccidia*

The next three genera of sporozoa belong to the subclass Coccidia. Schizogony occurs in various nucleated cells of many species of mammals and birds, and sporogony occurs in the intestinal mucosa of the definitive host. Infective oocysts are passed in feces. Infection occurs when a susceptible host ingests mature oocysts containing sporozoites.

DIAGRAM 5–12

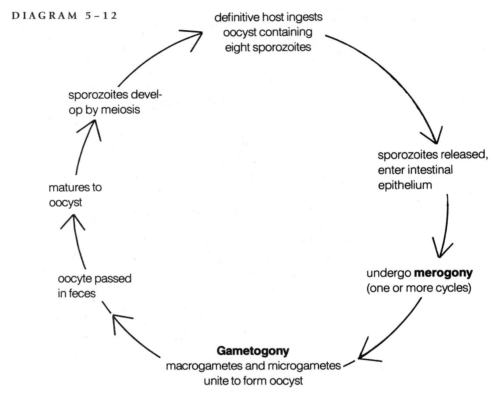

Life cycle of coccidian parasites

Toxoplasma gondii

Toxoplasma gondii is a sporozoan parasite that infects and undergoes schizogony in all nucleated cells of almost all animals and birds. The domestic cat and other members of Felidae, however, have been cited as the only definitive host for this parasite. In the cat, it is an intestinal parasite, with both schizogony and sporogony occurring in the intestinal mucosa (the enteric cycle). The cat becomes infected by eating infective oocysts (viable for up to 1 year in moist soil), by eating tissues of infected small animals, or by being infected transplacentally. Oocysts are shed in cat feces, and these become infective within several days for a variety of vertebrate intermediate hosts, including humans. Humans become infected by ingesting the infective oocyst in contaminated food or drink or by accidental hand-to-mouth transmission of contaminated soil or cat litter.

Initially, *Toxoplasma* divides mitotically in the tissues of humans as **tachyzoites,** which assume a crescentlike appearance when seen in tissue fluids. Infected tissue cells die, releasing free tachyzoites that invade new cells. In late or chronic infections, cysts (formerly called **pseudocysts**) form in brain and other tissues. These cysts contain *Toxoplasma* **bradyzoites** and may remain viable for long periods, being held in check by the host's immune system.

The infection in humans is usually asymptomatic; however, it may be highly symptomatic in early infections and can mimic several other infections, such as infectious mononucleosis. A serious concern is that *Toxoplasma* may be transmitted across the placenta to the fetus in a woman who acquires her first infection during the pregnancy. It can cause death of the fetus or mental retardation or blindness later in the child's life.

In addition to ingestion of oocysts from cat feces or from transplacental infection, the most common source of infection for humans is ingestion of undercooked meat (especially sheep, pigs, and rabbits) containing calcified cysts. Rarely, goat's milk containing tachyzoites can be a source of infection. Transmission can also occur through blood transfusions and organ transplantation. The latter event is more serious because the organ recipient will be immunocompromised and unable to respond to the disease.

METHOD OF DIAGNOSIS

1. Serologic testing: Sabin-Feldman dye test, latex agglutination, various fluorescent antibody methods, ELISA. A 16-fold increase in IgG antibody in a second sample taken 21 days later indicates an acute infection. Differentiation of acute and chronic infections is complex and requires testing for both IgG and IgM antibodies.
2. Tissue biopsy or impression smears stained with Giemsa stain. Bradyzoites are strongly periodic acid–Schiff (PAS) positive.

TREATMENT

1. Pyrimethamine and sulfadiazine (add folinic acid in an immunosuppressed host)
2. Spiramycin

Sarcocystis spp.

Two species of *Sarcocystis* (formerly known as *Isospora hominis* in humans)—*S. hominis* (from cattle) and *S. suihominis* (from pigs)—have a life cycle similar to that of *Toxoplasma*. Humans, dogs, or cats can become definitive hosts if they eat uncooked intermediate-host beef or pork tissue containing **sarcocysts.** Bradyzoites released from the sarcocyst invade intestinal cells in these definitive hosts and undergo gametogony, producing infective oocysts. These oocysts can be recovered in stool. When infected with this parasite, immunocompromised humans may have severe diarrhea, fever, and weight loss. Oocysts ingested from fecally contaminated food by the intermediate host (cattle or pigs) release sporozoites that go to muscle tissue and form sarcocysts. Humans can also be accidental intermediate hosts by ingesting oocysts and forming sarcocysts in muscle. Other species of *Sarcocystis* are found in wild animal reservoir hosts.

The broadly oval oocyst contains two sporocysts, each of which contains four mature sporozoites. The sporocysts, measuring 9 to 16 μm by 8 to 12 μm, are commonly seen free in feces. Intact oocysts and individual sporozoites are rarely seen.

Isospora belli

There is one pathogenic coccidian for which the human is the only definitive host and in which both schizogony and sporogony, accompanied by mild pathology, occur. This species is *Isospora belli*. There are no known intermediate hosts in this parasite's life cycle. Characteristic oocysts can be found in infected human feces. The oocysts of *I. belli* in a fresh fecal specimen are transparent, measuring 30 μm × 12 μm, and are immature (containing a single mass of protoplasm called the sporoblast) or, rarely, developing (containing two sporoblasts). Within 18 to 36 hours after feces are passed, each of the two sporoblasts develops a sporocyst wall and contains four sausage-shaped infective sporozoites. Full maturation takes 4 to 5 days.

This parasite is found worldwide, and transmission to humans is direct via sporulated oocysts in fecally contaminated food or water. Human infection can cause anorexia, nausea, abdominal pain, diarrhea, and possible malabsorption.

METHOD OF DIAGNOSIS

1. Oocysts are recoverable with zinc sulfate flotation technique, and they stain well with iodine.
2. Oocysts in polyvinyl alcohol-preserved sediment are difficult to see because the cyst wall is very thin and refractile.
3. Oocysts of *I. belli* are undeveloped in fresh feces and retain the oocyst wall. Although oocysts of *Sarcocystis* spp. resemble those of developed *I. belli*, *Sarcocystis* oocysts are smaller and often lose the cyst wall; single free sporocysts, each containing four mature sporozoites, can therefore be seen in stool samples in *Sarcocystis* spp. infections.

SPECIMEN REQUIREMENTS

Several routine fecal specimens are usually sufficient.

TREATMENT

Trimethoprim-sulfamethoxazole (TMP-SMX)

Cryptosporidium parvum

Cryptosporidium parvum differs from other coccidian protozoa because it forms an intracellular parasitophorous vacuole bounded by the host-cell membrane near the outer surface of a host intestinal cell. This parasite invades the gastrointestinal mucosal surface of many vertebrate hosts, including humans. Both trophozoites and schizonts are attached to the host-cell membrane. Eight merozoites develop within the schizont and, on maturation, are released to begin a new schizontic cycle or to initiate a sexual cycle in the intestinal mucosa. Macrogametocytes and microgametocytes join to become mature gametes. Sexual union forms an oocyte, which then develops into an oocyst. The entire life cycle can occur within a single host because oocysts are autoreinfective. External infection is probably acquired from food or water contaminated with oocysts from feces of animal reservoir hosts, such as calves. Human-to-human transmission occurs, and nosocomial infections have also been reported. The oocysts are immediately infective when passed in feces. The oocyst is 4 μm and contains four sporozoites.

Human infection, first reported in 1976, was thought to be uncommon and was found primarily in patients with compromised immune systems. Since then, many more cases have been reported in many populations worldwide. In 1987, an estimated 13,000 cases of gastroenteritis were reported in a 2-month period in Carroll County, Georgia. Of the patients tested, 34% were found to have *Cryptosporidium* oocysts. Follow-up studies suggested that this parasite caused as many as 54% of these cases. The source of infection was found to be the county's public water supply.

Outbreaks in 1993 and 1996 were associated with drinking unpasteurized apple cider. The apples were probably tainted by exposure to contaminated soil in the first outbreak and by washing apples in fecally polluted water in the second case. Another outbreak in 1995 was linked to chicken salad that may have been contaminated by a food handler in a home day-care center. Unwashed contaminated green onions were the probable source of another earlier outbreak. These events indicate that infections caused by this parasite are not rare and often are associated with improperly washed, fecally contaminated fruits and vegetables.

The symptom common to all reported cases is acute diarrhea. The disease is self-limited in patients with normal immune systems and lasts from 1 to 2 weeks; however, oocysts may be shed intermittently for up to 60 days after the diarrhea has ended. Meticulous handwashing after infection will reduce further transmission of oocysts. Immunodeficient patients, such as those with AIDS or people receiving immunosuppressant drugs, often develop chronic diarrhea after infection with *C. parvum*. Patients with AIDS have also developed respiratory cryptosporidiosis.

Cyclospora cayetanensis

Another coccidian parasite that resembles *C. parvum* is *Cyclospora cayetanensis* (formerly called cyanobacterium-like body). Infection by this parasite causes a self-limiting diarrhea that may last 3 or 4 days; however, relapses often occur over 2 to 3 weeks. Antidiarrheal preparations provide relief of symptoms, and treatment with TMP-SMX will reduce the possibility of relapse. Transmission of this organism appears to be indirect, through contaminated water or food, rather than by direct transfer from person to person. People of all ages can contract this disease.

Since 1990, several notable outbreaks have occurred in the United States. The first occurred among 21 staff members at a Chicago hospital. The source of this outbreak was associated with drinking tap water that was possibly contaminated by stagnant polluted water stored in a rooftop reservoir. The infection was confirmed in 11 of the 21 cases, and symptoms lasted up to 9 weeks. Later outbreaks reported from 1995 through 1997 were associated with imported raspberries raised on farms in Guatemala. Although the true cause of the contamination was not conclusively proven, there were definite links between contaminated soil, water, and the fruit. Other cases have been associated with vegetables, such as Mesclun lettuce and fresh basil. Further study is needed to completely clarify this parasite's epidemiology and life cycle.

It is important to differentiate this parasite from *C. parvum* and other sporozoa by careful measurement and observation of oocysts recovered in fecal specimens. Oocysts of *C. cayetanensis* measure 8 to 10 μm and are undeveloped, taking 5 to 14 days for sporozoites to develop in vitro.

METHOD OF DIAGNOSIS

1. Oocysts can be recovered using sedimentation techniques but are most easily recovered by flotation methods and can be observed using phase-contrast (preferred) or bright-field microscopy. Unstained *Cyclospora* spp. appear as glassy, wrinkled spheres. *C. cayetanensis* does not stain well with iodine, trichrome, or iron-hematoxylin. Oocysts autofluoresce when viewed under a fluorescent microscope, and this is a useful diagnostic characteristic.
2. Acid-fast stained smears of fecal material are also useful. (See p. 177 for modified acid-fast method.) Stained cells containing *Cryptosporidium* spp. appear as red spherical bodies measuring 3 to 6 μm in diameter, whereas those of *Cyclospora* spp. (8 to 10 μm in diameter) range from pink to red, and some may contain granules or have a bubbly appearance.
3. Trophozoites, schizonts, microgametocytes, and macrogametocytes of *C. parvum* can be distinguished when using the electron microscope to examine smears of biopsy material from the jejunum.

DIAGNOSTIC STAGE OF INTESTINAL COCCIDIA

TABLE 5–6 □ COCCIDIAN FORMS FOUND IN FECES

Parasite	Stage in Feces	Size (μm)	Appearence in Feces	Cyst
Sarcocystis spp.	Free sporocysts	9–16	Contains four sporozoites	
Isospora belli	Immature oocyst	20–33 × 10–19	Contains one or two immature sporoblasts	
Cryptosporidium parvum	Mature oocyst	4–6	Contains four sporoblasts	
Cyclospora spp. (CLB)	Immature oocyst	8–10	Contains immature sporoblast	

SPECIMEN REQUIREMENTS

Three fecal specimens collected on alternate days are usually sufficient.

TREATMENT

- *I. belli:* TMP-SMX
- *C. parvum:* paromomycin (experimental)
- *Sarcocystis* spp.: none for tissue disease; antidiarrheal for intestinal infection
- *C. cayetanensis:* TMP-SMX

DISTRIBUTION

Distribution is worldwide.

⇨ FOR REVIEW

1. Compare and contrast the life cycles and methods of diagnosis for T. gondii and Sarcocystis spp.:

_____

2. Explain how infection with C. parvum occurs, and contrast it with I. belli:

_____

3. Describe the appearance of the oocysts of C. parvum and C. cayetanensis:

_____

Microsporidia

The microsporidia have recently been recognized as tissue parasites in immunocompromised patients. In humans, they are small (1 to 2.5 μm), obligate intracellular parasites that can inhabit all body tissues. They consist of nine named genera and one "catch-all" genus (*Microsporidium africanum*), which is currently used for species that have not yet been fully described. Other genera include *Brachiola* spp., *Enterocytozoon bieneusi*, *Encephalitozoon hellem*, *Encephalitozoon* (*Septata*) *intestinalis*, *Nosema connori*, *Pleistophora* spp., *Vittaforma corneae*, and *Trachipleistophora hominis*. These organisms inject infective contents from the spore into the host cell through a small polar tube. The organism multiplies inside the host cell by binary fission (merogony) or multiple fission (schizogony) and sexual reproduction (sporogony). Spores are produced with thick walls and, for *E. bieneusi*, are released into the intestine and passed in stool. Other hosts become infected by ingesting spores. Spores are resistant to the environment, and some infections may be acquired by inhaling spores. Microsporidia have been found in the CNS, eyes, lungs, kidney, myocardium, liver, and adrenal cortex and have been found associated with other diseases, such as leprosy, tuberculosis, schistosomiasis, malaria, and Chagas' disease. Infection by *E. bieneusi* is the most common microsporidial infection found in patients with AIDS. *E. bieneusi* infections are also found in immunocompetent individuals, causing a self-limited diarrheal disease that resolves within 2 weeks. *Encephalitozoon cuniculi* and *E. hellum* are most frequently associated with eye infections.

METHOD OF DIAGNOSIS

1. Diagnosis is accomplished by histology on respective tissue using acid-fast and PAS stains or electron microscopy.
2. Modified trichrome-stained thin fecal smears may reveal spores. Positive controls are necessary.

SPECIMEN REQUIREMENTS

1. Tissue biopsy materials for processing in histology (best staining with PAS, methenamine silver, or acid-fast stains)
2. Three fecal collections on alternate days; thin smears are necessary

TREATMENT

No satisfactory treatment is generally available, except for *Encephalitozoon* (*septata*) *intestinalis*. Albendazole has been used successfully to treat these infections.

DISTRIBUTION

Distribution is worldwide.

OF NOTE

1. Double infections with Cryptosporidia and Microsporidia are common.
2. Table 5–7 compares the clinical manifestations of microsporidial species in immunocompetent and immunoincompetent patients.

FOR REVIEW

1. *State how microsporidia infections may be acquired:*

_____

2. *List body site(s) where microsporidia may be found in an infected host:*

_____

3. *State how microsporidia infections are diagnosed:*

_____

 Pneumocystis carinii

Pneumocystis carinii is the causative agent of atypical interstitial plasma-cell pneumonia (PCP). This organism has been included in parasitology texts for some time because it was long thought to be a protozoa. Pneumocystis is now classified as a fungus in the phylum Ascomycota, class Archiascomycetes, order Pneumocystidales. The reader should consult recent literature for details on this organism.

TABLE 5–7 □ CLINICAL MANIFESTATIONS OF MICROSPORIDIAL SPECIES PATHOGENIC IN HUMANS

Microsporidial Species	Immunocompromised Patients	Patients with Normal Immune Systems
Brachiola vesicularum	Myositis, corneal ulcer, keratitis	Keratitis
Enterocytozoon bieneusi	Chronic diarrhea, wasting syndrome, "AIDS cholangiopathy," cholangitis, chronic sinusitis, chronic cough, pneumonitis	Self-limiting diarrhea in adults and children, traveler's diarrhea, asymptomatic carriers
Encephalitozoon cuniculi	Disseminated infection	Not described
Encephalitozoon hellem	Disseminated infection, kerato-conjunctivitis, sinusitis, bronchitis, pneumonia, nephritis, cystitis, prostatitis, urethritis	Not described
Encephalitozoon intestinalis (formerly *Septata intestinalis*)	Chronic diarrhea, cholangiopathy, sinusitis, bronchitis, pneumonitis, nephritis, bone infection	Self-limiting diarrhea, asymptomatic carriers
Pleistophora spp.	Myositis	Not described
Trachipleistophora antropophtera	Brain, heart, kidney pathology	Not described
Trachipleistophora hominis	Myositis, nasal sinusitis	Not described
Nosema connori	Disseminated infection	Not described
Vittaforma corneae (formerly *Nosema corneum*)	Disseminated infection, corneal ulcer	Keratitis
*Microsporidium africanum**	Not described	Corneal ulcer, keratitis

Microsporidium is a collective genus name for Microsporidia that cannot be classified because available information is not sufficient.
Adapted from Manual of Clinical Microbiology, ed 7. ASM Press, Washington, DC, 1999 and Diagnostic Medical Parasitology, ed 4. ASM Press, Washington, DC, 2001.

Table 5–8 reviews the life cycles and other important information about the Protozoa. Consult Color Plates 72 to 133.

TABLE 5–8 □ PATHOGENIC PROTOZOA

Scientific and Common Name	Epidemiology	Disease-Producing Form and Its Location in Host	How Infection Occurs	Major Disease Manifestations, Diagnostic Stage, and Specimen of Choice
Entamoeba histolytica (amebic dysentery)	Worldwide	Trophozoites in large intestinal mucosa, liver, or other tissues	Ingestion of cyst in fecally contaminated food or water	Enteritis with abdominal pain and bloody dysentery; diagnosis: cysts and trophozoites in feces
Blastocystis hominis (none)	Worldwide	Protozoa in intestine	Ingestion of organisms in fecally contaminated food or water	Diarrhea, fever, abdominal pain, vomiting; diagnosis: central body form in feces
Acanthamoeba spp. (chronic meningo-encephalitis)	Worldwide	Trophozoites and cysts in tissues of brain, eye, skin, etc.	Accidental entrance through skin lesion	Slow disease development (over 10 days), chronic skin lesions, keratitis; diagnosis: trophozoites in CSF, trophozoite cysts in tissue or ocular samples
Naegleria fowleri (primary amebic meningo-encephalitis)	Worldwide	Amebic trophozoites in brain	Accidental entrance of free-living waterborne trophozoites through nasopharynx mucosa	Rapid death (4–6 days) following acute symptoms of meningitis; diagnosis: motile trophozoites in CSF. Never refrigerate the specimen before examination
Giardia lamblia (traveler's diarrhea)	Worldwide	Trophozoites in large intestinal mucosa	Ingestion of cysts in fecally contaminated food or water	Mild to severe dysentery, malabsorption syndrome; diagnosis: cysts and trophozoites in feces
Dientamoeba fragilis (none)	Worldwide	Trophozoites in large intestine	Ingestion of trophozoite (?)	Diarrhea; diagnosis: trophozoites in feces (no cysts formed)
Trichomonas vaginalis (trich)	Worldwide	Trophozoites in urethra or vagina	Sexual contact	Irritating, frothy vaginal discharge in women, men usually asymptomatic; diagnosis: trophozoites in urine or vaginal smear (no cysts formed)
Trypanosoma brucei gambiense (sleeping sickness)	West Africa	Trypomastigote in blood, lymph nodes, later in CNS	Bite of *Glossina* spp. (tsetse fly)	Fever, lymphadenopathy (Winterbottom's sign), enlarged spleen and liver, lethargy, and death; diagnosis: trypomastigotes in blood smear, CSF
Trypanosoma brucei rhodesiense (sleeping sickness)	East Africa	Trypomastigote in blood, lymph nodes, later in CNS	Bite of *Glossina* spp. (tsetse fly)	Fever, lymphadenopathy (Winterbottom's sign), enlarged spleen and liver, lethargy, and death, course more acute and fatal than *T. gambiense*; diagnosis: trypomastigotes in blood smear

Scientific and Common Name	Epidemiology	Disease-Producing Form and Its Location in Host	How Infection Occurs	Major Disease Manifestations, Diagnostic Stage, and Specimen of Choice
Trypanosoma cruzi (Chagas' disease)	South America	C-shaped trypomastigote and epimastigote forms early in blood; later, L.D. bodies in heart and other tissues	Infected feces of *Triatoma* spp. (kissing bug) rubbed into bite site	Fever, enlarged spleen and liver, Romana's sign (edema around eyes), chronic damage to heart and alimentary tract, acute death, especially in children; diagnosis: trypomastigotes in blood, xenodiagnosis
Leishmania tropica complex (Oriental boil)	Mediterranean area, Asia, Africa, Central America	Amastigotes in macrophages of skin lesion	Bite of *Phlebotomus* spp. (sandfly)	Self-healing skin lesion; diagnosis: amastigotes in macrophages around lesion
Leishmania braziliensis complex (New World leishmaniasis, espundia)	Central and South America, especially Brazil	Amastigotes in macrophages of skin lesion and mucocutaneous tissue	Bite of *Lutzomyia* spp. and *Psychodopygus* spp.	Self-healing skin lesion, later ulceration of cephalic mucocutaneous tissue; diagnosis: recovery of amastigotes from lesion
Leishmania donovani (kala-azar)	Mediterranean area, Asia, Africa, South America	Amastigotes in macrophages in skin lesion and somatic organs	Bite of *Phlebotomus* spp.	Initial skin lesion, later daily double-spiking fever, enlarged liver and spleen, death in late stages; diagnosis: L.D. bodies in early lesion, organ tissue biopsy later
Balantidium coli (balantidial dysentery)	Worldwide	Trophozoites in large intestinal mucosa	Ingestion of cysts in fecally contaminated food or water	Moderate or mild dysentery; diagnosis: trophozoites or cysts in feces
Plasmodium vivax (benign tertian malaria)	Tropics, subtropics, some temperate regions	Schizogony and gametocytes in RBCs	*Anopheles* spp. mosquito transmits sporozoites	Cyclic fever, chills, enlarged spleen, parasites in RBCs; diagnosis: malarial forms in blood smear
Plasmodium malariae (quartan malaria)	Tropics	Schizogony and gametocytes in RBCs	*Anopheles* spp. mosquito transmits sporozoites	Cyclic fever, chills, enlarged spleen, parasites in RBCs, relapses; diagnosis: malarial forms in blood smear
Plasmodium falciparum (malignant malaria)	Tropics	Trophozoites and gametocytes in peripheral RBCs	*Anopheles* spp. mosquito transmits sporozoites	Cyclic fever, chills, enlarged spleen, parasites in RBCs, blackwater fever from hemoglobin in urine, blockage of capillaries, death; diagnosis: malarial forms in blood smear
Plasmodium ovale (ovale malaria)	West Africa	Schizogony and gametocytes in RBCs	*Anopheles* spp. mosquito transmits sporozoites	Cyclic fever, chills, enlarged spleen, parasites in RBCs; diagnosis: malarial forms in blood smear
Toxoplasma gondii (toxoplasmosis)	Worldwide	Trophozoites intracellularly in all organs; pseudocysts in brain and other tissue	Ingestion of oocysts; ingestion of trophozoites or pseudocysts in undercooked meat; congenital passage of trophozoites	Fever, enlarged lymph nodes; in fetus or neonate: damage or death; can cause acute infection in immunosuppressed patient; diagnosis: serology

Continued on following page

TABLE 5–8 □ PATHOGENIC PROTOZOA (Continued)

Scientific and Common Name	Epidemiology	Disease-Producing Form and Its Location in Host	How Infection Occurs	Major Disease Manifestations, Diagnostic Stage, and Specimen of Choice
Isospora belli (none)	Worldwide	Schizogony and gametology stages in intestinal epithelium	Ingestion of infective oocysts	Diarrhea; diagnosis: oocyst and sporozoites in feces
Sarcocystis spp. (none) (zoonosis)	Worldwide	Sarcocyst in muscle, oocyst formation in intestine	Ingestion of sarcocyst from undercooked meat or oocyst from water or food contaminated by infected or pigs	Sarcocysts (Miescher's tubes) in muscle do not generally cause problems; diagnosis: tissue biopsy, oocysts in feces
Cryptosporidium parvum (none)	Worldwide	Invades gastrointestinal tract mucosa	Probably by ingestion of fecally contaminated food or water; human-to-human transmission	Diarrhea; diagnosis: tropho-zoites and schizonts in biopsy of jejunum
Cyclospora cayetanensis	Worldwide	Oocyst formation in intestine	Probably by ingestion of fecally contaminated food or water	Diarrhea; diagnosis: oocysts in feces, acid fast and autofluorescent
Babesia spp. (*B. microti* in the United States) (none) (zoonosis)	Worldwide	*Babesia* trophozoites in RBCs	Tick bite (*Ixodes scapularis*); rarely, via blood transfusion	Fever, symptoms can resemble malaria; diagnosis: trophozoites in blood smear

ABBREVIATIONS: CNS = central nervous system; CSF = Cerebrospinal fluid; RBCs = red blood cells.

CASE STUDY 5–1

A 22-year-old woman was admitted to the emergency department at 3:00 A.M. complaining of burning during urination and severe vaginal itching. The physician ordered a routine urinalysis and a vaginal swab for microscopic examination. The technologist observed many motile organisms measuring approximately 12 μm in diameter in both the urine microscopic wet mount and the vaginal wet-mount preparation.

1. What is the most likely organism (genus and species) seen in the wet preparation?
2. How is this infection acquired?
3. What symptoms are seen in men infected with this organism?
4. What should be done to prevent reinfection in this patient?

CASE STUDY 5–2

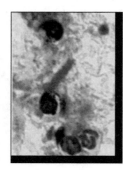

A mother, working outside the home, took her 2-year-old son on the third day of his illness to his pediatrician. The child had diarrhea and vomiting that became progressively worse over the 3-day period. The watery stool specimen sent to the laboratory revealed no white or red blood cells when examined for parasites, but the technologist noted many refractile organisms measuring approximately 5 μm that resembled yeast. A modified trichrome stain revealed the acid-fast organisms shown in the accompanying figure.

1. What is the identity of this parasite (genus and species)?
2. What is the usual course of this disease in immunocompetent individuals? How is the disease treated?
3. How did this child probably acquire the infection?
4. When can the child return to group day care?

CASE STUDY **5–3**

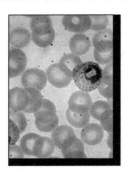

A 20-year-old woman arrived at an immediate-care medical facility with recurring fever and chills. She reported an episode that began about 30 minutes before her admission. She had had headaches, muscle aches, and nausea for 4 days before the beginning of the fever and chills. She told the physician that she had recently returned from a missionary trip to Honduras and thought she might have the flu. A complete blood count and urinalysis were ordered, but the results were unremarkable. The differential report, however, noted the parasite forms seen in the accompanying figure.

1. What is the probable parasite (genus and species)?
2. What characteristics allowed you to differentiate this parasite from others in the same genus?
3. How did the patient acquire this infection?
4. What steps could the patient have taken to avoid this infection?

CASE STUDY **5–4**

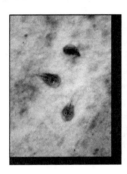

Two 16-year-old boys returned from a 4-week camping trip in the northwest United States. For 2 weeks after the trip, both boys experienced abdominal cramps and diarrhea, usually within 1 hour after eating. Foul-smelling flatulence was present as well. On questioning, the boys denied drinking water that was not treated with halazone tablets (a chloramine disinfectant used to purify water). Three of their stools were submitted for culture and identification of enteric bacterial pathogens and intestinal parasites. All the results were negative for bacterial pathogens, and only one trichrome stain from one sample revealed the parasite form seen in the accompanying figure.

1. What parasite (genus and species) do you report?
2. How did these boys become infected, assuming they correctly used their halazone tablets?
3. Why wasn't the parasite recovered in more of the specimens submitted?
4. What other tests are available for detecting this organism?

CASE STUDY **5–5**

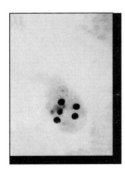

A young couple returned from a honeymoon trip to Mexico. Two weeks later, the young man began having diarrhea. After 3 days of up to six bowel movements per day, he went to the doctor. The physician ordered a stool culture and an examination for eggs and parasites. The technologist noted bloody mucus in the liquid specimen and prepared a wet mount from this material. An irregular motile organism measuring approximately 15 μm was observed. The parasite form in the accompanying figure was found in the permanently stained smear.

1. What parasite (genus and species) do you suspect?
2. What are the primary characteristics used to differentiate and identify this organism?
3. What other disease manifestations can occur if this infection progresses beyond the intestinal tract?
4. How could the patient have acquired this infection?

You have now completed the chapter on Protozoa. After reviewing this material carefully with the aid of your learning objectives, proceed to the post-test.

Word Puzzles

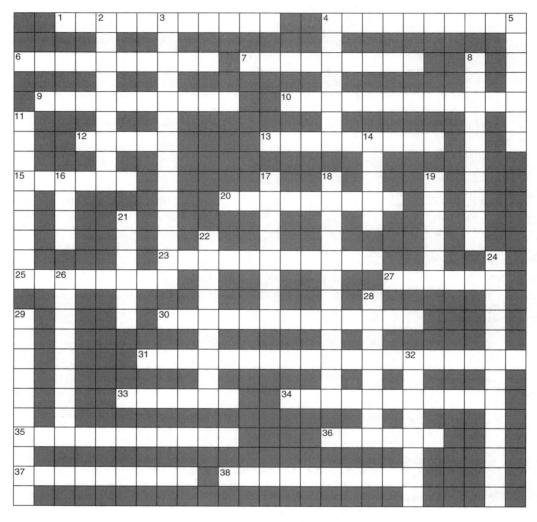

Across

1. Transformation from a cyst to a trophozoite after the cystic form has been swallowed by the host
4. A phylum containing protozoa that move by means of cilia; have two dissimilar nuclei
6. A sex cell that can produce gametes
7. An organism having a hard, segmented exoskeleton and paired, jointed legs
9. A long-surviving modified liver schizont of *P. vivax* that is the source of relapsing infections in this species
10. A flattened, spindle-shaped, flagellated form seen in the gut or salivary glands of the insect vectors in the life cycle of trypanosomes
12. A thin, firm, rodlike structure running along the base of the undulating membrane of certain flagellates
13. The fertilized oocyst in which the sporozoites of *Plasmodium* have developed
15. The encysted form of the ookinete that occurs on the stomach wall of *Anopheles* spp. mosquitoes infected with malaria
20. Basophilic nuclear DNA
23. The motile stage of protozoon that feeds and multiplies within the host
25. The small mass of chromatin within the nucleus; also termed karyosome
27. An object that can absorb and harbor organisms and can cause human infection by direct contact
30. The basal body origin of flagella that supports the undulating membrane in kinetoplastid flagellates
31. Small ovoid amastigote forms found in tissue macrophages in patients with *Leishmania donovani* infection (3 words)
33. On the outer edge
34. Slowly multiplying intracellular trophozoites of *Toxoplasma gondii*
35. The stage of *Plasmodium* spp. that develops in liver cells
36. A mature sex cell
37. Infective cyst containing banana-shaped bradyzoites
38. An infection that originates in and is acquired from a medical facility

Down

2. Pertaining to the skin
3. Similar to epimastigote except kinetoplast located posteriorly and undulating membrane extends along entire body
4. A host harboring and disseminating a parasite, but exhibiting no clinical signs or symptoms
5. The intracellular portion of a flagellum
8. The form of *Plasmodium* that develops inside the sporocyst
11. One of the trophozoites released from human red blood cells or liver cells at maturation of the asexual cycle of malaria
14. Multiple hairlike processes attached to a free surface of a cell; functions for motility
16. The immotile stage protected by a cyst wall formed by the parasite
17. A subkingdom consisting of unicellular eukaryotic animals
18. A subphylum containing organisms that move by means of one or more flagella
19. An opening
21. The fertilized cell resulting from the union of male and female gametes
22. The association of two different species of organisms in which one partner is benefited and the other is neither benefited nor injured
24. A condition seen in malarial infections; infected red blood cells and symptoms reappear after an apparent cure
26. A disorder marked by bloody diarrhea, mucus, or both in feces
28. The fever-chills syndrome in malaria
29. A cyst with as elastic membrane formed by the host following an acute infection with *Toxoplasma gondii*
32. The axial rod functioning as a support in flagellates

```
F  O  M  I  T  E  T  I  O  Z  O  T  P  Y  R  C  S  U  P  C
K  G  A  T  S  O  C  Y  E  T  I  O  Z  O  R  E  M  S  N  P
Q  E  T  A  C  H  Y  Z  O  I  T  E  S  A  O  U  U  Y  I  P
E  T  O  G  I  T  S  A  M  A  T  A  T  O  L  O  N  M  T  F
A  E  T  W  T  M  L  O  Q  J  X  S  C  L  E  O  U  I  A  N
I  M  N  V  N  E  A  Z  M  V  Y  Y  E  N  G  I  O  Q  M  O
L  A  E  Q  O  R  S  O  V  C  S  G  A  O  R  Y  S  B  O  I
I  G  T  E  Z  O  N  T  A  T  A  T  Z  T  T  N  L  W  R  T
C  S  A  T  I  G  E  O  J  L  U  I  A  F  S  O  T  D  H  A
E  E  P  O  H  O  M  R  F  C  H  T  J  R  Y  G  S  E  C  L
T  T  B  G  C  N  M  P  Y  C  J  S  D  E  C  O  A  T  L  L
I  I  U  I  S  Y  O  H  S  T  R  Y  F  L  O  T  L  E  A  E
O  O  S  T  S  Y  C  O  D  U  E  S  P  Y  R  E  P  N  I  G
Z  Z  M  S  Y  X  O  R  A  P  G  O  X  T  O  M  O  I  M  A
O  Y  H  A  J  R  E  I  R  R  A  C  N  S  P  A  T  K  O  L
H  D  I  M  T  S  Y  C  O  C  R  A  S  O  S  G  E  O  C  F
P  A  R  O  H  P  O  G  I  T  S  A  M  X  R  T  N  O  O  X
O  R  Y  R  E  T  N  E  S  Y  D  S  F  A  I  M  I  B  S  E
R  B  H  P  P  A  P  I  C  O  M  P  L  E  X  A  K  R  O  T
T  B  I  F  X  O  P  A  R  O  H  P  O  I  L  I  C  Z  N  N
```

amastigote	costa	kinetoplast	pseudocyst
Apicomplexa	cryptozoite	Mastigophora	sarcocyst
atrium	cutaneous	merogony	sporocyst
axostyle	cyst	merozoite	schizogony
bradyzoites	dysentery	nosocomial	schizont
carrier	exflagellation	oocyst	subpatent
chromatin	flagellum	ookinete	tachyzoites
cilia	fomite	paroxysm	trophozoite
Ciliophora	gamete	promastigote	
commensal	gametogony	protozoa	

Post-Test

1. Matching: Use each number as many times as appropriate: **(12 points)**

   a. _____ Malaria parasite with 6 to 12 merozoites in the schizont

   b. _____ C- or U-shaped body with a large kinetoplast

   c. _____ Large kidney-shaped nucleus

   d. _____ Trophozoite ingests red blood cells

   e. _____ Large glycogen vacuole

   f. _____ Schizonts not seen in peripheral blood

   g. _____ Pseudocysts in brain

   h. _____ Nonpathogenic

   i. _____ Oocysts found in human feces

   j. _____ Commonly causes relapses of malaria

   k. _____ Transmitted by tsetse fly

   l. _____ Pathogenic intestinal flagellate

   1. *Isospora belli*
   2. *Toxoplasma gondii*
   3. *Plasmodium vivax*
   4. *Plasmodium malariae*
   5. *Plasmodium falciparum*
   6. *Trypanosoma brucei gambiense*
   7. *Trypanosoma cruzi*
   8. *Entamoeba histolytica*
   9. *Entamoeba hartmanni*
   10. *Endolimax nana*
   11. *Iodamoeba butschlii*
   12. *Giardia lamblia*
   13. *Trichomonas vaginalis*
   14. *Balantidium coli*

2. How would you differentiate *Entamoeba histolytica* from *Entamoeba dispar* in a fecal smear? **(2 points)**

3. How would you differentiate *Entamoeba histolytica* from *Entamoeba coli* in a fecal smear? **(2 points)**

4. Define the following: **(20 points)**
   a. Trophozoite
   b. Cyst
   c. Sporozoite
   d. Schizogony
   e. Carrier
   f. Oocyst
   g. Pseudocyst
   h. L.D. body
   i. Paroxysm
   j. Atrium

5. State method of infection for each of the following diseases: **(20 points)**
   a. Kala-azar
   b. Giardiasis
   c. Chagas' disease
   d. Toxoplasmosis
   e. Trichomonal urethritis
   f. Balantidial dysentery
   g. Babesiosis
   h. Malaria
   i. Sleeping sickness
   j. Cutaneous leishmaniasis

6. Draw the ring form(s) in a red blood cell for each of the following: **(6 points)**
   a. *Plasmodium vivax*
   b. *Plasmodium malariae*
   c. *Plasmodium falciparum*

Each of the following multiple-choice questions is worth 2 points.

7. *Cryptosporidium parvum* oocysts are best detected in fecal specimens using the:
   a. Gram stain
   b. Iodine stain
   c. Methenamine silver stain
   d. Modified Ziehl-Neelson acid-fast stain
   e. Trichrome stain

8. The two parasitic organisms most commonly associated with waterborne outbreaks of diarrhea include:
   a. *Blastocystis hominis* and *Isospora belli*
   b. *Entamoeba coli* and *Giardia lamblia*
   c. *Entamoeba histolytica* and *Endolimax nana*
   d. *Giardia lamblia* and *Cryptosporidium parvum*
   e. *Trichomonas hominis* and *Toxoplasma gondii*

9. The malaria parasite characterized by the presence of multiple ring forms or "banana-shaped" gametocytes in red blood cells is:
   a. *Babesia* spp.
   b. *Plasmodium falciparum*
   c. *Plasmodium malariae*
   d. *Plasmodium ovale*
   e. *Plasmodium vivax*

10. The characteristic that most clearly differentiates cysts of *Iodamoeba butschlii* from other amebic cysts is(are):

    a. Chromatoid bars with rounded ends

    b. Eight nuclei with eccentrically located karyosomes

    c. Ingested bacteria and red blood cells

    d. A large glycogen vacuole

    e. Lemon-shaped cysts

11. A blood parasite that invades reticulocytes, is characterized by single ring forms and Schuffner's dots, and may cause a true relapse is:

    a. *Babesia* spp.

    b. *Plasmodium falciparum*

    c. *Plasmodium malariae*

    d. *Plasmodium ovale*

    e. *Plasmodium vivax*

12. A 44-year-old man was admitted to the hospital following a 2-week history of low-grade fever, malaise, and anorexia. Examination of a Giemsa-stained blood film revealed many intraerythrocytic parasites. Further history revealed frequent East Coast camping trips near Martha's Vineyard and Nantucket Island but no travel outside the continental United States. Most likely, this parasite is:

    a. *Babesia microti*

    b. *Leishmania donovani*

    c. *Plasmodium ovale*

    d. *Toxoplasma gondii*

    e. none of these

13. The coccidian parasite that produces mild intestinal pathology in humans and for which the human is the only definitive host is:

    a. *Toxoplasma gondii*

    b. *Sarcocystis hominis*

    c. *Isospora belli*

    d. *Cryptosporidium parvum*

    e. *Cyclospora cayetanensis*

14. While examining a fecal specimen, *Isospora belli* is suspected. The technologist would expect to see:

    a. Cysts (8 to 10 μm) containing sporozoites

    b. Oocysts (25 × 14 μm) that are acid fast

    c. Cysts with red blood cell inclusions

    d. Spores (2 μm) that are acid fast

15. Material from a gum lesion is stained with trichrome, revealing amoebae that have a single nucleus and contain partially digested neutrophils. The most likely identification is:

    a. *Entamoeba gingivalis*

    b. *Entamoeba dispar*

    c. *Entamoeba polecki*

    d. *Trichomonas tenax*

    e. *Entamoeba histolytica*

16. Concerning *Toxoplasma gondii*, all of the following are true EXCEPT:

    a. Congenital infections can occur

    b. Human infection occurs when oocysts are ingested

    c. They are diagnosed by serology tests

    d. Human infection occurs when sarcocysts are ingested in undercooked meat

    e. Domestic cats are definitive hosts

17. *Acanthamoeba keratitis* is usually associated with:

    a. Contaminated lens-cleaning solutions

    b. Hard contact lenses

    c. Soft contact lenses

    d. Wearing lenses while swimming

    e. Swimming without lenses

18. Concerning *Enterocytozoon bieneusi*, all of the following are true EXCEPT:

    a. It is the most frequent *Microsporidium* infection found in AIDS patients

    b. Infection occurs when spores are ingested

    c. Infection occurs when spores are inhaled

    d. Infection occurs when sporozoites are ingested

    e. Infection occurs from blood transfusion

19. The protozoa causing diarrhea that has been associated with raspberries, strawberries, herbs, and some vegetables is:

    a. *Balantidium coli*

    b. *Cyclospora cayetanensis*

    c. *Cryptosporidium parvum*

    d. *Dientamoeba fragilis*

    e. *Isospora belli*

20. Blackwater fever is caused by:

    a. *Plasmodium falciparum*

    b. *Plasmodium vivax*

    c. *Trypanosoma brucei gambiense*

    d. *Trypanosoma cruzi*

    e. *Leishmania donovani*

21. A 48-year-old man was admitted to the hospital after complaining of fever and shortness of breath. Radiographs revealed an enlarged heart, and complete blood count smear results revealed rare C-shaped trypomastigote forms. The patient was an active military duty years ago in the Panama Canal zone. The most likely parasite is:

    a. *Babesia microti*
    b. *Leishmania donovani*
    c. *Plasmodium falciparum*
    d. *Trypanosoma brucei gambiense*
    e. *Trypanosoma cruzi*

22. Winterbottom's sign is associated with:

    a. *Babesia microti*
    b. *Leishmania donovani*
    c. *Plasmodium falciparum*
    d. *Trypanosoma brucei gambiense*
    e. *Trypanosoma cruzi*

23. Fecal samples should be washed with saline only because washing with water will destroy:

    a. *Blastocystis hominis*
    b. *Cryptosporidium parvum*
    c. *Entamoeba* cysts
    d. *Isospora belli*
    e. *Acanthamoeba* spp.

24. A 25-year-old man was admitted to the hospital with a severe headache, fever, nausea, and vomiting. Symptoms began suddenly 2 days after vacationing at a summer cabin situated on an inland lake. A spinal tap revealed a purulent CSF with no bacteria. A motile form resembling a leukocyte was observed on direct examination of the fluid. The most likely causative organism is:

    a. *Acanthamoeba* spp.
    b. *Blastocystis hominis*
    c. *Entamoeba polecki*
    d. *Naegleria fowleri*
    e. *Entamoeba histolytica*

25. The parasite that may invade and multiply in the liver or spleen is:

    a. *Leishmania braziliensis*
    b. *Leishmania donovani*
    c. *Leishmania mexicana*
    d. *Leishmania tropica*
    e. *Trypanosoma brucei gambiense*

BIBLIOGRAPHY

Intestinal Protozoa
Arean, VM, and Koppisch, E: Balantidiosis: A review and report cases. Am J Pathol 32:1089, 1956.
Babb, RR, et al: Giardiasis: A cause of traveler's diarrhea. JAMA 217:1359, 1971.
Brandborg, LL, et al: Human coccidiosis—A possible cause of malabsorption. The life cycle in small bowel mucosal biopsies as a diagnostic feature. N Engl J Med 283:1306, 1970.
Centers for Disease Control. Foodborne Outbreak of Cryptosporidiosis—Spokane, Washington, 1997. Morb Mortal Wkly Rep 47:565, 1998.
Centers for Disease Control. Outbreak of Cyclosporiasis—Northern Virginia–Washington, DC–Baltimore, Maryland, Metropolitan Area, 1997. Morb Mortal Wkly Rep 46:689, 1997.
Centers for Disease Control. Update: Outbreaks of Cyclosporiasis—United States and Canada, 1997. Morb Mortal Wkly Rep 46:521, 1997.
Kuroki, T, et al: Isolation of Legionella and free-living amoebae at hot spring spas in Kanagawa, Japan. J Jpn Assoc Kansenshogaku Zasshi 72(10):1050–1055, 1998.
Mahmoud, AAF, and Warren, KS: Algorithms in the diagnosis and management of exotic diseases. II. Giardiasis. J Infect Dis 131:621, 1975.
Markell, ED, and Udkow, MP: *Blastocystis hominis*: pathogen or fellow traveler? Am J Trop Med Hyg 35:1023–1026, 1986.
Markell, EK. Is there any reason to continue treating *Blastocystis* infection? Clin Infect Dis 21:104–105, 1995.
Martinez-Palomo, A (ed): Amebiasis. In Human Parasitic Diseases, Vol 2. Elsevier, New York, 1986.
Meyer, EA (ed): Giardiasis. In Human Parasitic Diseases, Vol 3. Elsevier, New York, 1990.
Ong, SJ, Cheng, MY, Liu, KH, and Horng, CH: Use of the ProSpecT microplate enzyme immunoassay for the detection of pathogenic and nonpathogenic *Entamoeba histolytica* in faecal specimens. Trans R Soc Trop Med Hyg 90:248–249, 1996.

Pernin, P, et al: Comparative recoveries of Naegleria fowleri amoebae from seeded river water by filtration and centrifugation. Appl Environ Microbiol 64(3):955–959, 1998.
Pritchard, JH, et al: Diagnosis of focal hepatic lesions. Combined radioisotope and ultrasound techniques. JAMA 229:1463, 1974.
Rivera, WE, et al: Differentiation of *Entamoeba histolytica* and *E. dispar* DNA from cysts present in stool specimens by polymerase chain reaction: its field application in the Philippines. Parasitol Res 82:585–589, 1996.
Rohr, U, et al: Comparison of free-living amoebae in hot water systems of hospitals with isolates from moist sanitary areas by identifying genera and determining temperature tolerance. Appl Environ Microbiol 64(5):1822–1824, 1998.
Sanuki, J, et al: Identification of *Entamoeba histolytica* and *E. dispar* cysts in stool by polymerase chain reaction. Parasitol Res 83:96–98, 1997.
Silberman, JD, et al: Human parasite finds taxonomic home. Nature 380:398, 1996.
Singh, M, et al: Elucidation of the life cycle of the intestinal protozoan *Blastocystis hominis*. Parasitol Res 81:446–450, 1995.
Spice, WM, et al: Molecular and cell biology of opportunistic infections in AIDS. *Entamoeba histolytica*. Mol Cell Biol Hum Dis Ser 2:95–137, 1993.
Sterling, CR, and Ortega, YR: Cyclospora: An Enigma Worth Unraveling. Emerg Infect Dis 5(1):48–53, 1999.
Thompson, RCA, et al: *Giardia* and giardiasis. Adv Parasitol 32:71–160, 1993.
Troll, H, et al: Simple differential detection of *Entamoeba histolytica* and *Entamoeba dispar* in fresh stool specimens by sodium acetate-acetic acid-formalin concentration and PCR. J Clin Microbiol 35:1701–1705, 1997.
Walderich, B, et al: Differentiation of *Entamoeba histolytica* and *Entamoeba dispar* from German travelers and residents of endemic areas. Am J Trop Med Hyg 57:70–74, 1997.

Weiss, JB: DNA probes and PCR for diagnosis of parasitic infections. Clin Microbiol Rev 8:113–130, 1995.

Zierdt, CH: *Blastocystis hominis*—past and future. Clin Microbiol Rev 4:61–79, 1991.

Zuckerman, MJ, et al. *Blastocystis hominis* and intestinal injury. Am J Med Sci 308:96–101, 1994.

Atrial and Blood Protozoa

Almeida, IC, et al: A highly sensitive and specific chemiluminescent enzyme-linked immunosorbent assay for diagnosis of active *Trypanosoma cruzi* infection. Transfusion 37:850–857, 1997.

Atias, A, et al: Mega-esophagus, megacolon and Chagas' disease in Chile. Gastroenterology 44:433, 1963.

Avila, JC, and Harris, JR (eds): Subcellular Biochemistry, Vol 18. Intracellular Parasites. Plenum Press, New York, 1992.

Barry, JD: The relative significance of mechanisms of antigenic variation in African trypanosomes. Parasitol Today 13:212–218, 1997.

Berger, BJ, and Fairlamb, AH: Interactions between immunity and chemotherapy in the treatment of trypanosomiasis and leishmaniasis. Parasitology 105(suppl):71–78, 1992.

Bowman, S, et al; The Complete Nucleotide Sequence of Chromosome 3 of *Plasmodium falciparum*. Nature 400:532–538; 1999.

Britto, C, et al: Polymerase chain reaction detection of *Trypanosoma cruzi* in human blood samples as tool for diagnosis and treatment evaluation. Parasitology 110:241–247, 1995.

Brown, MT: Trichomoniasis. Practitioner 207:639, 1972.

Chang, KP, and Bray, RS (eds): Leishmaniasis. Elsevier, New York, 1985.

Cohen, S: Immunity to malaria. Proc R Soc Lond B Biol Sci 203:323, 1979.

Convit, J, et al: Diffuse cutaneous leishmaniasis: A disease due to an immunologic defect of the host. Trans R Soc Trop Med Hyg 66:603, 1972.

Cossio, PM, et al: Chagasic cardiopathy. Demonstration of a serum gamma globulin factor which reacts with endocardium and vascular structures. Circulation 49:13, 1974.

Dye, C, et al: Serological diagnosis of leishmaniasis on detecting infection as well as disease. Epidemiol Infect 110(3):647–656, 1993.

Eling, WM, et al: The need for live parasites for long-term immunity in malaria. Acta Leidensia 60(1):167–175, 1991.

Garnham, PCC: Malaria Parasites and Other Haemosporidia. Blackwell Scientific Publications, Oxford, 1966.

Goddard, J: Kissing Bugs and Chagas' Disease. Infect Med 16(3):172–180, 1999.

Goodwin, LG: The pathology of African trypanosomiasis. Trans R Soc Trop Med Hyg 65:797, 1970.

Grunwaldt, R: Babesiosis on Shelter Island. NY State J Med 77:1320–1321, 1977.

Hubsch, RM, et al: Evaluation of an autoimmune-type antibody in the sera of patients with Chagas' disease. J Parasitol 62:523–527, 1976.

Kaushik, A, et al: Malarial placental infection and low birth weight babies. J Commun Dis 24(2):65–69, 1992.

Komba, E, et al: Multicenter evaluation of an antigen-detection ELISA for the diagnosis of *Trypanosoma brucei rhodesiense* sleeping sickness. Bull WHO 70:57–61, 1992.

Luzzatto, L, et al: Glucose-6 phosphate dehydrogenase deficient red cells: Resistance to infection with malarial parasites. Science 164:839, 1969.

Mahmoud, AAF, and Warren, KS: Algorithms in the diagnosis and management of exotic diseases, IV. American trypanosomiasis. J Infect Dis 132:121, 1975.

Miller, LH, et al: Erythrocyte receptors for (*Plasmodium knowlesi*) malaria: Duffy blood group determinants. Science 189:561–563, 1975.

Murray, PR, and Baron, EJ (eds): Manual of Clinical Microbiology, American Society of Microbiology Washington, DC, 1999.

Nantulya, VM, et al: Diagnosis of *Trypanosoma brucei gambiense* sleeping sickness using an antigen detection enzyme-linked immunosorbent assay. Trans R Soc Trop Med Hyg 86:42–45, 1992.

Pepin, J, and Milord, F: The treatment of human African trypanosomiasis. Adv Parasitol 33:2–47, 1994.

Sherman, IW (ed): Malaria: parasite biology, pathogenesis, and protection. ASM Press, Washington, DC, 1998.

Szarfman, A, et al: Investigation of the EVI antibody in parasitic diseases other than American trypanosomiasis. An anti-skeletal muscle antibody in leishmaniasis. Am J Trop Med Hyg 24:19–24, 1975.

Targett, GA: Virulence and the immune response in malaria. Mem Inst Oswaldo Cruz 5(suppl):127–144, 1992.

Wahlgren, M, and Bejarano, MT: Malaria a Blueprint of "bad air." Nature 400:506–507, 1999.

White, NJ, and Ho, M: The pathophysiology of malaria. Adv Parasitol 31:84–173, 1992.

Other Protozoa

Aspock, H, and Pollak, A: Prevention of prenatal toxoplasmosis by serological screening of pregnant women in Austria. Scand J Infect Dis Suppl 84:32–37, 1992.

Babb, RR, et al: *Cryptosporidia enteritis* in a healthy professional athlete. Am J Gastroenterol 77(11):833–834, 1982.

Bonilla, HF, et al: Acanthamoeba Sinusitis and Disseminated Infection in a Patient with AIDS. Infect Med 16(6):397–400, 1999.

Bryan, RT, and Wilson, M: Clinical casebook: toxoplasmosis. Laboratory Management 26(8):40, 1988.

Bunyarartvej, S, et al: Human intestinal sarcosporidiosis: Report of six cases. Am J Trop Med Hyg 31:36–41, 1982.

Camargo, ME, et al: Immunoglobulin G and immunoglobulin M enzyme-linked immunosorbent assays and defined toxoplasmosis serological patterns. Infect Immun 21:55–58, 1978.

Centers for Disease Control and Prevention: Primary amebic meningoencephalitis: California, Florida, New York. Morb Mortal Wkly Rep 27:343, 1978.

Current, WL, and Barcia, LS: Cryptosporidiosis. Clin Microbiol Rev 4:325–358, 1991.

Cursons, RT, et al: Virulence of pathogenic free-living amebae. J Parasitol 64:744–745, 1978.

Didier, ES, et al: Comparison of three staining methods for detecting microsporidia in fluids. J Clin Microbiol 33:3138–3145, 1995.

Egger, MD, et al: Symptoms and transmission of intestinal cryptosporidiosis. Arch Dis Child 65:445–447, 1990.

Fayer, R (ed): Cryptosporidium and cryptosporidiosis. CRC Press, Boca Raton, FL, 1997.

Frenkel, JL: Toxoplasmosis and pneumocystosis: Clinical and laboratory aspects in immunocompetent and compromised hosts. In Prier, JE and Friedman, H (eds): Opportunistic Pathogens. University Park Press, Baltimore, 1974.

Garcia, LS: Intestinal coccidia and microsporidia in non-AIDS patients. Clin Microbiol Newslett 11:169–172, 1989.

Haase, G. *Pneumocystis carinii* Delanoe & Delanoe (1912) has been placed in the Archiascomycetales, a class of the Ascomycota. Infect Immun 65:4365–4366, 1997.

Hollister, WS, et al: Evidence for widespread occurrence of antibodies to *Encephalitozoon cuniculi* (microspora) in man provided by ELISA and other serological tests. Parasitology 102:33–45, 1991.

Ignatius, R, et al: Comparative evaluation of modified trichrome and Uvitex 2B stains for detection of low numbers of microsporidial spores in stool specimens. J Clin Microbiol 35:2266–2269, 1997.

Jackson, MH, and Hutchison, WM: The prevalence and source of *Toxoplasma* infection in the environment. Adv Parasitol 28:55–105, 1989.

Kinnig, P, et al: Sarcosporidiosis (*Sarcocystis suihominis*) in man. Immunol Infect 7:170–177, 1979.

Long, EG, et al: Morphologic and staining characteristics of a cyanobacterium-like organism associated with diarrhea. J Infect Dis 164:199–202, 1991.

Markus, MB: Sarcocystis and sarcocystosis in domestic animals and man. Adv Vet Sci Comp Med 22:159, 1978.

Metcalf, TW, et al: Microsporidial keratoconjunctivitis in a patient with AIDS. Br J Ophthalmol 76:177–178, 1992.

Moore, JA, and Frankel, JA: Respiratory and enteric cryptosporidiosis in humans. Arch Pathol Lab Med 115:1160–1162, 1991.

Murray, PR, and Baron, EJ (eds): Manual of Clinical Microbiology, American Society of Microbiology, Washington, DC, 1999.

Orenstein, JM: Microsporidiosis in the acquired immunodeficiency syndrome. J Parasitol 77:843–864, 1991.

Schuster, FL, and Visvesvara, GS: Axenic growth and drug sensitivity studies of *Balamuthia mandrillaris*, an agent of amebic meningoencephalitis in humans and other animals. J Clin Microbiol 34:385–388, 1996.

Tzipori, S: Cryptosporidiosis in perspective. Adv Parasitol 27:63–129, 1988.

Wakefield, AE, et al: *Pneumocystis carinii* shows DNA homology with the ustomycetous red yeast fungi. Mol Microbiol 6:1903–1911, 1992.

Webber, R, et al: Improved light-microscopical detection of microsporidia spores in stool and duodenal aspirates. N Engl J Med 326:161–166, 1992.

Wittner, Murray (ed) and Weiss, Louis M (contributing ed): The Microsporida and microsporidiosis. ASM Press, Washington, DC, 1998.

Zoonoses

Coatney, GR: The simian malarias: Zoonosis, anthroponosis or both? Am J Trop Med Hyg 20:795, 1971.

Levine, ND: Protozoan parasites of nonhuman primates as zoonotic agents. Laboratory Animal Care 20:371, 1970.

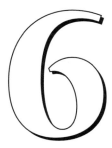

6 ARTHROPODA

LEARNING OBJECTIVES

ON COMPLETION OF THIS CHAPTER, THE STUDENT WILL BE ABLE TO:

1 State the criteria used for taxonomic classification of the **Arthropoda.**

2 State the general description of each order of Arthropoda that contains genera of medical importance.

3 State the definitions of the most commonly used terms specific for Arthropoda.

4 State the definitions of complete and incomplete metamorphosis, and give examples of each.

5 Identify Arthropoda to class by morphologic criteria.

6 Differentiate between Acarina and Insecta.

7 Describe the type of life cycle for each Arthropoda class.

8 Contrast the role of Arthropoda as intermediate hosts versus transport hosts for various parasites and microorganisms.

9 State the specific genus of Arthropoda serving as the required intermediate host for various helminth and protozoal infections.

10 Given an illustration or photograph (or actual specimen, with sufficient laboratory experience), identify diagnostic stages of Arthropoda.

11 Discuss problems caused by the Arthropoda that significantly affect humans, and propose solutions for these problems.

12 Discuss method(s) used to prevent infestations caused by arthropods.

13 Discuss methods used to control Arthropoda based on life cycles.

GLOSSARY

Arachnida. A class in the phylum Arthropoda containing ticks, mites, spiders, and scorpions.

Arthropoda. A phylum of the animal kingdom composed of organisms that have a hard, segmented exoskeleton and paired, jointed legs.

capitulum. A collective term referring to the mouth parts of ticks and mites that extend forward from the body.

chitin. A hard, insoluble polysaccharide that is the main compound in shells of crabs, exoskeletons of insects, and certain other insect structures.

Crustacea. A class in the phylum Arthropoda including crabs, water fleas, lobsters, shrimp, barnacles, and wood lice.

ctenidia (sing. ctenidium). Comblike structures found on the head region of fleas. These structures are useful in group classification. Genal ctenidia or combs are located just above the mouth parts. Pronotal combs are located immediately behind the head and extend posteriorly on the dorsal surface.

cypris. A larval resting stage in the life cycle of some crustaceans in which a metamorphosis occurs, comparable to a pupa.

ecdysis. Molting or shedding of an outer layer or covering and the development of a new one.

entomology. The branch of zoology dealing with the study of insects.

exoskeleton. A hard, chitinous structure on the outside of the body, providing support and protection for internal organs.

imago. The sexually mature adult insect or arachnid.

Insecta. A class in the phylum Arthropoda containing many insect types whose bodies are divided into three distinct regions: head, thorax, and abdomen.

instar. Any one of the nymphal or larval stages between molts.

invertebrates. Animals that have no spinal column.

metamorphosis. A change of shape or structure; a transition from one developmental stage to another. With incomplete metamorphosis, nymphs resemble adults; with complete metamorphosis, larvae and pupae are distinct and do not resemble adults.

myiasis. A condition caused by infestation of the body with fly larvae.

nauplius. The earliest and youngest larval form in the life cycle of crustaceans.

nymph. A developmental stage in the life cycle of certain arthropods that resembles a small adult.

pediculosis. Infestation with lice.

pupa (pl. pupae). The encased resting stage between the larva and imago stage (e.g., cocoon).

scutum. A chitinous shield or plate covering part (on the female) or all (on the male) of the dorsal surface of hard ticks.

temporary host. A host on which an arthropod (adult or larval form) resides temporarily to feed on blood or tissue.

● *Arthropods*

The Arthropoda is the largest phylum, containing more than 80% of all animal life. Arthropods directly cause or transmit more than 80% of all diseases. They are of major economic importance to agriculture, with both beneficial and destructive effects.

The phylum Arthropoda includes the segmented **invertebrates** that have a protective **chitinous exoskeleton** and bilaterally paired jointed appendages. The head has structures adapted for sensory and chewing or piercing functions. Eyes are single lens or compound. Digestive, respiratory, excretory, and nervous systems are present. The body cavity (the hemocele) is filled with a bloodlike substance.

The arthropods contain many members and are divided into five classes. Three classes (**Insecta, Arachnida,** and **Crustacea**) contain most of the medically important arthropods. The important disease-producing genera listed in Table 6–1 are members of various families.

Life Cycle

All Arachnida and most Insecta develop from egg to adult by a process called **metamorphosis** (Diagram 6–1). Incomplete or hemimetabolous metamorphosis has three stages: (1) egg, (2) **nymph,** and (3) **imago,** the sexually mature adult. The nymph, resembling a miniature adult, emerges from the eggs and molts several times before it becomes an imago. After each molt, the nymphal form is called an **instar.** Wings of flying insects increase in size with each instar. Lice, true bugs (Hemiptera), and arachnids develop through incomplete metamorphosis.

Complete metamorphosis has the egg, larva, **pupa,** and imago stages. An insect larva emerges from the egg as a segmented wormlike larva and matures through a series of larval instars until finally enclosing itself inside a pupa casing. After a time, the transformed imago emerges. Flies, mosquitoes, and fleas develop through complete metamorphosis.

Development of most crustaceans is by incomplete metamorphosis; however, the names of the stages are different. Eggs hatch and release free-swimming **nauplius** larvae that molt several times to become mature adults. However, some species undergo complete metamorphosis; the nauplius develops into a **cypris** larva (a stage similar to the pupa), and the transformed larva emerges as an adult.

Transmission of Disease

Although some insects are parasites of humans (e.g., ectoparasites including lice, mosquitoes, and ticks that feed on blood), other insects play an important role as vectors that transmit a variety of diseases. It is crucial that you understand the importance of the Arthropoda—both as ectoparasites and as potential vectors of other disease-causing microorganisms. Elimination of the vector is a commonly attempted method of disease control. Therefore, to understand proper measures of control, it is important to know which insect

TABLE 6–1 □ ARTHROPODS OF MEDICAL IMPORTANCE

Arthropod	Transmission Associations
	ORDER DIPTERA (FLIES AND MOSQUITOES)
FAMILY CULICIDAE (ALL MOSQUITOES)	
Aedes spp.	1. Viral—encephalitis, yellow fever, dengue fever, hemorrhagic fever 2. Nematoda—filariasis (*W. bancrofti*)
Anopheles spp.	1. Protozoa—malaria 2. Nematoda—filariasis (*W. bancrofti*—elephantiasis, *B. malayi*) 3. Viral—various fevers and encephalitides
Culex spp.	1. Nematoda—filariasis (*W. bancrofti*) 2. Viral—encephalitis
Mansonia spp.	1. Nematoda—filariasis (*W. bancrofti, B. malayi*) 2. Viral—various fevers
FAMILY CERATOPOGONIDAE (BITING MIDGES, PUNKIES, NO-SEE-UMS)	
Culicoides spp.	1. Nematoda—filariasis (*M. ozzardi, M. perstans, M. streptocerca*)
FAMILY SIMULIIDAE (BLACK FLIES, BUFFALO GNATS)	
Simulium spp.	1. Nematoda—filariasis (*O. volvulus, M. ozzardi*)
FAMILY PSYCHODIDAE (SANDFLY)	
Phlebotomus spp.	1. Protozoa—leishmaniasis (*Leishmania* spp.) 2. Viral—sandfly fever 3. Bacterial—*Bartonella bacilliformis*
FAMILY TABANIDAE (HORSEFLY)	
Tabanus spp.	1. Bacterial—anthrax and tularemia (*Bacillus anthracis, Francisella tularensis*) 2. Protozoa—trypanosomes (mechanical transmission)
Chrysops spp. (mango fly, deer fly)	1. Nematoda—filariasis (*Loa loa*)
FAMILY MUSCIDAE	
Musca spp. (house fly)	1. Bacterial—tularemia (*F. tularensis*) 2. Mechanical vector of many protozoan species
Stomoxys spp. (stable fly)	1. Mechanical vector of many protozoan species
Siphona spp. (horn fly)	1. Mechanical vector of many protozoan species
Glossina spp. (tsetse fly)	1. Mechanical vector of many protozoan species 2. Protozoa—trypanosomiasis (*Trypanosoma* spp.)
OTHER FLY FAMILIES	
Cochliomyia spp.	1. Myiasis—primary and secondary—screw worm
Other genera	1. Myiasis—maggots (fly larvae on skin wound), warbles (fly larvae inside tissues)

Continued on following page

TABLE 6–1 □ ARTHROPODS OF MEDICAL IMPORTANCE (Continued)

Arthropod	Transmission Associations
ORDER HEMIPTERA (BUGS)	
FAMILY REDUVIIDAE	
Triatoma spp. *Panstrongylus* spp. (kissing bugs)	1. Protozoa—visceral trypanosomiasis (*T. cruzi*)
FAMILY CIMICIDAE	
Cimex spp. (bedbugs)	1. Itchy bites
ORDER SIPHONAPTERA (FLEAS)	
FAMILY PULICIDAE	
Xenopsylla spp. (Oriental rat flea)	1. Bacterial—bubonic plague (black plague, *Yersinia pestis*) 2. Cestoda (*H. nana, H. diminuta*) 3. Rickettsial—murine typhus (*Rickettsia mooseri*)
Ctenocephalides spp. (cat or dog fleas)	1. Cestoda (*D. caninum*)
ORDER PARASITIFORMES	
FAMILY IXODIDAE (HARD TICKS)	
Dermacentor spp.	1. Tickettsial—Rocky Mountain spotted fever, Q fever (*R. rickettsii, Coxiella burnetii*) 2. Bacterial—tularemia (*F. tularensis*) 3. Viral—Colorado tick fever
Ixodes spp.	1. Protozoa—*Babesia* spp. 2. Tick fever—*R. rickettsii* 3. Viral—Colorado tick fever 4. Spirochete—Lyme disease (*Borrelia burgdorferi*)
FAMILY ARGASIDAE (SOFT TICKS)	
Ornithodoros spp.	1. Bacterial—relapsing fever (*Borrelia recurrentis*)
FAMILY SARCOPTIDAE (MITES)	
Sarcoptes spp. (mange mite)	1. Skin mange (*S. scabiei*)
FAMILY TROMBICULIDAE (MITES)	
Trombicula spp. (chigger)	1. Rickettsial—scrub typhus (*R. tsutsugamushi*)
ORDER ANOPLURA (BLOODSUCKING LICE)	
FAMILY PEDICULIDAE	
Pediculus spp. (body lice)	1. Spirochetes—louseborne relapsing fever (*B. recurrentis*) 2. Rickettsial—endemic typhus, trench fever (*R. prowazeki, R. quintana*)
Phthirus pubis (crab louse)	1. Itchy bites

Arthropod	Transmission Associations
FAMILY TRICHODECTIDAE	
Trichodectes spp. (biting lice of domestic mammals)	1. Cestoda—accidental infection *(D. caninum, H. diminuta)*
SUBCLASS COPEPODA	
Cyclops spp. (copepod, water flea)	1. Nematoda—Guinea worm (*D. medinensis*) 2. Cestoda—fish tapeworm (*D. latum*) 3. Sparganosis—*Spirometra* spp.
Diaptomus spp. (copepod, water flea)	1. Cestoda—fish tapeworm (*D. latum*)
Order Decapoda (crayfish, crab)	1. Trematoda—lung fluke (P. westermani)

species comprise an integral part of disease transmission and to understand the life cycle of the insect itself.

Mechanical Transfer

Insects can passively transfer infective organisms from feces or contaminated soil to food or utensils when they walk across or feed on inadequately protected food. This form of infective transmission is called mechanical transfer. Inadequate personal hygiene also provides a means by which a person may contract an arthropod-transmitted infection. Mechanical transfer implies that the insect is not required as part of a parasite's life cycle and that no further development or growth of the parasite occurs in the insect. This is true even if the parasite is carried inside the insect and is released in the insect's feces or is injected into the host by the biting insect.

Biological Transfer

A biological vector, by contrast, is a required part of the parasite's life cycle because growth and development of the parasite must occur inside the insect. Insects may serve as definitive or intermediate hosts. Infective parasites that develop in an insect generally are injected directly into a new host or, in a few species, are deposited on the host's skin.

Some pathogens can be passed from an adult insect to its offspring if the pathogen penetrates the insect egg(s) in utero. This is known as transovarial transmission. If the pathogen can survive in each part of the cycle (egg, nymph, adult), it has been transmitted transstadially. The term *vertical transmission,* used to describe these phenomena, means that parasites are passed from generation to generation within the same host species. Certain diseases are maintained by tick vectors via vertical transmission. For example, the tick *Ixodes scapularis* is the vector for *Babesia* spp. Merogony occurs inside the tick, and some of the merozoites invade tick eggs, causing the next generation to be infected and able to pass on the disease to humans when the tick takes a blood meal.

Insects as Parasites

In addition to mechanical or biological disease transmission, other major problems caused by insects include annoyance, delayed or immediate hypersensitivity reactions to bites (including fatal anaphylaxis), blood loss, secondary bacterial infections in open insect bite sites, and injection of toxins or venoms. Loss of food crops, loss of animal weight gain and productivity, and **myiasis** also cause profound economic losses.

Bites and Stings

Mechanical trauma is caused by a variety of insects, including bees, wasps, ants, spiders, scorpions, centipedes, and millipedes. Some people have severe allergic reactions to bee

DIAGRAM 6–1

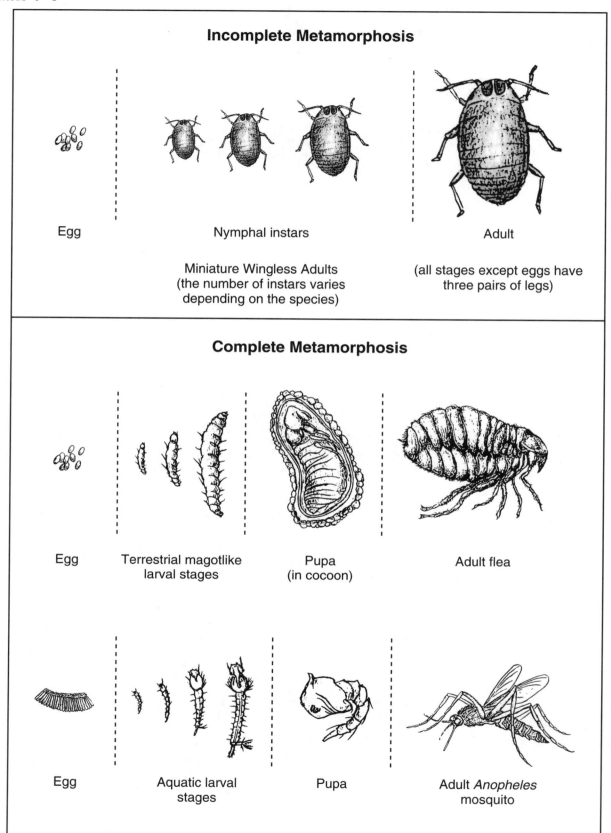

Incomplete Metamorphosis

Egg

Nymphal instars

Adult

Miniature Wingless Adults
(the number of instars varies
depending on the species)

(all stages except eggs have
three pairs of legs)

Complete Metamorphosis

Egg

Terrestrial magotlike
larval stages

Pupa
(in cocoon)

Adult flea

Egg

Aquatic larval
stages

Pupa

Adult *Anopheles*
mosquito

Life cycle of insects

and spider venoms. Bee toxins are similar to viperine snake venom because they have a he-molyzing factor; however, bee toxins also contain histamine. Allergic individuals may ex-hibit symptoms of anaphylaxis and may require antihistamine or epinephrine to stop the reaction if bronchospasm occurs. An estimated 50 to 100 people die each year from these reactions.

Wasps, hornets, and bumble bees are capable of multiple stings without losing their stinging apparatus. Honey bees can sting only once because they have a barbed stinger that detaches from the body as the bee flies away. Domestic honey bees are usually docile ex-cept when their hive is threatened, but a more aggressive honey bee known as the "African-ized" or "killer" honey bee was introduced to the Americas through Brazil in the 1950s. Since then, these bees have spread as far north as the southern United States and pose a greater threat to humans than their domestic cousins do.

Some members of the ant family Formicoidea can bite and sting humans and other animals. In the United States, harvester ants of the genus *Pogonomyrmex* and fire ants of the genus *Solenopsis* are the two groups of medical importance. At least 60,000 people are treated for fire ant bites annually. These ants defend their nests by attacking animals or hu-mans who disturb the surface mounds that top their nests. *Solenopsis invicta* is a particu-larly dangerous and prolific fire ant that was introduced into the United States in the 1930s. The fire ants are found in 16 states from Maryland to California, mainly throughout the southeast. The ant's aggressive behavior has adversely affected both wildlife and agricul-ture. Control has been difficult, and the economic impact has become significant in some locations. Farmers have had to stop farming some land because ants attack the workers and tractors cannot easily plow through 30-inch-high mounds found in the fields. Also, farm animals and wildlife suffer from attacking ants.

The two most troublesome spiders in the United States are the black widow *(La-trodectus mactans)* and the brown recluse violin spider *(Loxosceles reclusa)*. The black widow's neurotoxin rarely results in death and confers lasting immunity against future bites, but it produces severe complications, including abdominal cramps, hypertension, reduced heartbeat, feeble pulse, shock, convulsions, and delirium. Bites by the brown recluse cause painful, spreading, slow-healing necrotic wounds that require medical at-tention. Very large doses of venom can cause hemolytic anemia, fever, jaundice, hematuria, and death.

Scorpion stings are especially dangerous to children younger than 5 years of age. Symptoms resemble those of strychnine poisoning and include pain, numbness, muscle spasm, blindness, and twitching of toes and fingers. Death results from respiratory paral-ysis. Centipedes and millipedes generally are not considered dangerous, but a few centi-pedes can inflict painful bites, and some millipedes secrete a protective fluid that causes burns and brown discoloration to the skin.

Myiasis

The larvae (maggots) of nonbloodsucking flies invading tissue cause myiasis. Eggs or lar-vae may be deposited directly on skin or are transferred to the body from contaminated soil. The larvae of some fly species, however, must live in living tissue. This type of myiasis is called obligate myiasis.

Although obligate myiasis is more commonly seen in animals, humans may serve as hosts for several species. For example, the fly *Cochliomyia hominovorax* causes the disease known as primary screw worm. The fly is attracted to open wounds or nasal drainage, where it deposits its eggs. Larvae hatch in 11 to 22 hours, invade the skin, and begin feed-ing on tissue. Symptoms depend on the site of invasion; pain, swelling, and subcutaneous larval migration occur in most cases. Many other fly larvae cause similar problems world-wide, especially in children and livestock herders. Maggots of some species come out of soil at night to suck blood from a living host without burrowing into the skin. They later return to the soil. Others either invade skin lesions or penetrate unbroken tissue, where they remain and cause abscesslike lesions.

Facultative myiasis occurs when larvae enter living tissue after feeding on decaying tis-sue, such as that found in neglected wounds. The larvae need decaying tissue for food, and the myiasis in living tissue is only passive. Many filth flies are attracted to wounded, dead, or decaying animals. Nosocomial myiasis has been reported in elderly, immobile patients with open wounds. Larvae have been recovered from the ear, nose, and urogenital tract. Accidental ingestion of fly eggs or larvae may produce intestinal myiasis, resulting in various gastrointestinal symptoms.

Controlling Insects

Control of Arthropoda is difficult. Use of chemical sprays is still widespread, but it has very serious consequences for the environment and other life forms because synthetic chemicals are often carcinogenic, are nonbiodegradable, and remain in the food chain. In addition, many insecticide-resistant species of insects have evolved as a result of spraying.

Other arthropod control methods being tried include increasing natural predators (e.g., flies that lay eggs on fire ants, and hatching larvae eat the ant), destroying breeding grounds, controlling biologically (e.g., releasing artificially sterilized males, as was attempted with screw worm and fruit flies), using pheromones and other types of trap bait, introducing a faster-breeding competitive species, and removing host species on which the insect feeds. All of these methods often lead to only temporary control in local areas.

 FOR REVIEW

1. *Compare and contrast incomplete and complete metamorphosis. Give examples of insects included in each group.*

_____

2. *Compare and contrast mechanical and biological disease transmission. Give examples of each type of transmission.*

_____

3. *Explain how primary screw worm disease differs from the myiasis caused by filth flies.*

_____

4. *List three kinds of mechanical trauma caused by insects. Give examples of each type of trauma.*

_____

5. *Describe a possible type of control for each order of Arthropoda.*

_____

_____

_____

● *Insect Morphology*

Basic morphologic differences among the classes and orders of arthropods make ticks, mites, flies, mosquitoes, true bugs, lice, and fleas readily distinguishable from one another. The following section on insect morphology presents the major structural differences among the classes of medically important arthropods and provides some clinical and epidemiologic details. By studying Diagram 6–2 and the photos on pp. 153 and 154, you can review and recognize those important genera of arthropods that transmit infections to humans.

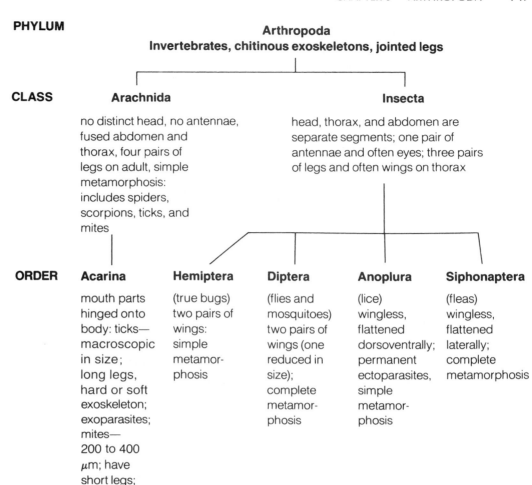

DIAGRAM 6-2

Classification of arthropods

Class Insecta

Order Diptera (Flies and Mosquitoes)

Diptera is the order of greatest medical importance; bloodsucking mosquitoes and flies may transmit many viral, protozoan, and helminthic diseases. Diptera are all ectoparasites as adults. One can differentiate among the dipteran insects by studying the characteristics of the parts listed here and by using an identification key in an **entomology** text or insect identification handbook. Examine the following:

1. Antennae—number of segments, presence or absence of hairs
2. Mouth parts—structures for piercing skin or sucking fluid
3. Coloration and hair distribution on body
4. Size and shape of the body and each of the three body segments (head, thorax, and abdomen)
5. Morphology of egg, larval, and pupal stages
6. Pattern of veins in the wings

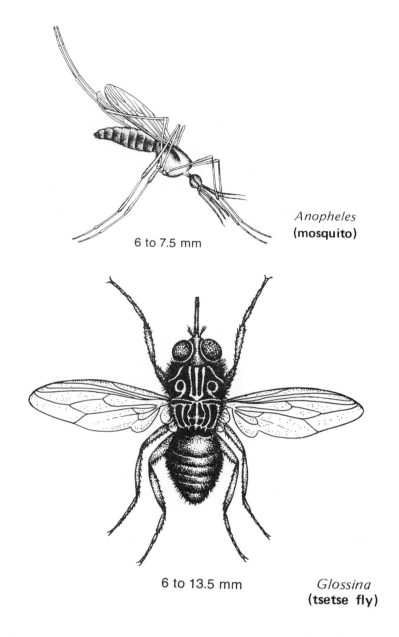

Anopheles
(mosquito)

6 to 7.5 mm

6 to 13.5 mm   *Glossina*
(tsetse fly)

OF NOTE

Because insect specimens submitted to the clinical laboratory are often in poor condition or do not exactly resemble specimens illustrated in handbooks, it may be necessary to enlist the expertise of an entomologist to obtain an accurate identification of the insect submitted.

Order Anoplura (Lice)   Lice are flattened dorsoventrally and have a three-segment body with antennae on the head and three pairs of legs extending from the middle (thorax) segment. The legs have claws on the ends for grasping body hair. Metamorphosis is simple, and the immature stages look like small adults. Lice are host specific. The lice are permanent ectoparasites and live only on the host, surviving just briefly in the environment. Eggs (nits) are deposited on hair shafts of the host. The order Anoplura includes bloodsucking lice; mouth parts are adapted for piercing the skin and sucking blood. The head is narrower than the thorax. *Phthirus pubis* (crab louse), *Pediculus humanus capitis,* and *Pediculus humanus humanus* (head and body lice, respectively) are endemic in the United States, with at least 6 to 12 million cases annually.

Lice are usually transferred directly from host to host. Eggs from louse-infested clothing or other personal articles also may be sources of infection; body lice may be acquired from sitting on cloth-covered seats in public places, such as theaters or waiting areas. Pubic lice are usually transferred via sexual intercourse, but infections may be acquired in locker rooms from towels and from mats on gymnasium floors.

Symptoms of **pediculosis** include itchy papules at the site of infestation. Saliva and fecal excretions of the louse often cause a local hypersensitivity reaction that leads to inflammation. If a secondary bacterial infection occurs, the lesion may resemble mange. Successful treatment requires that both the eggs and motile stages be killed.

During the 1996–1997 school year, approximately 80% of school districts in the United States reported at least one outbreak of head lice. Various commercial products such as Rid, Nix, Lice-Free, Clear, and AcuMed Comb can be used to treat head lice. (This list of products is not inclusive and does not constitute an endorsement by the authors for any product, supplier, or service.) However, numerous cases exhibited treatment resistance, prompting both physicians and parents to try home remedies. Home remedies include covering the hair with mayonnaise or margarine to smother the louse, followed by rinsing with a dilute vinegar solution (1:1 with water) and combing with a nit comb. Various combinations of plant oils have also been used successfully.

Another strategy being tested is the use of Ivermectin,* a drug normally used to treat roundworms. One study performed in Egypt showed that a single application of a liquid form of Ivermectin (0.8%) killed lice within 48 hours. Other studies have been favorable, but more testing is necessary before this treatment is shown to be safe and effective.

Body lice can transmit *Rickettsia* spp., causative agents of endemic typhus and trench fever. Louseborne relapsing fever caused by *Borrelia recurrentis* is also transmitted by *P. humanus humanus*. Body lice are sensitive to temperature and will leave the host who has a fever. The infected louse, which can survive in the environment for up to 1 week, will be able to infect a new host. As a result, rapid spread of disease among people in close quarters can occur. It is best to check clothing for lice because they can leave the skin when not feeding.

Treatment depends on the type of lice:

- *P. pubis:* 0.5% malathion lotion or 1% lindane
- *P. humanus capitis:* (1) permethrin, (2) pyrethrin with butoxide or 0.5% malathion or 1% lindane
- *P. humanus humanus:* regular bathing and decontamination of infested clothing by dry cleaning or washing at 50°C/122°F for 30 minutes

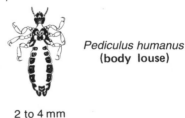

Pediculus humanus
(body louse)

2 to 4 mm

2 to 4 mm

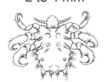

Phthirus pubis
(crab louse)

1 mm

Order Siphonaptera (Fleas)

Fleas are flattened laterally. They, too, have three pairs of clawed legs extending from the thorax; the rear pair is very long and adapted for jumping. One can differentiate the species of fleas by looking for the presence or absence of eyes and the genal and pronotal **ctenidia** (combs). Adult fleas suck blood and have mouth parts adapted for this purpose. Metamorphosis is complete; all stages develop to maturity in the external environment and are

---

*Available from the Parasitic Disease Drug Service, Centers for Disease Control and Prevention, U.S. Public Health Service, Atlanta, Georgia 30333; telephone (404) 639–3670.

on the host only for feeding. The adult flea takes a blood meal from a **temporary host** and then lays eggs in dark crevices. Treatment of a flea infestation therefore requires cleaning the environment and the host. Complete chemical control is difficult. Chemical treatment and control measures in the environment should be repeated 2 weeks later to kill larvae and adults that develop from resistant eggs.

Adult fleas may live as long as 1 year, and eggs may remain viable for even longer periods. Pet owners' homes can become flea infested. Eliminating fleas on pets and in the house is necessary to prevent further infestation. Sprays, powders, and dips have been used successfully, but continued treatment is required. A newer approach is Lufenuron, an oral preventive that is given to dogs and cats monthly. When fleas feed on the animal, the ingested chemical prevents development of eggs, thus breaking the life cycle. By following this protocol and avoiding new infestations, one can eventually eliminate fleas from the local environment.

The rat flea, *Xenopsylla cheopis*, is known to transmit *Rickettsia typhi*, the bacteria responsible for murine typhus. The rat flea is the primary vector for the causative agent of bubonic ("Black") plague, *Yersinia pestis*. Inasmuch as rats often live in colonies, fleas feed freely on various hosts. The disease is spread from rat to rat via flea bites. Infected fleas crushed on the host's body also allow the bacteria to gain entrance into the rat. Bubonic plague also can be found in squirrels and other small mammals. Management of the disease rests mainly on controlling rats and squirrels. Under suitable conditions, these bacteria may remain infective for 5 years in dried flea feces. These facts illustrate the difficulty of controlling fleas and the diseases they transmit.

As ectoparasites, fleas cause itchy bites when they feed. Repeated bites cause irritation with possible allergic reactions. Secondary bacterial invasion may also occur as itchy bites are scratched. Adult fleas usually feed several times in the same day and may move from host to host when several hosts are available. Furthermore, fleas are not very host specific. Dog and cat fleas readily take blood meals from humans. Although dog and cat fleas are not good transmitters of the plague bacillus, they can passively transmit tapeworms (*Hymenolepis nana*, *H. diminuta,* and *Dipylidium caninum*) to humans.

Ctenocephalides spp.
(flea)

1.5 to 4 mm

 FOR REVIEW

1. Discuss the various pathogens transmitted by lice. Include both mechanical problems and pathogens transmitted by these insects.

2. Compare and contrast the life cycles and methods of control of lice and fleas.

Class Arachnida

Order Acarina (Ticks and Mites)

Ticks can transmit at least one protozoal organism to humans and several bacterial, rickettsial, spirochetal, and viral organisms, as noted in Table 6–1. In fact, in the United States ticks transmit more vectorborne diseases than any other arthropod. Humans become infected with various organisms when the tick is feeding. Usually, the pathogen enters the bloodstream directly, but it may also be rubbed into a wound if the area around the wound is contaminated with tick feces. An infected tick that has been crushed while being removed from people or pets may provide an additional source of infection.

Furthermore, tick paralysis (tick-toxicosis) may occur if female ticks remain attached to susceptible hosts for at least 4 days. This lengthy attachment may occur if the tick attaches in areas such as the scalp that conceal it from view. Toxins in salivary secretions released by the tick (43 known species) affect nerve impulse transmission, causing acute ascending paralysis, which can lead to respiratory failure and death. Prompt removal of the tick usually prevents further progression of the paralysis and results in complete recovery within a few days. In some cases, epinephrine, antihistamines, or corticosteroids may be needed to arrest the process.

Tick bite wounds may become infected if mouth parts are left behind after tick removal. Ticks remain attached for extended feeding periods (for several hours or days), and the local skin reaction to the mouth parts and the tick's salivary secretions becomes inflamed and is often accompanied by edema and hemorrhage.

Adult ticks may live for 2 to 3 years or more and feed on several hosts. This longevity, coupled with the fact that most tickborne organisms may be transmitted vertically across generations (transstadial passage, transovarial passage, or both), makes them very good vectors of disease. Babesiosis is one example of a vertically transmitted disease.

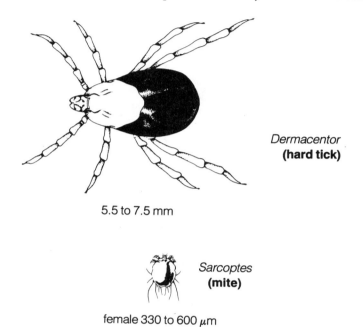

Dermacentor
(hard tick)

5.5 to 7.5 mm

Sarcoptes
(mite)

female 330 to 600 μm

The mite species *Sarcoptes scabiei* (the itch mite) causes the disease known as scabies (sarcoptic mange), which is diagnosed by finding the eggs, nymphs, or adults in skin scrapings of suspicious lesions. The diagnostic signs are red tunnels measuring from a few millimeters to several centimeters in length, which turn into extremely itchy papules. These mites have a relatively short life cycle, and newly hatched larvae within the skin reach adulthood in about 1 week. This short cycle allows infestations to become severe before treatment begins. *S. scabiei* is endemic in the United States and elsewhere.

House dust mites, *Dermatophagoides* spp., have been shown to cause house dust allergy. These mites feed on sloughed human skin cells, food particles, or other organic substances. Children are especially sensitive and may develop asthma or other respiratory symptoms. One study in Atlanta, Georgia, found that all houses inspected had dust mites and all the asthmatic children living in these houses had high titers of IgE antibody specific for *Dermatophagoides* spp. Symptoms may be aggravated when cockroach antigen is also present in the environment. Vacuum cleaning of furniture and carpets helps reduce house dust mite allergen. Frequent laundering of bedding will also aid in controlling this problem. Treatment can include pyrethrin, permethrin, 1% lindane, or 10% crotamiton.

MORPHOLOGY AND LIFE CYCLES

The mouth parts of ticks and mites are adapted for piercing and are attached directly on the body. The mouth parts are part of an anterior structure known as a **capitulum** (which should be grasped firmly with forceps when removing an embedded tick to avoid leaving mouth parts in the skin). The thorax is fused to a globular body; head and antennae are absent. The adults have four pairs of legs.

Acarid families include the following:

1. Ixodidae—a family containing the hard ticks that are temporary ectoparasites and are on the host only for feeding during larval, nymphal, and adult stages. Eggs hatch and emerging larvae migrate up blades of grass or twigs to wait for passing hosts. Larvae attach to hosts, feed for a few days, drop off, and then molt into nymphs. Nymphs will attach to new hosts, feed, return to the ground, and then molt to become adults. Adult females feed only once. After mating, eggs are laid and hatch in the environment.

   Three pathogenic organisms—*Borrelia burgdorferi* (the causative agent of Lyme disease), *Babesia microti*, and *Ehrlichia* spp. (a recently described rickettsial pathogen)—are all transmitted to humans through the bite of *Ixodes* spp. ticks. Mixed infections of *B. burgdorferi* and *B. microti* are occurring more frequently.

2. Argasidae—a family containing the soft ticks that are also temporary ectoparasites. The body of soft ticks is soft and leathery because it lacks the **scutum** found on the dorsal surface of hard ticks. With one important exception, they do not feed on humans. *Ornithodoros* spp., the vector for relapsing fever (*Borrelia* spp.) feed frequently for short periods, usually less than 30 minutes at a time. These ticks can sustain long periods (as long as 15 years) of starvation.

3. Sarcoptidae—a family containing mites that are permanent ectoparasites and live and reproduce in burrows in the skin. Mites are host specific and are usually transferred to new hosts in crowded quarters in which residents neglect personal hygiene. The morphologic characteristics of mites are similar to those in ticks except that mites are smaller and do not have a scutum. They are microscopic, and their four pairs of legs are shorter, with only the two anterior pairs extending past the margins of the body. Mites that normally infest other hosts may occasionally be temporary parasites of humans or other animals. For example, in the southern United States, *Ornithonyssus sylviarum*, a species of bird mite, migrates into homes from bird nests located in the eaves of houses. These insects attack cats, dogs, and humans, causing dermatitis, papules, vesicles, and even tissue necrosis at the bite site.

 FOR REVIEW

1. *Explain how ticks differ morphologically from other insects. Describe the life cycle of ticks.*

_____

2. *Compare and contrast the appearance of the Ixodidae and Argasidae ticks, and list the pathogens they can transmit to humans.*

_____

3. *Explain how diseases caused by mites differ from those caused by ticks.*

_____

4. *Discuss control of ticks and mites in the environment.*

_____

> **You have now completed the section on Arthropoda. After reviewing this material with the help of the learning objectives, proceed to the post-test.**

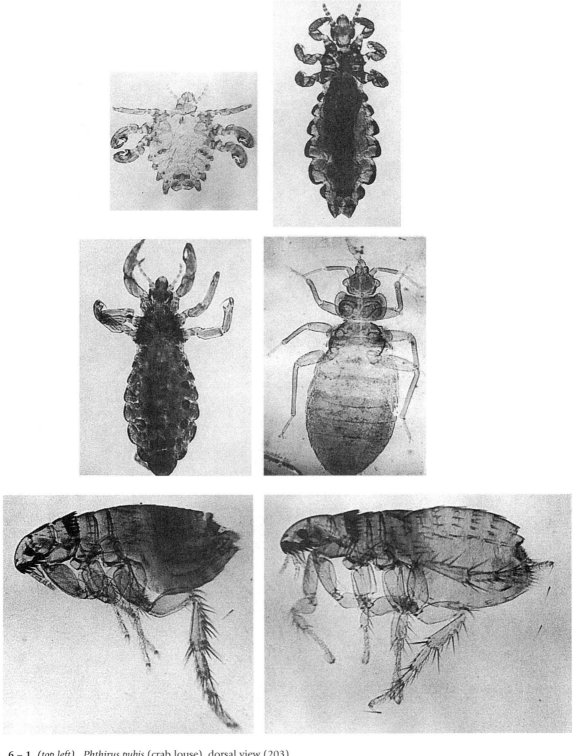

P H O T O   6 – 1 *(top left). Phthirus pubis* (crab louse), dorsal view (203).
P H O T O   6 – 2 *(top right). Pediculus corporis* (body louse), dorsal view (153).
P H O T O   6 – 3 *(middle left). Pediculus capitis* (head louse), dorsal view (203).
P H O T O   6 – 4 *(middle right). Cimex lectularius* (bedbug), dorsal view (203).
P H O T O   6 – 5 *(bottom left). Ctenocephalides* spp. (male dog or cat flea), lateral view (153).
P H O T O   6 – 6 *(bottom right). Ctenocephalides* spp. (female dog or cat flea), lateral view (153).

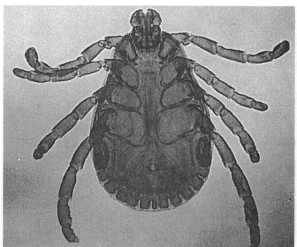
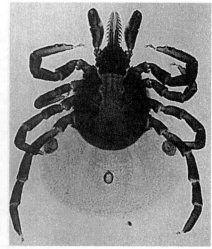
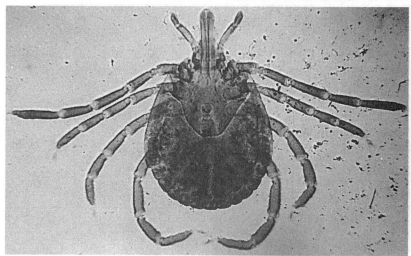
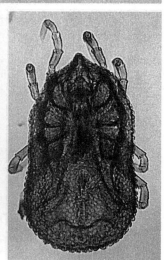
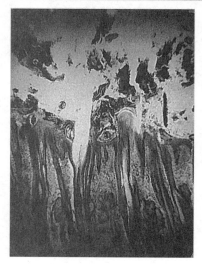

PHOTO 6–7 *(top left).* *Dermacentor andersoni* (hard tick), ventral view (103).
PHOTO 6–8 *(top right).* *Ixodes* spp. (hard tick), dorsal view (203).
PHOTO 6–9 *(middle left).* *Amblyomma americanum* (hard tick), dorsal view (103).
PHOTO 6–10 *(middle right).* *Ornithodoros* spp. (soft tick), ventral view (103).
PHOTO 6–11 *(bottom).* *Sarcoptes scabiei* (scabies in skin scraping) (403).

Word Puzzles

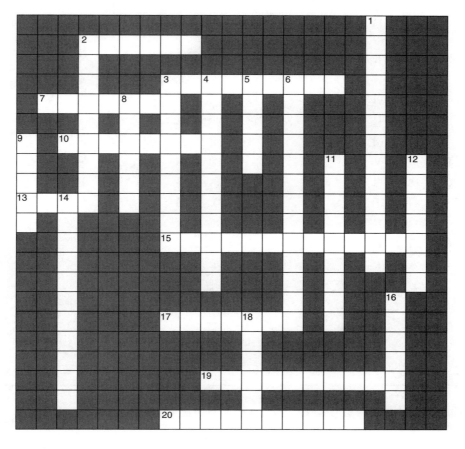

Across

2. Hard, insoluble polysaccharide; the main compound in shells of crabs and exoskeletons of insects
3. Comblike process found on the head region of fleas
7. Class in the phylum Arthropoda; includes many insect types; bodies divided into three regions—head, thorax, and abdomen
10. The earliest and youngest larval form in the life cycle of crustaceans
13. The encased resting stage between the larva and imago stage (e.g., cocoon)
15. A change of shape or structure; a transition from one developmental stage to another
17. The molting or shedding of an outer layer or covering and the development of a new one
19. Phylum composed of organisms having a hard, segmented exoskeleton and paired, jointed legs
20. The branch of zoology dealing with the study of insects

Down

1. A host on which an arthropod (adult or larval form) resides temporarily in order to feed on blood or tissue (2 words)
2. Class in the phylum Arthropoda; includes crabs, water fleas, lobsters, and shrimps
3. Term referring to the mouth parts of ticks and mites that extend forward from the body
4. A hard, chitinous structure on the outside of the body; provides support and protection for internal organs
5. The sexually mature adult insect or arachnid
6. Animals having no spinal column
8. Larval resting stage in the life cycle of some crustaceans in which a metamorphosis occurs
9. A developmental stage in the life cycle of certain arthropods that resembles a small adult
11. Class in the phylum Arthropoda; includes ticks, mites, spiders, and scorpions
12. A condition caused by infestation of the body with fly larvae
14. Infestation with lice
16. Any one of the nymphal or larval stages between molts
18. A chitinous shield or plate covering part (female) or all (male) of the dorsal surface of hard ticks

```
H   W   A   Y   F   K   U   P   N   I   T   I   H   C   B   V   O   C   N   M
A   R   R   A   S   U   I   L   P   U   A   N   T   V   I   V   S   A   S   X
G   F   T   Q   M   U   L   U   T   I   P   A   C   H   B   I   O   K   E   I
A   O   H   W   D   O   I   N   Z   W   L   I   P   M   S   C   N   M   T   P
E   T   R   N   D   A   I   I   A   H   K   M   M   A   V   Z   R   C   A   R
C   Y   O   Y   G   H   P   J   F   R   Y   R   I   A   Z   V   A   N   R   E
A   F   P   Q   E   G   N   U   L   N   A   Y   B   I   G   V   T   V   B   J
T   N   O   T   H   R   H   T   P   C   M   C   P   C   H   O   S   E   E   N
S   F   D   T   E   M   P   O   R   A   R   Y   H   O   S   T   N   Q   T   I
U   O   A   R   P   V   D   K   O   P   U   G   D   N   S   T   I   J   R   M
R   W   A   U   M   U   T   U   C   S   K   I   I   H   I   K   C   G   E   J
C   S   F   F   N   I   J   F   R   G   V   U   L   F   Q   D   L   G   V   N
F   W   W   Q   Q   N   O   T   E   L   E   K   S   O   X   E   A   D   N   I
O   A   T   C   E   S   N   I   C   M   B   O   W   D   X   V   S   B   I   A
L   D   J   L   K   P   Y   Y   J   K   P   A   R   G   C   Y   P   R   I   S
S   I   S   O   H   P   R   O   M   A   T   E   M   N   E   H   Q   V   P   F
D   D   C   F   X   U   X   M   A   S   I   S   Y   D   C   E   T   B   C   E
A   M   B   Q   I   G   A   K   G   B   G   M   U   I   D   I   N   E   T   C
M   D   D   W   Q   D   O   E   N   T   O   M   O   L   O   G   Y   V   C   T
B   U   W   J   D   C   S   I   S   O   L   U   C   I   D   E   P   Z   I   H
```

arachnida	cypris	instar	pediculosis
arthropoda	ecdysis	invertebrates	pupa
capitulum	entomology	metamorphosis	scutum
chitin	exoskeleton	myiasis	temporary host
crustacea	imago	nauplius	
ctenidium	insecta	nymph	

Post-Test

1. Matching: Enter the single best number choice for parasite transmission: **(20 points)**

   a. _____ *Aedes*   1. *Onchocerca volvulus*
   b. _____ *Anopheles*   2. *Trypanosoma gambiense*
   c. _____ *Simulium*   3. *Leishmania donovani*
   d. _____ *Phlebotomus*   4. *Giardia lamblia*
   e. _____ *Glossina*   5. *Brugia malayi*
                              6. *Plasmodium vivax*

2. Indicate the type of Arthropoda that causes each of the following conditions or transmits the causative agent for the listed diseases. Use each number as many times as appropriate. **(30 points)**

   a. _____ Myiasis   1. Bug (hemipteran)
   b. _____ Blood loss   2. Mosquito
   c. _____ Crabs   3. Tick
   d. _____ Scabies   4. Louse
   e. _____ Sleeping sickness   5. Fly
   f. _____ Babesiosis   6. Mite
   g. _____ Rocky Mountain   7. Flea
            spotted fever
   h. _____ Chagas' disease
   i. _____ The Black plague
   j. _____ Malaria

3. Based on your knowledge of the life cycle of fleas and lice, discuss control measures necessary to prevent the spread of each. **(10 points)**

4. State at least five ways in which Arthropoda are harmful to humans. **(10 points)**

*Each multiple-choice question is worth **2 points**.*

5. The arthropod vector associated with the transmission of the fish tapeworm is:
   a. *Aedes* spp.
   b. *Simulium* spp.
   c. *Phlebotomus* spp.
   d. *Cyclops* spp.
   e. *Pediculus* spp.

6. Obligate myiasis is associated with:
   a. *Triatoma* spp.
   b. *Cochliomyia* spp.
   c. *Cyclops* spp.
   d. *Glossina* spp.
   e. *Pediculus* spp.

7. The organism responsible for Lyme disease is transmitted to humans by:
   a. *Ixodes* spp.
   b. *Dermacentor* spp.
   c. *Borrelia burgdorferi*
   d. *Mansonia* spp.
   e. *Phthirus pubis*

8. The nematode *Loa loa* is transmitted to humans by:
   a. *Triatoma* spp.
   b. *Sarcoptes* spp.
   c. *Musca* spp.
   d. *Mansonia* spp.
   e. *Chrysops* spp.

9. The mange mite is a:
   a. *Ornithodoros* spp.
   b. *Pediculus* spp.
   c. *Sarcoptes* spp.
   d. *Trichodectes* spp.
   e. *Trombicula* spp.

10. The developmental stage *not* found in holometabolous metamorphosis is the:
    a. Egg
    b. Larva
    c. Imago
    d. Nymph
    e. Pupa

11. The free-swimming larval form found in the crustacean life cycle is called the:
    a. Cypris
    b. Imago
    c. Nauplius
    d. Nymph

12. *Babesia* spp., transmitted by a tick, is maintained in the tick population by:
    a. Lateral transmission
    b. Mechanical transmission
    c. Transmytotic transmission
    d. Vertical transmission

13. Fly larvae were recovered from an open wound on the arm of a nursing home patient. This finding is called:
    a. Facultative myiasis
    b. Intestinal myiasis
    c. Mechanical myiasis
    d. Obligate myiasis

14. Pediculosis is caused by:

    a. Fleas
    b. Lice
    c. Scorpions
    d. Ticks

15. The family that contains hard ticks is:

    a. Arachnida
    b. Argasidae
    c. Ixodidae
    d. Sarcoptidae

16. *Yersinia pestis* is transmitted by:

    a. *Dermacentor* spp.
    b. *Pediculus* spp.
    c. *Sarcoptes scabiei*
    d. *Xenopsylla* spp.

17. A larva was removed from a bedridden hospital patient's nose. This condition is referred to as:

    a. Mechanical transmission
    b. Nosocomial myiasis
    c. Primary screw worm disease
    d. None of these

18. The mite associated with asthma and respiratory symptoms is:

    a. *Cimex* spp.
    b. *Dermatophagoides* spp.
    c. *Sarcoptes* spp.
    d. *Trombicula* spp.

19. An 8-year-old girl with respiratory symptoms comes to the emergency department. Her mother tells the physician that her daughter has been more clumsy than usual over the past 3 days. On physical examination, an engorged tick is found on the child's neck. Her temperature is 37°C, and her complete blood count levels are normal. These symptoms suggest that the child has:

    a. Babesiosis
    b. Colorado tick fever
    c. Lyme disease
    d. Tick paralysis

BIBLIOGRAPHY

Alexander, JOD: Mites and skin diseases. Clin Med 79:14, 1972.
Alexander, JOD: Arthropods and Human Skin: Berlin, Springer-Verlag, 1984.
Baker, EW, et al: A Manual of Parasitic Mites of Medical or Economic Importance. National Pest Control Association Technical Publication, New York, 1956.
Barnes, RD: Invertebrate Zoology, ed 3. WB Saunders, Philadelphia, 1974.
Beaver, PC, and Jung, RC: Animal Agents and Vectors of Human Disease, ed 5. Lea & Febiger, Philadelphia, 1985.
Borror, DJ, et al: An Introduction to the Study of Insects, ed 4. Holt, Rinehart & Winston, New York, 1976.
Brown, HW, and Neva, FA: Basic Clinical Parasitology, ed 5. Appleton-Century-Crofts, New York, 1983.
Burgess, I: Sarcoptes scabiei and scabies. Adv Parasitol 33:235–292, 1994.
Centers for Disease Control and Prevention. Tick paralysis—Washington, 1995. Morb Mortal Wkly Rep 45:325–326, 1996.
Davies, JE, et al: Agromedical approach to pesticide management. Annu Rev Entomol 23:353, 1978.
Donabedian, H, Khazan, U: Norwegian scabies in a patient with AIDS. Clin Infect Dis 14(1):162–164, 1992.
Elgart, ML: Scabies. Dermatol Clin 8(2):257–263, 1990.
Fain, A: The pentastomida parasitic in man. Ann Soc Belg Med Trop 55:59, 1975.
Faust, EC, et al: Animal Agents and Vectors of Human Disease, ed 4. Lea & Febiger, Philadelphia, 1975.
Fleas of Public Health Importance and Their Control. CDC-DHEW Publication, U.S. Government Printing Office, Washington, DC, 1973.
Forsman, KE.: Pediculosis and scabies. What to look for in patients who are crawling with clues. Postgrad Med 98(6):89–100, 1995.
Goddard, J: Physician's Guide to Arthropods of Medical Importance, ed. 2. CRC Press, Boca Raton, FL, 1996.
Haag, ML, et al: Attack of the scabies: What to do when an outbreak occurs. Geriatrics 48:45–53, 1993.

Harves, AD, and Millikan, LE: Current concepts of therapy and pathophysiology in arthropod bites and stings, part 2. Insects: Review. Int J Dermatol 14:621, 1975.
Horen, PW: Insect and scorpion stings. JAMA 221:894, 1972.
Introduction to the Epidemiology of Vector-Borne Diseases, CDC-DHEW Publication, U.S. Government Printing Office, Washington, DC, 1947.
James, MT: The Flies That Cause Myiasis in Man. Miscellaneous Publication No. 631, U.S. Government Printing Office, Washington, DC, 1960.
James, MT, and Harwood, RF: Hermes' Medical Entomology, ed 6. Macmillan, New York, 1969.
Lane, AT: Scabies and head lice. Pediatr Ann 16:51–54, 1987.
Lane, RP, and Crosskey, RW: Medical Insects and Arthropods, Chapman & Hall, London, 1993.
Lice of Public Health Importance and Their Control. CDC-DHEW Publication, U.S. Government Printing Office, Washington, DC, 1973.
Meinking, TL, et al. The treatment of scabies with ivermectin. N Engl J Med, 333:26–30, 1995.
National Communicable Disease Center. Pictorial Keys: Arthropods, Reptiles, Birds, and Mammals of Public Health Significance. Communicable Disease Center, Atlanta, 1969.
National Institute of Allergy and Infectious Diseases. NIAID Fact Sheet: Tick-Borne Diseases: An Overview for Physicians, June 1996.
Nicholls, PH: When your resident has scabies. Geriatr Nurs 15(5): 271–273, 1994.
Orkin, J, et al: Scabies and Pediculosis. JB Lippincott, Philadelphia, 1977.
Orlin, M, and Maibach, HI (eds): Cutaneous Infestations and Insect Bites. Marcel Dekker, New York, 1985.
Pest Control: An Assessment of Present and Alternative Technologies, Vol V. Pest Control and Health. Environmental Studies Board, National Research Council, National Academy of Science, Washington, DC, 1976.
Rasmussen, JE: Scabies. Pediatr Rev 110–114, 1994.
Ruppert, EE, and Barnes, RD: Invertebrate Zoology, ed 6. Saunders College Publishing, Philadelphia, 1994.

Smart, J: A Handbook for the Identification of Insects of Medical Importance. British Museum, London, 1956.

Smith, KGV (ed): Insects and Other Arthropods of Medical Importance. British Museum (Natural History), London, 1973.

Sonenshine, DE: Biology of Ticks, Vol 2. Oxford University Press, New York, 1994.

Spach, DH, et al: Tick-Borne Diseases in the United States. N Engl J Med 329:936, 1993.

Steere, AC, et al: Erythema chronicum migrans and Lyme arthritis: Epidemiologic evidence for a tick vector. Am J Epidemiol 108:312, 1978.

Taplin, D, Meinking, TL: Scabies, lice, and fungal infections. Prim Care 16(3):551–576, 1989.

Ticks of Public Health Importance and Their Control. CDC-DHEW Publication, U.S. Government Printing Office, Washington, DC, 1974.

Youssef MYM, et al. Topical application of ivermectin for human ectoparasites. Am J Trop Med Hyg 53:652–653, 1995.

Zumpt, F: Myiasis in Man and Animals in the Old World: A Textbook for Physicians, Veterinarians, and Zoologists. Butterworth, London, 1965.

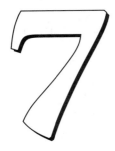

CLINICAL LABORATORY PROCEDURES

ON COMPLETION OF THIS TEXT AND SUFFICIENT EXPERIENCE IN A CLINICAL LABORATORY, THE STUDENT WILL BE ABLE TO:

1 Recognize potential sources of error in laboratory procedures.

2 Recognize and sketch the important morphologic features of parasites present in clinical specimens that are routinely examined microscopically.

3 Calibrate and correctly use an ocular micrometer to measure parasites.

4 Demonstrate the proper technique for handling and disposing of contaminated materials.

5 State the proper procedures for collection and transport of fecal specimens.

6 Select proper procedures for performing a routine fecal examination to detect the presence of parasites.

7 Properly prepare fecal smears.

8 Properly prepare iodine-stained and unstained wet mounts of fecal material.

9 Correctly perform the trichrome stain on fecal material.

10 Properly scan a microscope slide (wet mount or permanently stained) for the presence of parasites, and identify by the scientific name, when possible, any parasites found therein.

11 Select the appropriate concentration technique for the recovery of any given parasite.

12 Correctly perform the zinc sulfate flotation and the formalin-ethyl acetate sedimentation concentration techniques for recovery of intestinal parasites.

13 Correctly prepare thin and thick blood smears.

14 Correctly perform the Giemsa staining technique for blood smears.

15 Identify parasites in a stained blood smear.

16 Select proper procedures and use the proper protocol for the identification of filarial infections.

17 Identify parasites present on a cellophane tape preparation for pinworms.

18 Name the media that may be used for in vitro cultures of protozoa.

19 Prepare all solutions used routinely in the laboratory.

20 Prepare serum for parasite serology.

21 List the types and principles of serologic tests used in the diagnosis of parasitic infections, including commercially available reagents and procedures offered through the Centers for Disease Control and Prevention (CDC) reference laboratories.

22 Demonstrate correct procedures and protocol for quality-control (QC) measures.

● *Introduction*

This chapter explains, in detail, the various diagnostic procedures performed in a clinical laboratory to recover and identify parasites. These techniques provide the information used by the physician to treat and manage patients with parasitic diseases. Topics include the following:

1. Specimen collection and worker safety
2. The routine fecal examination (ova and parasites)
   a. Macroscopic examination
   b. Microscopic examination

      Direct wet mount
      Ocular micrometer calibration

   c. Fecal concentration procedures

      Sedimentation method
      Flotation method

   c. Permanent staining procedures

      Trichrome stain
      Iron hematoxylin stain

3. Other diagnostic procedures
   a. Cellophane tape test for pinworm disease
   b. Modified acid-fast stain
   c. Giemsa or other stain for blood smears
   d. Knott technique
   e. Culture media
4. Immunodiagnostic methods

Reagent preparation and tables listing some vendors of supplies and reagents and contacts for information relating to parasitology are included.

● *Specimen Transport Procedures*

Many laboratories in small hospitals, private clinics, or physicians' offices do not routinely perform examinations for ova and parasites; instead, they send specimens to larger laboratories. Successful diagnosis of intestinal parasitic diseases requires "fresh" stool specimens. Therefore, when examinations must be delayed, it is important to preserve the integrity of the specimen by placing it in a proper transport medium either immediately after passage by the patient using a collection kit or as soon as the specimen arrives in the laboratory.

A two-vial system is currently accepted as a standard means of transport. One vial should contain 8 to 10 mL of polyvinyl alcohol (PVA) fixative,* and a second vial should contain 8 to 10 mL of 10% formalin. Added to this are 2 to 3 mL of feces (most systems have fill lines marked on the vial). Be sure to select appropriate (e.g., bloody, slimy, watery) specimen areas. Sample material should be taken from the outer edge, ends, and middle of formed stools. One must thoroughly break up and mix the sample using applicator sticks. The vial should be capped tightly. The specimen is now ready for transport.

NOTE: Single-vial systems are available (see Table 7–5, p. 188). These systems offer the advantages that most procedures, including many immunoassays, can be performed from one vial and no mercury compounds are included in the formulation. The disadvantage of these systems is that staining characteristics of protozoa are not consistent. It is important to verify with the manufacturer the capabilities of the system to ensure that no formula ingredients will interfere with any procedures performed in the laboratory. Table 7–1 summarizes the advantages and disadvantages of commonly used preservatives.

The receiving laboratory then processes the sample. Smears for trichrome* or other staining should be made from the PVA tube. Direct wet mounts made from the 10% formalin vial can be examined, and either tube may be used as source material for the for-

---

*Methods of preparation of reagents noted in this chapter and marked by asterisks are described on pages 186 to 192.

TABLE 7–1 □ GENERAL PRESERVATIVES FOR STOOL SPECIMENS

Preservative	Advantages	Disadvantages
10% Formalin	1. All-purpose fixative 2. Easy to prepare 3. Long shelf life 4. Good preservation of morphology of helminth eggs, larvae, protozoan cysts 5. Suitable for concentration procedures 6. Suitable for acid-fast, safranin, and chromotrope stains 7. Compatible with immunoassay kits	1. Not suitable for some permanent stained smears such as trichrome 2. Inadequate preservation of morphology of protozoan trophozoites 3. Can interfere with polymerase chain reaction (PCR), especially after extended fixation time
MIF (merthiolate-iodine-formaldehyde)	1. Components both fix and stain organisms 2. Easy to prepare 3. Long shelf life 4. Useful for field surveys 5. Suitable for concentration procedures	1. Not suitable for some permanent stained smears such as trichrome 2. Inadequate preservation of morphology of protozoan trophozoites 3. Iodine interferes with other stains and fluorescence 4. Iodine may cause distortion of protozoa
PVA (polyvinyl-alcohol)	1. Good preservation of morphology of protozoan trophozoites and cysts 2. Easy preparation of permanent stained smears such as trichrome (solution both preserves organisms and makes them adhere to slides) 3. Preserved samples remain stable for several months	1. Inadequate preservation of morphology of helminth eggs and larvae, coccidia, microsporidia 2. Contains mercuric chloride 3. Difficult to prepare in the laboratory 4. Less suitable for concentration procedures 5. Cannot be used with immunoassay kits 6. Not suitable for acid-fast, safranin, and chromotrope stains
SAF (sodium acetate-acetic acid-formalin)	1. Suitable for both concentration procedures and preparation of permanent stained smears 2. Easy to prepare 3. Long shelf life 4. Suitable for acid-fast, safranin, and chromotrope stains 5. Compatible with immunoassay kits	1. Requires additive (e.g., albumin-glycerin) for adhesion of specimens to slides 2. Permanent stains not as good as with PVA or Schaudinn solution
Schaudinn solution	1. Good preservation of morphology of protozoan trophozoites and cysts 2. Easy preparation of permanent stained smears	1. Less suitable for concentration procedures 2. Contains mercuric chloride 3. Inadequate preservation of morphology of helminth eggs and larvae, coccidia, Microsporidia 4. Poor adhesion of liquid or mucoid specimens to slides

Adapted from Department of Parasitic Disease (CDC) material.

malin-ethyl acetate concentration method. The zinc sulfate flotation method can be performed using the 10% formalin vial.

● *Fecal Examination*

General considerations for a routine fecal examination in the clinical laboratory include the following:

1. Naturally passed stools are preferred for examination. Specimens can be passed into a clean, wide-mouthed cardboard container or a bedpan. Samples collected in a bedpan must not be contaminated with urine and must be promptly transferred to an appropriate container before being submitted to the laboratory. All specimen containers must be correctly and completely labeled. A single label should be attached to the side of the container (not the lid alone), or both the lid and container may be labeled. Necessary information includes the following:
   a. Patient's full name (last, first, middle initial; no abbreviations)
   b. Hospital or other identification number
   c. Attending physician's name
   d. Date and time of collection
   e. Time of specimen arrival in the laboratory
   Because specimens may also be infected with other pathogens such as viruses, fungi, or bacteria, it is best to place all specimen containers in plastic zipper-locking bags before delivering them to the laboratory so that all workers handling the samples are adequately protected from infective agents. Protocols for handling infectious materials must be followed at all times.
2. For a routine parasitic workup, it is recommended that patients submit stools from three normal bowel movements, one every other day, or within a 10-day period.

NOTE: One or two specimens are often sufficient for the recovery and identification of helminth eggs.

3. Fresh specimens should be processed according to the following time guideline:
   a. Liquid stool within 30 minutes
   b. Semisolid stool within 1 hour
   c. Formed stool within 24 hours of collection
   Formed stools may be refrigerated for 1 to 2 days if their examination must be delayed, although this practice does not guarantee the recovery of all parasites. Hookworm eggs mature and hatch if allowed to remain at room temperature, and they may be confused with *Strongyloides* larvae unless carefully observed. (See also p. 162 for preservation materials and transport procedures.)
4. Protozoan cysts may be found more commonly than trophozoites in formed stools and are often easier to identify than trophozoites. Trophozoites are found more commonly in liquid stools. Because trophozoites do not survive long, all specimens must be examined in a timely manner. For this reason, it is important to require and verify collection and arrival times for all fecal specimens; otherwise, reported results may be invalid. If transportation to the laboratory or examination is to be delayed, part of the specimen should be preserved, when collected, in PVA-fixative* or in 10% aqueous formalin.* Formalin preserves eggs, cysts, and larvae for wet-mount examination and for concentration. PVA-fixative preserves cysts and trophozoites for permanent staining.
5. When amebiasis or giardiasis is suspected, several specimens (at least three) should be examined, one every other day. Additional specimens are examined when necessary. For each specimen received, a direct wet mount (fresh liquid or soft stool only), a fecal concentration technique, and a permanently stained smear should be prepared and examined. Purged specimens must be examined immediately or they are worthless. Saline purges using Epsom salt, sodium sulfate, or Fleet Phospho-Soda are satisfactory, but castor oil, mineral oil, and suppositories make examination for protozoa impossible. Although using purged specimens increases the probability of recovering trophozoites, proper facilities for collection and examination must be available. These conditions make this procedure impractical for routine use.

6. Feces containing x-ray contrast media such as barium salts should be rejected because they make a proper examination impossible. If barium salts have been given, it is necessary to wait from 5 to 10 days before submitting a specimen for parasitic examination.

7. All specimens for parasitic studies should be collected before beginning treatment with any antibiotics. If antibiotics have been given, new fecal collections should not begin until 2 weeks after therapy has ended.

8. For growth of *Entamoeba histolytica*, culture media such as Balamuth, Boeck and Drbohlav, McQuay, or Cleveland-Collier may be useful. The techniques are time-consuming, and success depends on knowledge and experience with the technique. These media cannot differentiate *E. histolytica* from *Entamoeba dispar*. For these reasons, culture techniques should be used only in laboratories that have sufficient volume to justify maintaining the procedure. Various authorities express conflicting views on the relative usefulness of culture media, inasmuch as the number of cysts needed for viable cultures may be so great that they should be detectable in feces at that number by ordinary microscopic methods.

9. The Occupational Safety and Health Administration's (OSHA) Final Rule on Bloodborne Pathogens requires all laboratories to be in compliance. In part, the rule states that: "The standard for reducing worker exposure to bloodborne pathogens is based on the adoption of Universal Precautions as a method of infection control. *Universal precautions* is defined as a method of infection control in which all human blood and certain body fluids are treated as if known to be infectious for HIV, HBV, and other bloodborne pathogens."[†] Although the rule does not specifically refer to parasitic diseases found in other body locations, the same procedures needed to protect a worker from bloodborne pathogens provide protection from virtually all infectious agents.

   From other information presented in the OSHA ruling, the following specific safety guidelines are suggested:

   a. Gloves and a protective coat or apron must be worn when handling feces or other specimens.

   b. Hands should be washed with disinfectant soap on entering and leaving the laboratory and after removing gloves.

   c. Laboratory garments (including gloves) should never be worn outside the laboratory.

   d. Nothing should be placed in the mouth when in the laboratory.

   e. Avoid touching your face with your hands, and do not place personal articles, such as eyeglasses, clothing, or books, on the workbench.

   f. Care should be taken to maintain all working space in a neat and clean condition. The workbench should be cleaned before and after each work period with disinfectant such as 2.5% Amphyl (soap, *o*-phenylphenol, and alcohol) or a 50% bleach solution made with water and commercial bleach.

   g. All contaminated materials should immediately be placed in a disinfectant or other appropriate container for disposal.

   h. Spills should be overlaid with Amphyl or a 50% commercial bleach solution and absorbent towels or sand. After 10 minutes, the contaminated material should be disposed in a plastic biohazard bag or other suitable container.

   i. If spills create aerosols, especially from a centrifuge accident, all personnel should leave the laboratory at once and remain away for 1 hour. The person responsible for cleaning up the spill should wear protective clothing, gloves, and a mask.

Macroscopic Examination

The process of macroscopic examination, a routine component of a fecal examination for parasites, involves the following procedures:

1. Note the consistency of the specimen. Mushy or liquid stools suggest possible trophozoites of intestinal protozoa. Protozoan cysts are found more frequently in formed stools. Helminth eggs and larvae may be found in either liquid or formed stools.

[†]The OSHA Bloodborne Pathogens Standard is available from the Government Printing Office (GPO Order #069-001-0004-8), Superintendent of Documents, Washington, DC 20402.

2. Examine the surface (top and bottom) of the specimen for parasites (e.g., tapeworm proglottids or, less commonly, adult pinworms).
3. Break up the stool with applicator sticks to check for the presence of adult helminths (e.g., *Ascaris*).
4. Examine the stool for blood, mucus, or both.
   a. Fresh blood (bright red) indicates acute lower intestinal tract bleeding.
   b. Bloody mucus suggests ulceration, and some of this material should be preferentially examined microscopically for trophozoites.
5. Sieve feces after drug treatment for tapeworms to ensure recovery of the scolex. Current therapies have greatly reduced the need for this procedure.

Of Note

1. Adult worms, if recovered, are examined and identified directly.
2. Tapeworms are differentiated by examining gravid proglottids. Because eggs of *Taenia solium* are infective for humans, great care must be exercised when handling these specimens. When examining a gravid proglottid, it should be fixed in 10% formalin (eggs within the uterine structures are still viable) and then cleared by immersing it in glycerin or lactophenol solution (1:1). Uterine branches may be made more visible by injecting a small amount of India ink into the uterine or genital pore. A 1-mL syringe with a 25-gauge needle should be used to inject the ink. The segment should then be flattened by gently pressing it between two glass slides.

Microscopic Examination

The routine microscopic examination of fecal specimens for ova and parasites consists of three distinct procedures. These include a direct saline wet mount, a fecal concentration technique, and a permanently stained fecal smear. The direct wet mount is a rapid-screening technique and is used to study trophozoite motility. The concentration method increases the chance for recovering parasitic forms. The various staining procedures are used to study and confirm the identity of small parasites, such as protozoa, by staining intracellular organelles. Each of these procedures is described in the following sections.

Direct Wet Mount

Direct wet mounts, using fresh stool only, are prepared by using an applicator stick to thoroughly mix a small amount of feces with a drop of saline placed on a microscope slide. To perform, one should apply a 22-mm cover glass so that air bubbles are not trapped under the glass. A smear should be thin enough that a printed page can be read through it. The entire preparation should be examined for the presence of eggs, larvae, and protozoa. Systematic examination, using the 10× lens, may be accomplished by starting at the lower edge of the slide and observing each field until reaching the upper edge (Diagram 7–1).

DIAGRAM 7–1

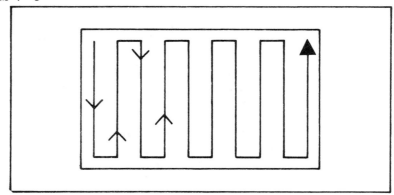

The preparation is then moved one field to the right while continuing to examine each field and moving downward until reaching the lower edge. The examiner should move right one field and repeat in this manner until the entire slide has been examined. Next, at least one-third of cover-slipped area should be examined randomly using the high dry objective lens because protozoa may have been overlooked at 10× magnification.

Care must be used when adjusting the light on the microscope. A common error is the use of too much light, which prevents proper contrast. Because protozoa are translucent and colorless when unstained, they are not visible unless the light is reduced. A drop of iodine* may be used to help demonstrate eggs and cyst structures more clearly, but this kills and distorts trophozoites so that motility cannot be observed. A saline mount and an iodine mount can be prepared at opposite ends of the same slide, using separate coverslips.

RESULTS AND REPORT FOR DIRECT WET MOUNTS

1. Any observed parasites are reported by their scientific name, including both the genus and species names when possible, and the specific stage (e.g., eggs, trophozoites, larvae) seen.
2. Certain cellular elements, such as blood cells or yeast, and *Blastocystis hominis* should be reported semiquantitatively as few, moderate, or many red blood cells (RBCs), white blood cells (WBCs), yeast, or other cells if they are clearly identifiable. *Trichuris trichiura* and trematode infections should also be quantitated in this manner.
3. Charcot-Leyden crystals may be reported semiquantitatively as few, moderate, or many.

QUALITY-CONTROL CONSIDERATIONS

1. Verify weekly that the iodine solution is clear and not contaminated with bacteria or fungi and that it has the dark brown color of strong tea.
2. Positive control material can be prepared by adding fixed human buffy coat cells to negative stool specimens. The cytoplasm of WBCs has a yellow-gold color, similar to that of protozoan trophozoites. A preserved known-positive fecal specimen can also be used for QC. The control specimen should be examined at least quarterly or whenever new stain is prepared.
3. The ocular micrometer and microscope should be calibrated at least annually when the microscope is used heavily or when it is moved frequently. Yearly recalibration may not be necessary if the microscope is used infrequently; however, if in doubt, recalibrate.
4. QC results should be recorded, and the action plan for "out-of-control" results should be followed if needed.
5. The laboratory name should be on the report.

Of Note

1. Many artifacts and other formed structures can be seen when examining a wet mount. These include RBCs, WBCs, macrophages, mucosal epithelium, yeast, undigested vegetable cells, pollen grains, and hair. To the untrained eye, any of these may be mistaken for parasites. It is important to become familiar with these artifacts.
2. Eosinophils may be present, indicating an allergic immune response that may be related to a parasitic infection or to another allergen, such as pollen or food. Breakdown products of degenerating eosinophils form Charcot-Leyden crystals, which appear as slender crystals with pointed ends. These stain red-purple with trichrome stain. Their presence indicates that an allergic immune response has occurred.
3. Free-living amoeba, flagellates, or even ciliates may be found in specimens that have been contaminated with water from sewage, stagnant ponds, or soil. These organisms may be difficult to differentiate from pathogens.
4. Wet mounts for screening can also be made from fecal specimens preserved in formalin or PVA, but no motility of organisms will be present, and this step can be omitted if a preserved specimen is the only specimen received.

Ocular Micrometer Calibration

Whenever a microscopic examination is performed, a calibrated ocular micrometer should be used because size differences of various internal structures and of whole organisms are important in a differential diagnosis. Artifacts and other fecal debris can resemble parasites; these can often be excluded based on their size.

PROCEDURE

1. Install an ocular micrometer disk in the eyepiece of the microscope by placing it underneath the eyepiece lens.
2. Place a stage micrometer on the microscope's stage and, using the 10× objective, focus on the stage scale. The stage scale is 1 mm long (some brands have different lengths) and is calibrated in hundredths (each 0.01 mm = 10 μm).

3. Line up the left edge of the ocular scale with the left edge of the stage scale (Diagram 7–2).

DIAGRAM 7-2

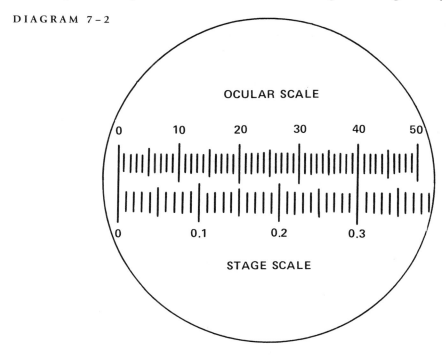

4. Find a place at the farthest point to the right where a line on the ocular micrometer is exactly superimposed on a line of the stage micrometer.
5. Calculate the number of micrometers indicated by each division on the ocular scale, using the following formula:

$$\frac{\text{Number of stage micrometer spaces} \times 10\ \mu\text{m}}{\text{Number of ocular micrometer spaces}} = \mu\text{m/ocular space}$$

For example, in Diagram 7–2, note that the 40th ocular scale line is exactly superimposed over the 30th stage scale line (0.3 mm). Use the following formula: 30 × 10/40 = 7.5 μm per ocular space

6. Repeat steps 2 through 5 for each objective lens. Record the calibration equivalent for each objective so that parasites may be measured when viewed at any magnification. It is convenient to post these values on the microscope. Approximate sizes/space are as follows:

   10× = 7.5 μm
   40× = 3.0 μm
   100× = 1.0 μm

The ocular micrometer and microscope should be calibrated annually, but calibration may be required more or less often depending on the microscope's use.

7. To measure a parasite, line up the left edge of the egg or cyst with the zero on the ocular scale, count the number of ocular spaces to the other edge, and multiply by the appropriate lens factor. For example, an egg that occupied four ocular spaces under low power would actually be 30 μm wide if the multiplier was 7.5 μm per space.

Concentration Techniques for Parasite Stages in Feces

A fecal concentration technique increases the possibility of detecting parasites when few are present in feces, and it is a routine part of the clinical procedures. A single concentrate from one fecal specimen is often sufficient to detect helminth infections. Additional specimens may be required to find and identify protozoa. A permanent stained smear is recommended to confirm protozoan morphology.

Two general types of methods are used: sedimentation and flotation. The formalin-ethyl acetate sedimentation concentration method is the most commonly used technique for concentrating eggs and cysts and is more efficient than flotation methods.

Sedimentation Method   This method concentrates parasite stages present in a large amount of feces into about 2 g of sediment.

PROCEDURE FOR THE FORMALIN-ETHYL ACETATE METHOD

1. Add 5 to 15 g ($^1/_2$ to 1 teaspoon) of fresh feces to a suitable container and use applicator sticks to mix with 10 to 15 mL of 10% formalin. Allow the mixture to stand for 30 minutes for fixation. This step kills and preserves protozoa, larvae, and most eggs. However, some eggshells, such as *Ascaris,* are impervious to formalin.
2. Strain the mixture through two layers of dampened surgical gauze into a 15-mL glass conical centrifuge tube and add enough saline to nearly fill the tube.
    a. Do not use more than two layers of surgical gauze or more than one layer of the newer "pressed" gauze because thicker layers trap mucus that may contain *Cryptosporidium* spp. oocysts or microsporidia.
    b. Do not strain any specimen that contains a large amount of mucus. Instead, centrifuge the mixture for 10 minutes at 500 g, decant into disinfectant, and continue the procedure with step 7.
3. Centrifuge the suspension at 500 g (1500 rpm) for 10 minutes. Decant the supernatant into disinfectant. Resuspend the sediment in saline or formalin and recentrifuge if the sample contains excessive debris. (The rpm values are noted so that workers may more easily adjust speeds to reach the appropriate gravity when using common tabletop centrifuges, but proper calibration steps should be performed to verify speeds.)
4. Resuspend the washed stool sediment in 7 mL of 10% formalin and add 4 mL of ethyl acetate. Cap the tube with a rubber stopper, and shake it vigorously for 30 seconds. This step extracts fats from the feces and reduces bulk; do not use if a very small amount of debris is present or if the original specimen contains much mucus. Carefully remove the stopper away from the face because organic vapor may cause spurting of fecal debris.
5. Centrifuge the tube for 10 minutes at 500 g. Four layers should result (see Diagram 7–3).

DIAGRAM 7–3

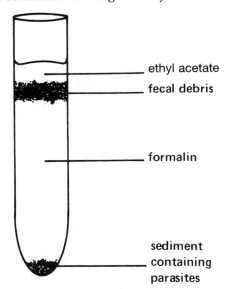

ethyl acetate
fecal debris

formalin

sediment
containing
parasites

6. Rim the upper debris layer with an applicator stick, and decant the entire supernatant into disinfectant. Invert the centrifuge tube completely in one smooth motion, but do it *only once.* If excess ethyl acetate is left inside the tube or if the tube is plastic, use a cotton-tipped applicator stick to swab the inside of the tube while the tube is still inverted. Excess ethyl acetate appears as bubbles when the slide preparation is made and may dissolve plastic tubes.
7. Mix together a small drop of fecal sediment and 1 drop of iodine stain on a slide. Add

a cover glass and carefully examine the entire preparation microscopically for parasites. Also examine an unstained preparation of the concentrate because cysts are refractile and more easily detected unstained and because the morphology of unstained larval forms is more characteristic.

OF NOTE

1. The sedimentation procedure can be used to concentrate PVA-fixed material as follows. Thoroughly mix the PVA-stool suspension with applicator sticks, add about 4 mL of the mixture to a test tube containing 10 mL of saline, and mix well. Filter the mixture through gauze as in step 2, and continue the procedure as described. Sodium acetate-acetic acid-formalin (SAF)-preserved specimens can be processed beginning directly at step 2. *Isospora belli* is usually missed in PVA-preserved concentrates, although it is found in a formalin-preserved specimen. Reasons for this discrepancy are unknown. Some authorities do not recommend concentrating PVA-fixed materials because protozoa become so distorted that they are not recognizable.

2. Ethyl acetate has replaced the earlier use of ether. Ethyl acetate is nonflammable; therefore, it is a much safer chemical for laboratory use. Recovery of *Hymenolepis nana* eggs and cysts of *Giardia lamblia* is enhanced with ethyl acetate. Some workers consider Hemo De to be even safer than ethyl acetate.

3. Centrifugation speeds and times are important because *Cryptosporidium* oocysts and microsporidian spores may not be recovered if centrifugation is insufficient.

4. If water is used to rinse the sediment in step 3, *B. hominis* cysts rupture, leading to a false-negative report for this organism.

5. Extra washing of fixed sediment may be necessary because iodine causes precipitation of excess mercuric chloride. If precipitation is noted when the slide is examined, simply rewash the sediment once or twice and prepare a new slide. Do not wash the sediment more than twice because organisms may be lost, which may lead to a false-negative result.

RESULTS AND REPORT FOR SEDIMENTATION PROCEDURES

1. Any observed parasites are reported by their scientific name, including both the genus and species names, when possible, and the stage present.

2. Certain cellular elements, such as blood cells, may be reported semiquantitatively as few, moderate, or many RBCs, WBCs, or other cells if they are clearly identifiable. Yeast is noted, but quantitation is determined from the permanently stained smear.

3. Charcot-Leyden crystals may be reported semiquantitatively as few, moderate, or many.

QUALITY-CONTROL CONSIDERATIONS

1. Verify weekly that all solutions are clear and are not visibly contaminated.

2. Known-positive specimens should be concentrated and organisms should be identified to verify technique at least quarterly or whenever the centrifuge is calibrated.

3. QC results should be recorded, and the action plan for "out-of-control" results should be followed if needed.

Flotation Methods

Flotation methods use liquids with a higher specific gravity than that of eggs or cysts so that parasites float to the surface and the concentrate can be skimmed from the top of the tube. The concentrating solution should have a final specific gravity of 1.18 (1.20 can be used with formalin-preserved specimens). The most commonly used reagent is zinc sulfate, and a description of the procedure using this solution follows. It is important to note that this method does not easily recover operculated eggs or infertile *Ascaris* eggs. In addition, the high specific gravity kills trophozoites and causes distortion of certain other fragile eggs, such as *H. nana*. For these reasons, it is recommended that if only a single concentration procedure is to be used, it should be the formalin-ethyl acetate sedimentation technique.

PROCEDURE FOR THE ZINC SULFATE* FLOTATION METHOD
The procedure should be performed as follows:

1. Prepare fixed and washed feces in a 13- × 100-mm round-bottom tube as described in steps 1 and 2 of the procedure for the formalin-ethyl acetate concentration method.
2. Wash once or twice in saline (centrifuge each time at 500 g [1500 rpm] for 10 minutes) to obtain 1 mL or less of sediment.
3. Resuspend and thoroughly mix the sediment in 12 mL of zinc sulfate solution (specific gravity 1.18 to 1.20 as verified with a hydrometer).
4. Centrifuge for 2 minutes at 500 g (1500 rpm), allowing the centrifuge to stop without vibration. Gently and carefully place the tube in a rack in a vertical position without shaking it, and slowly add enough zinc sulfate down the side of the tube with a dropper pipette to fill the tube so that an inverted meniscus forms (Diagram 7–4).

DIAGRAM 7–4

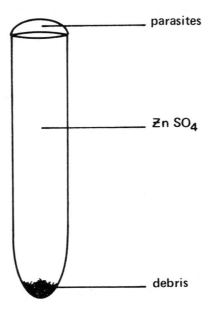

parasites

Zn SO$_4$

debris

5. Without shaking the tube, carefully place a 22- × 22-mm cover glass on top of the tube so that its underside rests on the meniscus. The meniscus should not be so high that fluid runs down the side of the tube, carrying parasitic forms away from the cover glass.
6. Allow the tube to stand vertically in a rack with the coverslip suspended on top for 10 minutes.
7. Carefully lift the cover glass with its hanging drop containing parasites on the underside and mount on a clean slide, liquid side down. You may place a small drop of iodine stain on the slide before adding the cover glass. Gently rotate the slide after adding the cover glass to ensure a uniform mixture. Thoroughly examine the coverslip preparation microscopically, using the procedure outlined on page 165.

OF NOTE
Gravity flotation is not particularly effective in concentrating organisms. Many workers prefer the following variation:

1. After washing as in step 1, resuspend sediment in 12 mL of zinc sulfate solution. Then fill the tube to within 0.5 mL of its top.
2. Centrifuge for 2 minutes at 500 g (1500 rpm) and allow the centrifuge to stop without vibration.
3. Use either a sterile Pasteur pipette or a flamed and cooled wire loop (bent at a right angle to the stem) to transfer 2 or 3 drops of the surface film to a clean glass slide. Add a drop of iodine stain, mix, and add a cover glass. Examine microscopically.
4. Oocysts of *I. belli* and some other organisms are so lightweight that they float very near the top of the liquid.

5. You may also examine the wet mount when unstained by using a phase-contrast microscope or when stained with Kinyoun modified acid-fast stain to help detect *Cryptosporidium, Cyclospora,* and *Isospora.*

6. Some thin-shelled helminth eggs and protozoan cysts are distorted by prolonged exposure to the high specific gravity of the zinc sulfate solution; therefore, microscopic examination of these samples must be done within 5 minutes after the centrifuge stops.

7. If flotation is the only concentration technique used, be sure to also examine the sediment because heavy operculated eggs and infertile *Ascaris* eggs do not float.

RESULTS AND REPORT FOR FLOTATION PROCEDURES

1. Any observed parasites are reported by their scientific name, including both the genus and species names, when possible.

2. Certain cellular elements, such as blood cells, may be reported semiquantitatively as few, moderate, or many RBCs, WBCs, or other cells if they are clearly identifiable. Yeast is noted, but quantitation is determined from the permanently stained smear.

3. Charcot-Leyden crystals may be reported semiquantitatively as few, moderate, or many.

QUALITY-CONTROL CONSIDERATIONS

1. Verify weekly that all solutions are clear and are not visibly contaminated.

2. Known-positive specimens should be concentrated, and organisms should be identified to verify technique at least quarterly or whenever the centrifuge has been calibrated.

3. The ocular micrometer and microscope should be calibrated at least annually.

4. QC results should be recorded, and the action plan for "out-of-control" results should be followed if needed.

Permanent Staining Procedures

Trichrome Stain for Intestinal Protozoa

The Wheatley trichrome* technique is a rapid procedure that gives good results for routine identification of intestinal protozoa in fresh fecal specimens. It is to be the final part of a complete fecal examination. This procedure is the confirmation step for all identifications of protozoan parasites.

The cytoplasm of *E. histolytica* trophozoites and cysts appears light blue-green or light pink. *Entamoeba coli* cysts are slightly more purplish. Nuclear structure is clearly visible; karyosomes of nuclei stain ruby red. Degenerated organisms stain pale green. Background material stains green, providing a good contrast with the protozoa. The procedure requires that fecal smears be fixed with either PVA* or Schaudinn* solution.

Cryptosporidium, Cyclospora, Isospora, and Microsporidia do not stain well using this technique. However, modifications of this method, such as those of Kokoskin, Ryan, or Weber, allow microsporidia to be visualized. These parasites will appear refractile and pink-red when using any of these modifications. *Cryptosporidium, Cyclospora,* and *Isospora* can be recognized when acid-fast stains are used (see p. 177).

TRICHROME STAINING PROCEDURE

1. Using an applicator stick, place a thin film of fresh feces on a microscope slide and, while the smear is wet, place it in Schaudinn fixative solution (without acetic acid) for 5 minutes at 50°C or for 1 hour at room temperature. Rinse in 70% alcohol for 5 minutes to remove excess fixative. (Omit this fixation if smears have been preserved in PVA.) Diarrheic stools should be mixed with PVA fixative. The PVA fixative then acts as an adhesive for the slide preparation. When using PVA-fixed material from a transport vial, follow this procedure:

   a. Transfer some of the well-mixed PVA-fixed material to several layers of paper towel. Let the mixture stand for 3 minutes to absorb excess PVA. *This step must be performed.*

   b. Using an applicator stick, spread some of the specimen onto a clean glass slide. Adherence to the slide is improved if the material is spread to the edges of the slide.

   c. Slides should be dried either overnight at room temperature or for 2 to 3 hours on a slide warmer at 37°C or in an incubator at 37°C. Morphologic distortion may result if slides are dried too rapidly. The slide must be dried thoroughly to avoid washing off the film during staining.

2. Place slide in the 70% ethanol solution (with enough iodine added to turn the alcohol to the color of strong tea) for 2 minutes (10 minutes for PVA-fixed smears).
3. Place slide successively in two changes of 70% solutions of ethanol for 5 minutes in each solution. Place in trichrome* stain for 10 to 20 minutes.
4. Rinse in acidified 90% ethanol* for 1 to 3 seconds. Usually a brief dip in and out is sufficient. Drain immediately.

NOTE: Inasmuch as the acid alcohol continues to destain as long as it is in contact with the material, the time allowed should include the few seconds between the time the slide is removed from the destain and the subsequent rinse in absolute alcohol in step 5.

5. Rinse quickly with several dips each in two changes of absolute ethanol. These alcohol solutions should be changed frequently to prevent them from becoming so acid that the destaining process continues. Prolonged destaining in acid alcohol may cause the organisms to be poorly differentiated. Larger trophozoites, particularly those of *E. coli,* may require slightly longer periods of staining.

NOTE: If several slides are stained simultaneously, they should be destained separately. Remove only one slide at a time from the stain. Destain it, rinse it in the 100% alcohols, and continue at step 6. Place in two changes of absolute ethanol for 5 minutes each.

6. Place in clean xylene (or xylene substitute) for 5 minutes.
7. Mount slides using a mounting medium (e.g., Permount) and a No. 1 cover glass. An alternate method for examining the smear is as follows:
   a. Remove the slide from the last xylene solution. Place face up on a paper towel and allow it to dry completely. (Xylene substitutes take longer to dry.)
   b. Fifteen minutes before examining the slide, add a drop of immersion oil to the dry fecal film. Let the oil penetrate the film for 10 to 15 minutes. If the material appears refractile at the end of the waiting period, either add more oil or wait a few more minutes before examining the slide.
   c. Add a No. 1 cover glass to the smear just before viewing the film, and examine under oil immersion using the 100× objective. Examine at least 200 to 300 individual oil immersion fields before reporting a negative result.

RESULTS AND REPORT FOR THE TRICHROME STAIN PROCEDURE

1. Trophozoites and cysts, human tissue or blood cells, and yeast (single, budding, or pseudohyphae) are easily identified, but helminth eggs and larvae often retain excessive stain, making them difficult to identify.
2. Any observed parasites are reported by their scientific names, including both the genus and species names when possible, and the stage observed.
3. Certain cellular elements, such as blood cells or yeast, may be reported semiquantitatively as few, moderate, or many RBCs, WBCs, yeast, or other cells, such as macrophages, if they are clearly identifiable.
4. Charcot-Leyden crystals may be reported semiquantitatively as few, moderate, or many.
5. All reportable objects may be quantitated using the following scheme:

Average Number of Organisms, Cells, or Other Artifacts Counted in 10 Oil Immersion Fields	*Quantity Reported*
≤2	Few
3–9	Moderate
≥10	Many

QUALITY-CONTROL CONSIDERATIONS

1. Because trichrome stains are quite stable, it is usually necessary only to check each new batch of stain. If staining is done infrequently, it is advisable that periodic checks be made at least monthly. The College of American Pathologists (CAP) checklist can also be consulted for current recommendations.
2. Positive control material can be prepared by adding human buffy coat cells to negative stool specimens. From this mixture, smears are made and stained along with unknown slides. Known-negative slides should be processed with each set of unknowns. If positive fecal material is available from patients or QC survey samples, control slides may be made from PVA-fixed material. Check WBCs and known parasites for color.
3. The 70% ethanol-iodine solution should be changed at least weekly or more often if slides are too green.
4. QC results should be recorded, and the action plan for "out-of-control" results should be followed if needed.

Modified Trichrome Stain for Microsporidia

Microsporidia are not visualized in the routine Wheatley trichrome method because the stain does not penetrate the cell. The modified trichrome* technique of Weber and Green uses a much higher concentration of chromotrope 2R dye and longer staining time to overcome this problem. This procedure will reveal microsporidia in any fecal specimen, fresh or preserved in formalin, SAF, or from a zinc-based single-vial system.

MODIFIED TRICHROME STAINING PROCEDURE

1. Using a 10-μm aliquot of fresh or preserved unconcentrated liquid fecal material, prepare a smear on a clean glass slide covering an area measuring 45 × 25 mm.
   a. This procedure may also be performed using concentrated fecal material. *Be sure* to use only two layers of gauze to filter the specimen because spores may be trapped if more layers are used. Unpublished data generated at the University of California–Los Angeles Clinical Microbiology Laboratory suggests that centrifugation at 500 × g for 10 minutes (approximately 1500 rpm) will increase the number of spores in the sediment.
   b. Spread a 10-μL aliquot of concentrated sediment onto a clean glass slide covering an area measuring 45 × 25 mm.
2. Dry the slides either overnight at room temperature or for 2 to 3 hours on a slide warmer at 37°C or in an incubator at 37°C. Morphologic distortion may result if slides are dried too rapidly. The slide must be dried thoroughly to avoid washing off the film during staining.
3. Place the slide in absolute methanol for 5 minutes.
4. Allow the smear to air-dry.
5. Place the slide in the trichrome stain for 90 minutes.
6. Rinse the slide in acid-alcohol for no more than 10 seconds.

NOTE: If several slides are stained simultaneously, they should be destained separately. Remove only one slide at a time from the stain. Destain it, rinse it in the 95% alcohols (step 7), and continue at step 8.

7. Rinse quickly with several dips each in two changes of 95% ethanol.

NOTE: These alcohol solutions should be changed frequently to prevent them from becoming so acid that the destaining process continues. Prolonged destaining in acid alcohol may cause the organisms to be poorly differentiated.

8. Place the slide in 95% ethanol for 5 minutes.
9. Place the slide in absolute ethanol for 10 minutes.
10. Place in clean xylene (or xylene substitute) for 10 minutes.
11. Mount slides using a mounting medium (e.g., Permount) and a No. 1 cover glass. Examine under oil immersion using the 100× objective. Examine at least 200 to 300 individual oil immersion fields before reporting a negative result.

RESULTS AND REPORT FOR THE MODIFIED TRICHROME STAIN PROCEDURE
Spore walls stain pink to red with a clear interior, or the polar tube may appear as a red horizontal or diagonal bar. Bacteria, some yeasts, and some debris will also stain pink to red. Background material stains green. Before reporting a positive result, you must carefully measure all suspicious forms and compare them with other red color shapes and examine control smears.

NOTE: Watery specimens will yield smears with less debris and larger numbers of spores.

QUALITY-CONTROL CONSIDERATIONS

1. Because trichrome stains are quite stable, it is usually necessary to check only each new batch of stain. If staining is done infrequently, it is advisable to make periodic checks at least monthly. The CAP checklist can also be consulted for current recommendations.
2. Positive control smears should be stained along with test smears each time the procedure is performed. Because the spores are small (1 to 2 μm in diameter), it is necessary to use only actual microsporidial spores. It may be difficult to obtain positive control material. If positive fecal material is available from patients or QC survey samples, control slides may be made from formalin-preserved material. Known-negative slides also should be processed with each set of unknowns.
3. QC results should be recorded, and the action plan for "out-of-control" results should be followed if needed.

Iron Hematoxylin Stain for Intestinal Protozoa

There are many variations of the iron hematoxylin technique. The Tompkins-Miller method gives excellent results and is a good alternative to the Wheatley trichrome method for completing the fecal examination. This method may be used with freshly fixed feces (Schaudinn fixative solution) or with feces preserved in PVA or SAF solutions.

Protozoan trophozoites and cysts stain blue-gray. The nuclei, karyosomes, and other cell inclusions stain darker than the cytoplasm. Yeast, RBCs and crystals stain blue-gray to black. Detail is clear, but without contrasting colors. The background material appears a lighter shade of blue-gray.

Cryptosporidium, Cyclospora, Isospora, and Microsporidia do not stain well using this technique. However, a modification of this method adds acid-fast reagents to this procedure, thus allowing *Cryptosporidium, Cyclospora,* and *Isospora* to be visualized. These parasites will appear refractile and pink-red in color when using any of these modifications. The modified Trichrome stain of Kokoskin, Ryan, or Weber also can be used to reveal microsporidia.

IRON HEMATOXYLIN STAINING PROCEDURE

1. Prepare smears as described for the Wheatley trichrome stain method (see p. 171).
   a. If using SAF-fixed feces, mix one drop of Mayer's albumin with one drop of SAF-fixed fecal sediment on a clean glass slide using an applicator stick and then spread the mixture evenly.
   b. Allow the slide to air-dry. Do not blot. Begin staining at step 4.
2. Place thoroughly dried fecal smears into 70% ethanol for 5 minutes.
3. Place slides for 2 to 5 minutes in a mixture of 70% ethanol containing sufficient D'Antoni iodine solution so that the solution is the color of strong tea (usually several drops are needed).
4. Place slides in 50% ethanol for 5 minutes.
5. Wash slides with running tap water for 3 minutes. (Allow a constant stream to run into the staining container.)
6. Place slides in 4% aqueous ferric ammonium sulfate* mordant for 5 minutes.
7. Place slides in tap water for 1 minute.
8. Place slides in 0.5% aqueous hematoxylin working stain* solution for 10 minutes.
9. Place slides in tap water for 1 minute.
10. Place slides in 2% aqueous phosphotungstic acid* solution for 2 to 5 minutes to decolorize smears.

11. Wash slides in running tap water for 10 minutes.
12. Add a few drops of saturated aqueous solution of lithium carbonate* to 70% ethanol. Place slides in this solution for 3 minutes.
13. Rinse slides briefly in 80% ethanol.
14. Place slides in 95% ethanol for 3 minutes.
15. Place slides in two changes of 100% ethanol for 5 minutes each.
16. Place slides in two changes of xylene or xylene substitute for 5 minutes each.
17. Mount slides using a mounting medium (e.g., Permount) and a No. 1 cover glass. The alternative mounting method presented previously may be used if desired (see p. 172).

RESULTS AND REPORT FOR IRON HEMATOXYLIN STAIN PROCEDURE

1. Trophozoites and cysts, human tissue or blood cells, and yeast (single, budding, or pseudohyphae) are easily identified, but helminth eggs and larvae often retain excessive stain, making them difficult to identify.
2. Any observed parasites are reported by their scientific names (including both the genus and species names, when possible) and life-cycle stage.
3. Certain cellular elements may be reported semiquantitatively as few, moderate, or many; this includes RBCs, WBCs, yeast, or other cells, such as macrophages, if they are clearly identifiable.
4. Charcot-Leyden crystals may be reported semiquantitatively as few, moderate, or many.
5. All reportable objects may be quantitated using the following scheme:

Average Number of Organisms, Cell, or Other Artifacts Counted in 10 Oil Immersion Fields	*Quantity Reported*
≤2	Few
3–9	Moderate
≥10	Many

QUALITY-CONTROL CONSIDERATIONS

1. Because iron hematoxylin stains are stable for several months, it is usually necessary to check each new batch of stain. If staining is done infrequently, it should be checked at least monthly. The stain should be checked by dropping one drop of stain into 100 mL of alkaline tap water. If the resulting color is light purple, the stain is satisfactory for use. The CAP checklist can also be consulted for current recommendations.
2. Positive control material can be prepared by adding human buffy coat cells to negative stool specimens. From this mixture, smears are made and stained along with unknown slides. Known-negative slides should be processed with each set of unknowns. If positive fecal material is available from patients or QC survey samples, control slides may be made from PVA-fixed material. Check WBCs and known parasites for color.
3. The 70% ethanol-iodine solution should be changed at least weekly or more often if slides are staining too blue.
4. QC results should be recorded, and the action plan for "out-of-control" results should be followed, if needed.

 FOR REVIEW

1. Describe the information derived from the macroscopic and direct wet-mount fecal examination:

_____

2. Compare and contrast the principal advantages and concerns with the use of the sedimentation and flotation concentration techniques:

_____

3. Describe the proper protocol for reporting the results of stained fecal smear examination:

_____

4. List the specific types of organisms that might be missed in each step of the fecal examination:

_____

5. List and discuss the special procedures or stains used to reveal missed organisms:

_____

Cellophane Tape Test for Pinworm

As the female pinworm *(Enterobius vermicularis)* migrates out of the anus to deposit her eggs on the perianal region, eggs may be easily recovered for identification.

Procedure

The following test should be performed in the morning before the patient has washed or defecated because the eggs are generally deposited in the perianal region at night.
1. Fold the edges of a 3- × ³/₄-inch piece of clear cellophane tape around the end of a tongue depressor so that the sticky side is out. Alternatively, a pinworm paddle kit can be used.
2. Spread the buttocks and apply the tape face or paddle to the anal area, using a rocking motion to touch as much of the perianal mucosa as possible. Remove the tape and apply it to a microscope slide, sticky side down. Press firmly so that no air bubbles are trapped (Diagram 7–5).

DIAGRAM 7–5

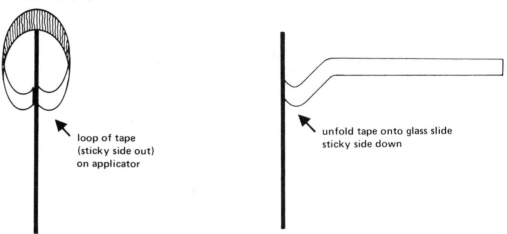

loop of tape (sticky side out) on applicator

unfold tape onto glass slide sticky side down

3. Examine the slide or the pinworm paddle for pinworm eggs under low power, using low light as described in the microscopic examination on page 165. Be sure to examine the entire area under the tape. The eggs are colorless; therefore, good focus on the area between the tape and the slide and low-light contrast are critical.

Of Note

A parent can collect the specimen from a young child at home using a pinworm paddle kit supplied by the doctor. The paddle is then returned to the laboratory for examination.

1. Wear gloves when performing the examination because pinworm eggs are usually infective.
2. Pinworm infection should not be ruled out until at least five consecutive daily negative preparations have been examined.
3. Cellophane tape can be cleared by lifting one edge of the tape from the slide and then placing 1 or 2 drops of xylol or toluol under the tape before examination. Disperse the liquid by carefully pressing the tape down onto the slide.
4. If opaque (Magic) tape is submitted erroneously, add a drop of immersion oil to the top of the tape to clear it sufficiently for microscopic examination.

Results and Report for Cellophane Tape Preparation

Pinworm eggs are reported as found or not found.

● Other Diagnostic Procedures

Several other procedures are commonly used in the laboratory and are presented in this section. Table 7–2 summarizes procedures used to recover and identify parasites from various types of bodily specimens.

Modified Kinyoun Acid-fast Stain (Cold Method)

In recent years, *Cryptosporidium parvum*, *Cyclospora*, *I. belli*, and the Microsporidia have caused severe diarrheal diseases, especially in immunocompromised patients. Because these parasites may be difficult to detect and identify by routine methods, it is necessary to use modified acid-fast and modified trichrome stains to confirm their identity.

This procedure may be used on fresh, formalin-preserved, or SAF-preserved fecal sediment or on other clinical specimens, such as duodenal fluid, bile, or any type of pulmonary specimen. PVA-preserved specimens are not acceptable for this staining technique.

1. Smear 1 to 2 drops of concentrated specimen on each of two slides and allow them to air-dry. Do not make the smears too thick. (A wet smear should be thin enough so that a printed page can be read through it.)
2. Fix slides by placing them in absolute methanol for 1 minute.
3. Flood slides with Kinyoun carbolfuchsin, and stain for 5 minutes.
4. Rinse briefly (3 to 5 seconds) with 50% ethanol.
5. Rinse thoroughly with water.
6. Decolorize with 1% sulfuric acid for 2 minutes or until no more color runs from the slide.
7. Rinse with water. Drain.
8. Counterstain with methylene blue for 1 minute.
9. Rinse with water, and allow to air-dry.
10. Examine the slide using the low and high dry objective. Use oil immersion to observe internal detail.

Results and Report for Kinyoun Acid-fast Stain Procedure

1. The color range of *C. parvum* (4 to 6 μm), *Cyclospora* (8 to 10 μm), *Sarcocystis* (9 to 12 μm), and *I. belli* (25 × 15 μm) oocysts or sporocysts is from pink to deep purple. Depending on the species (see p. 125), sporozoites or sporoblasts may be visible within the oocyst. The background color is blue.
2. Microsporidia spores (1 to 2 μm) stain red and may resemble small yeast or bacteria. Identification must be confirmed using the modified trichrome stain, fluorescent antibody, or other antibody techniques.
3. Immunoassay antibody techniques may be needed to confirm the identity of light infections with *C. parvum*.
4. *Cyclospora* are acid-fast variable, have no definite internal morphology, and are larger than *C. parvum*. Oocysts autofluoresce (green—450 to 490 DM excitation filter, blue—365 DM excitation filter) and stain orange with safranin.
5. Any parasites detected are reported by their scientific name, including both genus and species name, when possible.
6. Three fecal specimens from alternate days should be examined.

Quality-control Considerations

1. Positive control slides should be made from 10% formalin-preserved *C. parvum* specimens. A positive control slide should be stained with each batch.
2. Check macroscopically to be sure the specimen adhered to the slide.
3. QC results should be recorded, and the action plan for "out-of-control" results should be followed if needed.

Blood-smear Preparation and Staining for Blood Parasites

These procedures are used for the recovery and identification of *Plasmodium*, trypanosomes, microfilaria, *Babesia* spp., and *Leishmania donovani*. Both thin and thick smears should be prepared, stained, and examined. Thin smears offer the advantage of very little distortion of the parasite, but the disadvantage is that many fields must be examined to detect parasites when they are few in number. At least 200 to 300 thin film fields should be examined under oil immersion before reporting a negative smear. Although thick-smear

TABLE 7–2 □ MISCELLANEOUS SPECIMEN PROCESSING

Specimen Source	Collection Procedure Used	Parasites	Laboratory Examination
Duodenum	Entero-Test*	*Giardia lamblia* *Isospora* spp. *Clonorchis sinensis* *Strongyloides stercoralis* *Fasciola hepatica* *Encephalitozoon intestinalis* *Enterocytozoon bieneusi*	Wet mount and/or permanent stains made from "washed" string
Cornea	Scrapings sent to the laboratory in airtight container	*Acanthamoeba* spp. *Naegleria* spp. *Loa loa* Microsporidia *Vittaforma corneae*	Wet mount and /or permanent stains
Cerebrospinal fluid (CSF) and other body fluids from sterile sites	Collect according to established procedure for each fluid type	*Naegleria fowleri* *Acanthamoeba* spp. *Toxoplasma gondii* *Taenia solium* (cysticercosis) *Trypanosoma* spp. Microsporidia	Wet mount and /or permanent stains
Liver abscess	Aspiration	*Entamoeba histolytica* *Fasciola hepatica* *Leishmania donovani* *Echinococcus* spp. Microsporidia	Wet mount and /or permanent stains, culture techniques
Urine	Clean-catch urine sample	*Schistosoma hematobium* *Trichomonas vaginalis* Microsporidia	Examine sediment microscopically
Lymph node	Surgical biopsy	*Leishmania donovani*	Impression smears
Skin	Surgical biopsy Skin snips	*Leishmania* spp. *Onchocerca volvulus*	Permanent stains Wet mount
Mouth	Scrapings at the gum line	*Entamoeba gingivalis* *Trichomonas tenax*	Wet mount and /or permanent stains
Nose	Discharge	*Naegleria fowleri* *Trachipleistophora hominis*	Wet mount and /or permanent stains
Genital secretions (prostate, urethra, vaginal)	Swabs submitted in sterile saline	*Trichomonas vaginalis* Microsporidia	Wet mount on fresh specimen
Sigmoidoscopy	Aspirates, scraping, or biopsy	*Isospora* spp. *Cyclospora* spp. *Cryptosporidium parvum* *Schistosoma mansoni* Microsporidia	Wet mount and /or permanent stains, histology
Sputum	Early-morning deep cough	*Paragonimus* spp., also *Strongyloides* spp. *Ascaris* spp., *Entamoeba gingivalis*, hookworm Microsporidia	Wet mount and /or permanent stains Similar mounts following concentration with NaOH or *N*-acetyl-cysteine for mucoid specimens

*Available from "Hedeco" Health Development Corp. East Palo Alto, California.

preparations often distort the parasite's morphology, the chances of detecting parasites are improved. Because the thick-smear technique concentrates blood, the same volume of blood can be screened about three times faster than that in a thin smear. If improperly made, however, thick smears are useless. Fresh or ethylenediaminetetraacetic acid (EDTA)-preserved specimens are preferred. Slides made from capillary blood must be made from a free-flowing drop that is not squeezed out or contaminated with alcohol.

Smear Preparation   Prepare thin smears by touching a clean, grease-free slide to a small drop of blood so that the drop is near one end of the slide. Hold a second spreader slide on edge at a 30-degree angle on the slide, which is also holding the specimen, and draw back into the drop, allowing it to spread along the edge of the spreader slide (Diagram 7–6). Then, smoothly and rapidly push the spreader slide forward so that the blood spreads out and trails in a flat sheet. The

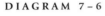

DIAGRAM 7–6

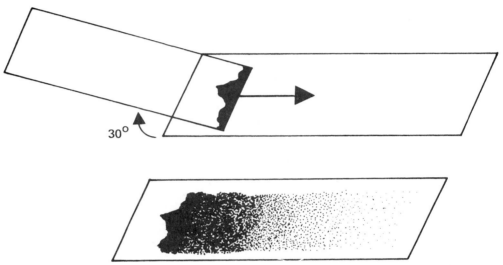

30°

amount of blood should be small enough that it is all spread before the spreader reaches the end of the specimen slide. Allow to air-dry and stain as described in the Giemsa staining procedure. Screen the thin film for 30 minutes under 100×, and examine 300 microscopic fields of the thick film under oil immersion before reporting a specimen as negative.

Prepare thick smears by touching a clean slide to a large drop of blood. Using a corner of another slide, spread the blood evenly in a circular film about the size of a dime or nickel (1.8 to 2.0 cm in diameter). Allow to air-dry overnight, and lake the blood by placing the slide in Giemsa-buffered water for 10 minutes. (Laking may be omitted if a 1:50 Giemsa stain is used.) Laking causes RBCs to break open (i.e., lyse), which causes hemoglobin's red color to disappear, leaving the blood spot translucent. The lysed blood smear should be stained according to the description that follows. Thin and thick smears can be made at opposite ends of the same slide. Only the thin smear should be fixed before staining in methanol. (Some authorities believe that better results are obtained when smears are prepared on separated slides.)

If filariasis is suspected, both diurnal and nocturnal blood samples are drawn to account for the periodicity of microfilariae. A concentration test for microfilaria is performed as described on page 180. In cases of suspected malaria, if the first specimens are negative, the patient's blood should be retested every 6 to 8 hours for at least 3 days to account for the periodicity of schizogony. Unstained and stained blood smears should be stored protected from insects and light in slide storage boxes. QC, known-positive, and known-negative slides should be used routinely for all staining procedures on blood and feces. Universal Precautions should be used at all times when handling blood or other body fluids.

GIEMSA STAINING PROCEDURE

For thin smears, the blood smear is immersed briefly in absolute methyl alcohol (two dips). The slide is then placed in working Giemsa stain (made by diluting stock Giemsa*

1:100 with pH 7.0 working buffer*) for 2 hours. The time may be reduced to 45 minutes if a 1:50 dilution is used or to 20 minutes if a 1:20 dilution is used. The smear is gently rinsed in buffer (two dips), drained, and air-dried. *Do not blot.* Examine under oil immersion as described previously.

For thick smears, unlaked smears are placed in a 1:50 dilution of stock Giemsa for 50 minutes. *Do not use a 1:20 dilution.* Smears are gently washed with buffer for 3 to 5 minutes. Excessive washing decolorizes the film. Air-dry and examine under oil immersion.

OF NOTE

1. Three-minute quick stains for blood smears are available. Each laboratory should carefully compare results with standard staining methods.
2. Although parasites may be seen when stained with Wright's stain, it is not recommended for parasitologic use.

RESULTS AND REPORT FOR GIEMSA STAINING PROCEDURE

1. To detect stippling, smears should be prepared within 1 hour after EDTA specimens are drawn.
2. Malaria, *Babesia* spp., trypanosomes, and leishmania cytoplasm stains blue, with nuclear material staining red. Schüffner's dots stain red. A microfilaria sheath may not stain, but the nuclei in the organism stain blue to purple.
3. RBCs stain pale red; WBCs, purple; eosinophilic granules, bright purple-red; and neutrophilic granules, deep pink-purple.
4. Any detected parasites are reported by their scientific name, including both the genus and species names, when possible.

QUALITY-CONTROL CONSIDERATIONS

1. Because Giemsa stains are quite stable, it is usually necessary to check each new batch of stain only. If staining is done infrequently, it is advisable that periodic checks be done at least monthly. The CAP checklist can be consulted for current recommendations.
2. The stain should be filtered if sediment appears on blood films. Known-negative slides should be processed with each set of unknowns. If positive blood specimens are available from patients or QC survey samples, control slides may be made and preserved by dipping them in absolute methanol. Check WBCs and known parasites for color.
3. QC results should be recorded, and the action plan for "out-of-control" results should be followed if needed.

Knott Technique for Concentrating Microfilariae

When filariasis is suspected, it may be useful to concentrate blood to increase the possibility of finding microfilariae.

Procedure

1. Obtain 2 mL of whole blood by venipuncture and immediately place it in a centrifuge tube containing 10 mL of 2% formalin.
2. Stopper the tube and mix thoroughly by inverting and shaking the tube. The formalin lyses RBCs, fixes blood protozoa, and kills and straightens the bodies of microfilariae.
3. Centrifuge the tube for 5 minutes at 500 g (1000 rpm), or let it stand stoppered overnight in the refrigerator.
4. Decant the supernatant.
5. Remove the sediment with a Pasteur pipette and spread in a thick film on a slide.
6. The sediment may be examined wet for microfilariae, or the slide may be allowed to dry overnight, followed by staining with Giemsa for 45 minutes. (See thick-smear staining procedure described previously.) Destain in buffered water (pH 7.2) for 10 to 15 minutes, allow to dry, and examine.

Of Note

1. Although not routinely performed, it may be useful to examine whole blood collected in EDTA, heparin, or sodium citrate anticoagulant when trypanosomes or microfilariae are suspected. To perform this technique, centrifuge the sample at $100 \times$ g for 15 minutes, place a drop of fresh buffy coat on a slide, add a coverslip, and examine under low power ($10\times$) for microfilariae or high dry power ($40\times$) for trypanosomes. Parasites may be detected by their characteristic motility. The undulating motion of the trypanosome and the whiplike motion of the microfilariae are easily spotted because they cause movement of surrounding blood cells. This method may shorten the examination time needed for a positive diagnosis.

2. Other concentration techniques are available, including filtering lysed blood through a fine-pore filter and then staining the filter for microfilariae or passing blood through Sephadex filters, which selectively attach trypanosomes that can be later eluted. Stained blood films also must be examined to correctly identify the species of parasite.

Protozoa Culture Media

Routine diagnosis of protozoan infections is usually possible without using culture methods, and few clinical labs offer culture techniques; however, several media are available that support growth of many protozoan species. Commonly used media for intestinal protozoa are either a semisolid base set up as slant tubes with a liquid overlay (Boeck and Drbohlav medium, Cleveland-Collier, and McQuay diphasic charcoal medium) or a nutritive fluid (Balamuth medium). The axenic culture medium of Diamond is a useful diphasic medium in which a chick embryo extract is used as a liquid overlay for a slanted nutrient agar base. Diamond medium is used primarily in research centers and is most useful when stock cultures of *E. histolytica* must be maintained. Details for the in-house preparation of these basic media can be found in the bibliography in this chapter.

Regardless of the medium chosen, careful handling of the culture is important to obtain successful results. Only fresh fecal specimens (less than 6 hours old) should be used, and at least two wet mounts made from the sediment should be examined after incubation, inasmuch as growth is slow and numbers may be few.

Procedure

1. To any of the tubes of prepared media listed previously, add a 5-mm loop of sterile rice powder.
2. Add about 1.5 mL of fluid or semifluid feces to each tube that is used; if the stool is formed, add a pea-sized portion to the tube and mix gently.
3. Incubate at 37°C for 24 hours; examine at least 0.1 mL of the surface of the semisolid sediment for trophozoites. PVA-fixed smears may be made from the surface material and stained with trichrome if desired.
4. All cultures not showing trophozoites should be transferred to new media by transferring the top half of the sediment to a tube containing fresh media. The new tube is then incubated at 37°C for 24 hours, after which the culture surface is examined as in step 3. No further transfers are needed. The culture is considered negative at this point if parasites are not recovered.
5. To culture *Leishmania* and *Trypanosoma cruzi*, use Novy-MacNeal-Nicolle (NNN)* medium at room temperature. Thirty percent defibrinated rabbit blood in the agar and antibiotics in the fluid overlay are preferred. Aspirated material, bone marrow, chancre, or blood may be used as specimens for culture. Check condensate at the bottom of the slant for 1 month for the presence of organisms.

 FOR REVIEW

1. *List the reason for performing each of the following tests:*

   a. *Cellophane tape test:*

   _____

   b. *Modified Kinyoun acid-fast stain:*

   _____

    c. Thick and thin blood films:

_____

    d. Protozoal culture media:

_____

  2. *What procedures constitute a fecal examination for parasites? How are these performed?*

_____

  3. *What precautions should you take when handling or mailing infectious material?*

_____

● Immuno-diagnostic Methods

With few notable exceptions, such as tuberculosis, leprosy, and spirochetal diseases, the host usually responds to microbial and viral infections in a relatively timely and straight-forward manner. By contrast, the host's response to parasitic disease is much more complex and time-extended. Elaborate life cycles and complex, often-changing antigenic structures create complex responses and control problems for the host. Parasitic infections are often chronic because the host is unable to eliminate the source of infection, which forces the immune system to remain continually responsive. Various parasitic antigens have been shown to lead to host immunosuppression, improper processing of antibody-antigen complexes by macrophages, disruption of normal B- and T-lymphocyte functions, and hypersensitivity responses. Immune complexes may also form, leading to problems such as the autoimmune anemia or intravascular coagulation seen in American trypanosomiasis (Chagas' disease). Each of these complicated mechanisms can either cause or enhance the pathology seen in parasitic diseases.

Immune Response

All parasites elicit immune responses inducing the formation of multiple classes of antibodies and cellular responses. The entire range of immunologic responses can be seen in parasitic diseases. Many protozoan parasites are effectively reduced or eliminated by macrophages that have become activated by sensitized T cells, but many are not. Multicellular helminths add additional complexity.

High levels of IgE antibody and T-cell–dependent eosinophilia are commonly found in helminth infections. The IgE binds to mast cells, basophils, and eosinophils, causing the release of chemotactic factors, histamine activators, prostaglandins, and other mediators that produce various hypersensitivity reactions. Infections caused by small parasites, such as protozoa, often induce delayed hypersensitivity responses. Reactions such as immediate hypersensitivity, anaphylaxis, and delayed hypersensitivity may be related to metabolic byproducts, changing surface antigens, or other substances released by the parasite.

During the migration phase of many helminths, including schistosomes, the host responds to the infection by producing protective antibodies against the larval form. These antibodies provide resistance to reinfection by new larvae, resulting in a condition called concomitant immunity; this means that the host can harbor the adult and, at the same time, be resistant to reinfection by the larval stage of the same parasite.

Destruction of the Parasite

A helminth's large size creates problems for the immune system. A helminth is too large to be destroyed by antibodies or by white cells, as are unicellular organisms. It appears that a common mechanism for destroying these parasites requires that the surface of the adult be coated with antibody, which, in turn, attracts and binds WBCs that release enzymes that damage the outer surface membrane of the parasite. Later, after the initial damage has been done, macrophages may become involved. Alternatively, organisms can be walled off by granulomatous responses. In intestinal helminth infections in which adults are spontaneously eliminated, the level of IgE antibody often is increased. It has been proposed that expulsion of adult worms results from a localized anaphylactic reaction mediated by the antibodies and substances released by eosinophils and/or mast cells. Others believe that intestinal goblet cells (stimulated by cytokines released from activated T cells) secrete mucus that coats the damaged worm. This action, coupled with mast cell activation, increases gut motility to expel the parasite.

Immunologic/ Serologic Techniques

Although antibodies are often detectable in serum and may be useful guides when diagnosing diseases caused by parasites, they often have little or no correlation with the course or prognosis of the disease (toxoplasmosis is one exception). Subsequent protection from reinfection by the parasite cannot be predicted based on circulating antibody levels. The clinical picture of parasitic diseases—such as amebiasis of the liver, echinococcosis, trichinellosis, toxoplasmosis, and schistosomiasis—is not always clear-cut, but when the antibody titer reaches a detectable level in serum, it is often possible to confirm the diagnosis of these diseases serologically. Serology can also help definitively identify a parasite's presence when it is in organs or other deep-tissue sites, such as the brain or muscle, when no parasite stages are recoverable in blood, urine, or feces.

Toxoplasmosis serology can be used to differentiate acute, recent, and long-term infections in adults by comparing IgG and IgM serum antibody results. Infections of the fetus and newborn can be evaluated using IgG, IgM, and IgA antibody studies.

Antigen Detection

Serologic testing is becoming more useful, particularly as commercial products become more readily available. Current methods fall into two general groups: detecting antigens or detecting antibodies. There are a variety of procedures that use labeled antibodies that directly combine with a parasite or its soluble antigen. For example, *C. parvum*, *E. histolytica*, *E. histolytica/E. dispar*, *G. lamblia*, and *Trichomonas vaginalis* can be identified in clinical specimens by immunologic procedures. Indirect immunofluorescent (IIF), enzyme immunoassay (EIA), and enzyme-linked immunosorbent assay (ELISA) reagent test kits are available to test for these organisms. The IIF methods use monoclonal antibody against the parasite's cell wall and a fluorescein isothiocyanate-labeled anti-immunoglobulin to visualize the initial antibody-parasite complex. An EIA must have an enzyme conjugated (attached) to either an antigen or an antibody, depending on the assay being performed. After the antigen-antibody reaction has occurred and excess materials have been removed, a suitable substrate is added to react with the remaining enzyme. The amount of product formed is proportional to the concentration of the unknown antibody or antigen being measured. The ELISA methods capture organisms or soluble antigen by adding specimen samples to antibody-coated wells. Subsequent reactions cause a chromogen to change color to indicate the presence of bound antigen.

New diagnostic procedures can be expected in the future, especially as DNA probe technology develops. A DNA probe kit is available for detecting *T. vaginalis*. Polymerase chain reaction (PCR) techniques are used to identify *Naegleria fowleri*, *G. lamblia*, *T. cruzi*, and *Toxoplasma gondii*. Table 7–3 lists commercially available immunodiagnostic kits and reagents.

Antibody Testing

The second group of serology tests includes many different methods used to recover and measure levels of circulating antibodies. Current methods include IIF antibody tests; slide, tube, and agar precipitin tests; complement fixation; particle agglutination tests; and ELISA. Most commercial kit systems are based on an ELISA system. DNA probes are used in immunoblot methods at the CDC to diagnose cysticercosis, echinococcosis, paragonimiasis, and schistosomiasis. In underdeveloped countries where parasitic infections are common, high cost and other problems of technology limit the benefits from the availability of these procedures.

Potential Errors

Errors in serologic diagnosis may be related to errors in technique, mixed infections, cross-reacting antigens shared with other parasites or other microorganisms, or even to non–parasite-related diseases or to host antigens. Positive serology test results do not preclude previous infections because immune responses are often long lasting; nor do they rule out false-positive results or cross-reactions. QC tests using known-positive and

TABLE 7–3 □ COMMERCIALLY AVAILABLE KITS FOR IMMUNODETECTION OF SPECIFIC PARASITES

Organism and Kit Name	Manufacturer and/or Distributor	Type of Test
CRYTOSPORIDIUM PARVUM		
ProSpecT	Alexon-Trend	EIA
Microplate Assay		EIA
Rapid Assay		EIA
Color Vue		EIA
Kit also detects *Giardia lamblia*		
MeriFluor	Meridian Diagnostics	DFA
Kit also detects *Giardia lamblia*		EIA
Premier EIA		
Cryptosporidium	Novocastra	DFA
Rim Cryptosporidium	Remel	EIA
Triage Parasite Panel	Biosite Diagnostics, Inc.	Cartridge device, EIA
Kit also detects *Giardia lamblia* and *Entamoeba histolytica/ Entamoeba dispar* group		
ColorPAC *Giardia/Cryptosporidium* Rapid Assay	Genzyme/Becton-Dickinson	Cartridge device, IA
TechLab *Crypto/Giardia* IF Test TechLab *Cryptosporidium* Test	TechLab	DFA EIA
ENTAMOEBA HISTOLYTICA/ENTAMOEBA DISPAR		
ProSpecT Microplate Assay (will not differentiate between *E. histolytica* and *E. dispar*)	Alexon-Trend	
TechLab *Entamoeba* Test (will differentiate between *E. histolytica* and *E. dispar*)	TechLab	EIA
TechLab *Entamoeba/E. dispar* Test (will not differentiate between *E. histolytica* and *E. dispar*)		EIA
Entamoeba histolytica/E. dispar (will not differentiate between *E. histolytica* and *E. dispar*)	Remel, Wampole	EIA

Organism and Kit Name	Manufacturer and/or Distributor	Type of Test
GIARDIA LAMBLIA		
ProSpecT	Alexon-Trend	EIA
Microplate Assay		EIA
Rapid Assay		EIA
Color Vue		EIA
Combination with *Cryptosporidium*		
MeriFluor	Meridian Diagnostics	DFA
Combination with *Cryptosporidium*		EIA
Premier EIA		
Giardia	Novocastra	DFA
Rim Giardia	Remel	EIA
Wampole Giardia	Wampole	EIA
Triage Parasite Panel Combination with *Giardia lamblia* and *Entamoeba histolytica/E. dispar* group	Biosite Diagnostics, Inc.	Cartridge device, EIA
ColorPAC *Giardia/ Cryptosporidium* Rapid Assay	Genzyme/Becton-Dickinson	Cartridge device, IA
TechLab *Crypto/Giardia* IF Test	TechLab	DFA
TechLab Giardia Test		EIA
TRICHOMONAS VAGINALIS		
Affirm VP$_{III}$	MicroProbe/Becton-Dickinson	DNA Probe
Quik-Trich	Integrated Diagnostics	Latex Agglutination
Quik-Tri/Can (combination with *Candida*)		Dual Latex Agglutination
T. VAG DFA kit	Light Diagnostics— Chemicon Intl.	DFA
PLASMODIUM SPP.		
Consult manufactures—may not be available in the United States		
ICT Malaria P.f. ICT Malaria P.f/P.v	Chemicon Intl.	Rapid
ParaSightF	Becton-Dickinson	Rapid
OptiMAL	Flow	Rapid

Continued on following page

TABLE 7–3 □ COMMERCIALLY AVAILABLE KITS FOR IMMUNODETECTION OF SPECIFIC PARASITES (Continued)

Organism and Kit Name	Manufacturer and/or Distributor	Type of Test
HELMINTHS		
ICT Filariasis— *Wuchereria bancrofti*	Chemicon Intl.	Rapid
TropBio—Filariasis	JCU Tropical	Rapid EIA

Adapted from Diagnostic Medical Parasitology, ed 4. ASM Press, Washington, DC, 2001.

ABBREVIATIONS: DFA = direct fluorescent antibody; EIA = enzyme immunoassay.

VENDOR KEY
1. Alexon-Trend-Seradyn, 14000 Unity Street, NW, Ramsey, MN 55303-9115
1a. Becton-Dickinson Advanced Diagnostics, 2350 Qume Drive, San Jose, CA 95131-1087
2. Biosite Diagnostics, Inc., 11030 Roselle Street, San Diego, CA 38121
3. Chemicon International, Inc., 28835 Single Oak Drive, Temecula, CA 925990
4. Flow, Inc., 6127 SW Corbett, Portland, OR 97201
5. Genzyme Diagnostics, 1531 Industrial Road, San Carlos, CA 94070
6. Integrated Diagnostics, 1756 Sulphur Springs Road, Baltimore, MD 21227
7. Meridian Diagnostics, Inc., 3471 River Hills Drive, Cincinnati, OH 45244
8. MicroProbe Corporation, 1725 220th Street, NE, Bothell, WA 98021
9. Novocastra, 30 Ingold Road, Burlingame, CA 94010
10. Remel, 12076 Santa Fe Drive, Lenexa, KS 66215
11. TechLab, Inc., 1861 Pratt Drive, Suite 1030, Blacksburg, VA 24060-6364
12. TropBio Pty Ltd., James Cook University, Townsville, Queensland 4811, Australia
13. Wampole Laboratories, Half Acre Road, P.O. Box 1001, Cranbury, NJ 08512

NOTE: Because changes in products and companies are inevitable, the reader should contact each company to verify product availability. Also, other companies may offer products that may have been unintentionally omitted from this table. This table is provided as a resource only and not a specific recommendation for any particular product or company.

known-negative sera should always be performed. Direct detection methods require that known-positive antigens or organisms for controls be tested as well.

Support Services and Commercial Resources

In the United States, serum for such studies is commonly sent for serologic testing to a State Public Health Reference Laboratory or to the CDC. Samples for CDC processing must be sent via state laboratories because CDC does not accept specimens sent directly by private laboratories or physicians. Most serum specimens may be shipped frozen or preserved with thimerosal (1:10,000 final concentration). The vial, containing at least 2 mL of serum, should indicate the preservative used. Table 7–4 lists the antibody detection tests performed at CDC. For state public health testing availability, consult locally. For more specific details about test procedures, consult the bibliography at the end of this chapter.

At this time, several companies offer reagents and supplies for individual laboratories that want to perform their own procedures. Table 7–5 lists materials available from commercial suppliers. Table 7–6 lists several Websites that provide information related to parasitology and other professional, governmental, and regulatory sites. These resource guides are not inclusive and do not constitute an endorsement by the authors for any product, supplier, or service.

● *Reagent Preparation*

The following preparation instructions are provided for laboratory workers who wish to prepare their own reagents. Bulk materials and prepared products are available from vendors listed in Table 7–5.

D'Antoni Iodine Stain

1. Use when preparing wet-mount preparations of fresh or concentrated feces.
2. Reagents:
   a. 1 g potassium iodine.
   b. 1.5 g powdered iodine crystals.
   c. Add reagents to 100 mL of distilled water and shake it well. Store in brown stoppered bottles; filter daily.

TABLE 7–4 □ ANTIBODY DETECTION TESTS OFFERED AT THE CENTERS FOR DISEASE CONTROL AND PREVENTION*

Disease	Organism	Test
Amebiasis	*Entamoeba histolytica*	Enzyme immunoassay (EIA)
Babesiosis	*Babesia microti* *Babesia* spp. WA1	Immunofluorescence (IFA)
Chagas' disease	*Trypanosoma cruzi*	IFA
Cysticercosis	Larval *Taenia solium*	Immunoblot (blot)
Echinococcosis	*Echinococcus granulosus*	EIA, blot
Leishmaniasis	*Leishmania braziliensis* *L. donovani* *L. tropica*	IFA
Malaria	*Plasmodium falciparum* *P. malariae* *P. ovale* *P. vivax*	IFA
Paragonimiasis	*Paragonimus westermani*	Blot
Schistosomiasis	*Schistosoma* spp. *S. mansoni* *S. haematobium* *S. japonicum*	FAST-ELISA Blot Blot Blot
Strongyloidiasis	*Strongyloides stercoralis*	EIA
Toxocariasis	*Toxocara canis*	EIA
Toxoplasmosis	*Toxoplasma gondii*	IFA-IgG, EIA-IgM
Trichinosis	*Trichinella spiralis*	EIA, Bentonite flocculation

*For additional information about these tests or how to submit specimens for testing or for test results and interpretation, call the Division of Parasitic Diseases at (770) 488–4431.

Polyvinyl Alcohol (PVA) Fixative

1. Use to preserve feces for transport or staining.
2. Reagents*:
   a. Ethyl alcohol, 95% 156 mL.
   b. Mercuric chloride, aqueous (saturated) 312 mL.
   c. Glacial acetic acid 25 mL.
   d. PVA powder 20 mL.
   e. Glycerol 7.5 mL.
   f. Mercuric chloride is prepared by dissolving 130 to 140 g of the salt in 1000 mL of distilled water. Heat to dissolve, then cool, filter, and store in a stock bottle.
   g. Add the PVA powder to the alcohol slowly and stir. Heat to 75°C, and stir until the solution is clear. Add the other reagents and allow to cool. Store in a closed container, and use as needed. Decant the solution without disturbing the sediment.
3. Between 2 and 3 mL of feces per 8 to 10 mL of PVA solution are adequate for transport. (Check government regulations on mailing.) Slides may be made from the transport vial. PVA also can be used by mixing one drop of a liquid or very mucoid stool in three drops of PVA solution on a slide and allowing it to dry overnight at 37°C before staining.

10% Formalin

1. Use with the formalin-ethyl acetate sedimentation concentration method.
2. Reagents:
   a. Formaldehyde 1 part.
   b. Physiologic saline 9 parts.

TABLE 7–5 □ COMMERCIAL SOURCES OF REAGENTS AND SUPPLIES

Reagent or Supply	Vendor
SPECIMEN COLLECTION KIT(S)	
Formalin/PVA	1, 2, 3, 4, 5, 6, 7, 8, 11
PVA modified (copper base)	1, 3, 4, 5, 6, 7, 8, 10, 11
PVA modified (zinc base)	1, 2, 3, 4, 5, 6, 7, 8, 9, 10, 11
MIF	1, 2, 3, 4, 5, 6, 7, 8, 11
SAF	1, 2, 3, 4, 8, 11
Pinworm paddles	3, 4, 9
PRESERVATIVES (BULK)	
Schaudinn fixative solution	1(+,−), 3(+), 4(+), 5(+), 6(+), 8(−), 10(−)
PVA fixative solution	1, 2, 3, 4, 5, 6, 7, 8, 9, 10, 11
PVA powder*	3
MIF solution	1, 3, 4, 5, 6
SAF solution	1, 7
CONCENTRATION SYSTEMS	
Formalin-ethyl acetate	1, 2, 3, 4, 5, 6, 11
Zinc sulfate (sp. gr, 1.18/1.20)	1, 4, 5, 9
STAINS	1, 2, 3, 4, 5, 6, 7, 8, 9, 10, 11
Trichrome solution	1(w), 3(w), 4(w), 5(w), 6(w), 7, 8(w), 9(w), 10(w,g), 11(w)
Trichrome, modified†	1, 2, 3, 4, 5, 6, 7, 8, 9, 10, 11
Chromotrope 2R	11
Fast green FCF	3, 11
Light green SF yellowish	3, 11
Hematoxylin solution	4, 5, 7, 10
Hematoxylin powder	3, 11
Giemsa solution	3, 4, 5, 10, 11
Giemsa powder	3, 11
Carbol fuchsin-Kinyoun	1, 3, 4, 5, 7, 8, 10, 11
Modified acid-fast with DMSO	1, 7, 10
Auramine-rhodamine	3, 7, 10, 11
Acridine orange	7, 8, 10, 11
MISCELLANEOUS	
Lugol's iodine (dilute 1:5)	1, 3, 4, 7, 8, 10, 11
Dobell & O'Connor's iodine	1, 3, 4, 8, 11
Mayer's albumin	1, 4, 11

Reagent or Supply	Vendor
MISCELLANEOUS	
Bacto Entamoeba medium	12
Rice powder	12
Control slides or suspensions	1, 7

Adapted from Diagnostic Medical Parasitology, ed 4. ASM Press, Washington, DC, 2001.
*Use the grade with high hydrolysis and low viscosity for parasite studies.
†Used for the identification of microsporidia spores in stool or other specimens.

ABBREVIATIONS: w = Wheatley; g = Gomori; + = with acetic acid; − = without acetic acid

VENDOR KEY
1. Alpha-Tec Systems, Inc., P.O. Box 5435, Vancouver, WA 98668, (800) 221–6058
2. Evergreen Scientific, 2300 East 49th Street, Los Angeles, CA 90058, (800) 42–6261
3. Fisher Health Care (Chicago), 4500 Turnberry Drive, Hanover Park, IL 60103, www.fisherscientific.com
4. Hardy Diagnostics, 1430 West McCoy Lane, Santa Maria, CA 93455, (800) 266–2222
5. Medical Chemical Corp., 1909 Centinela Avenue, Santa Monica, CA 90404, (310) 829–4304, www.med-chem.com
6. Meridian Diagnostics, Inc., 3741 River Hills Drive, Cincinnati, OH 45244, (800) 543–1980
7. PML Microbiologicals, P.O. Box 459, Tualatin, OR 97062, (800) 547–0659
8. Sanofi Diagnostics Pasteur, 1000 Lake Hazeltine Drive, Chaska, MN 55318, (800) 666–5111
9. Scientific Device Lab., Inc., 411 E. Jarvis Avenue, Des Plaines, IL 60018, (847) 803–9495
10. Volu-Sol, Inc. (a Division of Biomune, Inc.), 5095 West 2100 South, Salt Lake City, UT 84120, (800) 821–2495
11. VWR Scientific, Inc., P.O. Box 7900, San Francisco, CA 94120, (415) 468–7150 (North California), (213) 921–0821 (South California), www.vwr.com
12. Advanced Diagnostics, 2350 Qume Drive, San Jose, CA 95131-1087, (800) 223-8226, www.bdfacs.com

NOTE: Because changes in products and companies are inevitable, the reader should contact each company to verify product availability. Also, other companies may offer products that may have been unintentionally omitted from this table. This table is provided as a resource only and not as a specific recommendation for any particular product or company.

Zinc Sulfate Solution

1. Use with the zinc sulfate flotation concentration method.
2. Reagents:
   a. 330 g zinc sulfate (reagent grade).
   b. Distilled water (final volume—1 L).
   c. Add reagent to the water with heat and stirring, and adjust the specific gravity to between 1.18 (for fresh stool) and 1.20 (for formalin preserved stool) using a hydrometer.

TABLE 7–6 ☐ USEFUL WEBSITES

PARASITOLOGY INFORMATION
American Society of Parasitologists: www.museum.uni.edu/asp/photo.htm Centers for Disease Control and Prevention: www.dpd.cdc.gov/dpdx/ Medical Chemical Corp. ParaSite: www.med-chem.com/para/index.htm Parasitology Resources: www.uchaswv.edu/library/parasites.html
ELECTRONIC IMAGES
Parasite Image Library: www.dpd/cdc.gov/dpdx/html/image_library.htm Parasites and Parasitological Resources: www.biosci.ohio-state.edu/~parasite/home.html Pictorial Presentation of Parasites: http://parasite.biology.uiowa.edu/image
ALLIED HEALTH PROFESSIONAL SITES
American Society of Clinical Laboratory Scientists: www.ascls.org American Society of Clinical Pathologists: www.ascp.org College of American Pathologists: www.cap.org National Committee for Clinical Laboratory Standards: www.nccls.org
GOVERNMENT WEBSITES RELATED TO HEALTH CARE REGULATIONS
Health Care Financing Administration: www.hcfa.gov Compliance Program, Fraud Alerts, Advisory Opinions, Red Book, Work Plan: www.dhhs.gov/proporg/oig Office of the Inspector General (OIG) Compliance Documents for Clinical Laboratories, Hospitals, and Third Party Billing: www.access.gpo.gov/su_docs/aces/aces|40.html

Giemsa Stain

1. Use to stain blood parasites.
2. Reagents:
   a. Giemsa stain may be purchased as a concentrated stock, or stock Giemsa can be prepared as follows:

      Powdered Giemsa 1 g
      Glycerol 66 mL
      Methanol (absolute) 66 mL

   b. Grind the stain in a mortar containing 5 to 10 mL of glycerol. Add the remaining glycerol and heat to 55°C in a water bath until the stain is dissolved. Cool and add the methanol. Let stand for 2 to 3 weeks. Filter and store in a brown bottle away from light.
3. Before use, dilute with Giemsa buffer.

Giemsa Buffer

1. Use with stock Giemsa stain.
2. Reagents:
   a. 0.067 M Na_2HPO_4 (disodium phosphate). Add 9.5 g to 1000 mL of distilled water. This is stock buffer No. 1.
   b. 0.067 M $NaH_2PO_4 \cdot H_2O$ (monosodium phosphate). Add 9.2 g to 1000 mL of distilled water. This is stock buffer No. 2.
3. Working buffer, pH 7.0, is prepared from stock buffers weekly and filtered before use. To 900 mL distilled water, add 61.1 mL of stock buffer No. 1 and 38.9 mL of stock buffer No. 2.

Trichrome Stain

1. Use to stain fecal smears for intestinal protozoa.
2. Reagents:
   a. Schaudinn solution: Saturated aqueous mercuric chloride; 130 to 140 g of mercuric chloride is added to 1000 mL of distilled water. Heat to dissolve, then cool and filter into a stock bottle. Working solution is prepared by mixing two parts of mercuric chloride solution with one part of 95% ethanol before use. Discard after use.
   b. Alcohol solutions: Various solutions may be prepared by diluting the appropriate volume of absolute (100%) ethanol with distilled water (e.g., a 70% solution is made by adding 30 mL of water to 70 mL of absolute alcohol). All alcohol solutions should be prepared fresh daily and kept tightly covered to prevent evaporation or absorption of atmospheric water.
   c. Trichrome stain:

      Chromotrope 2R 0.6 g
      Light green SF 0.15 g
      Fast green FCF 0.15 g
      Phosphotungstic acid 0.7 g
      Acetic acid (glacial) 1.0 mL
      Distilled water 100.0 mL

      Mix the dry components and add the acetic acid; allow to stand for 30 minutes, then add to water. The stain should be purple. Staining more than 14 smears daily tends to weaken the stain. Strength returns if the stain is exposed to air for 3 to 8 hours.
   d. Acid alcohol is prepared by adding 1 mL acetic acid to 99 mL 90% ethanol.

Modified Trichrome Stain for Microsporidia (Weber, Green)

1. Use to stain fecal smears for intestinal microsporidia.
2. Reagents:
   a. Alcohol solutions: Various solutions may be prepared by diluting the appropriate volume of absolute (100%) ethanol with distilled water (e.g., a 70% solution is made by adding 30 mL of water to 70 mL of absolute alcohol). All alcohol solutions should be prepared fresh daily or kept tightly covered to prevent evaporation or absorption of atmospheric water.

b. Trichrome stain:

> Chromotrope 2R 6.0 g (10 times normal formula)
> Fast green FCF 0.15 g
> Phosphotungstic acid 0.7 g
> Acetic acid (glacial) 3.0 mL
> Distilled water 100.0 mL
> Mix the dry components and add the acetic acid; allow to stand for 30 minutes, then add to water. The stain should be purple.

c. Acid alcohol is prepared by adding 4.5 mL acetic acid to 999.5 mL 90% ethanol.

NOTE: 1. Kokoskin's modification shortens the staining time to 10 minutes by raising the staining temperature to 50°C.
2. Ryan's modification uses aniline blue in place of fast green FCF; the background color is blue.

Iron Hematoxylin Stain

1. Use to stain fecal smears for intestinal protozoa.
2. Reagents:
   a. Schaudinn solution: Saturated aqueous mercuric chloride; 130 to 140 g of mercuric chloride is added to 1000 mL of distilled water. Heat to dissolve, then cool and filter into a stock bottle. Working solution is prepared by mixing two parts of mercuric chloride solution with one part of 95% ethanol before use. Discard working solution after each use.
   b. Alcohol solutions: Various solutions may be prepared by diluting the appropriate volume of absolute (100%) ethanol with distilled water. All alcohol solutions should be prepared fresh daily.
   c. Iron hematoxylin stain: 10% stock solution; 10.0 g of hematoxylin (crystals or powder) is added to 100 mL of 95 or 100% alcohol. Dissolve in a flask using gentle heat. Plug the flask with cotton and allow it to stand in sunlight to ripen for 6 weeks. Shake frequently to hasten the ripening process. Store the ripened stain in a glass-stoppered bottle and refrigerate. The stain is usable for at least 1 year. Working solution is prepared by mixing 5 mL of the 10% stock stain with 95 mL of distilled water. Discard after each use.
   d. Ferric ammonium sulfate (4% solution): Dissolve 4 g of ferric ammonium sulfate in 100 mL of distilled water.
   e. Phosphotungstic acid (2% solution): Dissolve 2 g of phosphotungstic acid in 100 mL of distilled water.
   f. Lithium carbonate (saturated aqueous solution): Dissolve 2 g of lithium carbonate in 100 mL of distilled water.

NNN Medium

1. Use to culture blood, aspirates, bone marrow, biopsy, or other tissue material for *Leishmania* spp. and *T. cruzi*.
2. Mix and bring to boiling the following ingredients:
   a. Agar 14 g
   b. Sodium chloride 6 g
   c. Distilled water 900 mL
3. Distribute medium to test tubes and sterilize in the autoclave.
4. Cool medium to 48°C and to each tube add one-third of its volume of sterilized defibrinated rabbit blood.
5. Mix thoroughly by rotation and allow to cool in a slanted position. Cooling is best done in an ice bath because rapid cooling promotes water condensation in the tube. Organisms develop most rapidly in the supernate at the bottom of the tube.
6. Check for sterility by incubating the medium overnight at 37°C.

Kinyoun Carbolfuchsin

1. Dissolve 4 g of basic fuchsin in 20 mL of 95% ethanol (solution A).
2. Dissolve 8 g of phenol crystals in 100 mL of distilled water (solution B).

3. Mix solutions A and B together. Store at room temperature. The solution is stable for 1 year.

1% Sulfuric Acid

1. Add 1 mL of concentrated sulfuric acid to 99 mL of distilled water. Store at room temperature. The solution is stable for 1 year.

Loffler Alkaline Methylene Blue

1. Dissolve 0.3 g of methylene blue in 30 mL of 95% alcohol.
2. Add 100 mL of dilute (0.01%) potassium hydroxide. Store at room temperature. The solution is stable for 1 year.

> You have now completed the section on clinical laboratory procedures. After reviewing this material with the aid of your learning objectives, proceed to the post-test.

Post-Test

Mark True (T) or False (F) for each of the following: (2 points each) Explain your answer.

_____ 1. In general, six sequential fecal specimens should be examined for the presence of any intestinal parasites.

_____ 2. Liquid or soft stools should be examined within 1 hour because trophozoites die rapidly.

_____ 3. Formed stools need not be refrigerated because protozoa have already formed cysts.

_____ 4. Wet mounts should be made when bloody mucus is noted in a stool specimen.

_____ 5. A castor oil enema may be used if only helminths are suspected.

_____ 6. It is not necessary to examine the whole slide if eggs or cysts are noted within the first few fields examined.

Discussion questions: (5 points each)

7. How should the microscope's light be adjusted for successful microscopic examination of wet mounts? Why?

8. When should a cellophane tape test be done? Why?

9. Name two types of concentration methods, explaining the principles and writing the procedure for each method.

10. What is the specific gravity of the solution used in the zinc-sulfate concentration method? How is it checked?

11. Which eggs are not easily recovered by flotation methods?

12. What is used to extract fats in the sedimentation method?

13. List the advantages and disadvantages of thin and thick smears for blood parasites.

14. How is blood laked in the preparation of thick blood smears?

15. List the expected staining reactions for protozoa, using trichrome stain.

16. Working Giemsa buffer is prepared from two stock solutions. What are the salts in each solution? What is the pH of the working buffer?

17. Explain how microsporidia may be visualized when recovered in feces.

18. Compare and contrast the antibody and antigen-based immunodiagnostic methods used in parasitology.

Match the reagents with the chemical components given: (2 points each). (Choices may be used more than once or not at all. Some answers may require multiple choices.)

19. a. _____ Iodine crystals
    b. _____ Mercuric chloride
    c. _____ Rice powder
    d. _____ Light green SF
    e. _____ Ethyl acetate
    f. _____ Phospho-tungstic acid
    g. _____ 10% formalin
    h. _____ 70% alcohol

   1. PVA
   2. D'Antoni stain
   3. Giemsa stain
   4. Trichrome stain
   5. Schaudinn solution
   6. Balamuth medium
   7. Sedimentation
   8. Flotation

Each multiple choice question is worth 2 points.

20. Charcot-Leyden crystals may be noted when examining fecal preparations. These crystals are associated with the immune response and are thought to be breakdown products of:
    a. Eosinophils
    b. Lymphocytes
    c. Macrophages
    d. Monocytes
    e. Neutrophils

21. The formalin-ethyl acetate concentration method for feces is used to demonstrate:
    a. Formation of amebic pseudopodia
    b. Hatching larval forms
    c. Motility of helminth larvae
    d. Protozoan cysts and helminth eggs
    e. Trophozoites

22. One of the following diagnostic procedures can be considered an urgent procedure (stat). That procedure is a(n):
    a. Ova and parasite examination for giardiasis
    b. Culture for amebic keratitis
    c. Blood film for malaria
    d. Baermann concentration for strongyloidiasis
    e. None of these

23. The best test procedure for correctly identifying *Enterobius vermicularis* infections is the:

   a. Formalin-ethyl acetate concentration method
   b. Cellophane tape test
   c. Zinc sulfate flotation method
   d. Entero-Test capsule
   e. Knott concentration

24. Amoeba trophozoite motility is best observed using a(n):

   a. Iodine-stained wet mount
   b. Unstained saline wet mount
   c. Unstained zinc sulfate flotation preparation
   d. Concentrated wet mount
   e. Giemsa stain

25. White blood cells may be used as a positive control material for all of the following procedures EXCEPT the:

   a. Direct wet mount
   b. Giemsa stain for trypanosomes
   c. Iron hematoxylin stain
   d. Trichrome stain

BIBLIOGRAPHY

Diamond, LS: Axenic culture of *Entamoeba histolytica*. Science 134:336, 1961.

Difco Manual of Dehydrated Cultural Media and Reagents for Microbiological and Clinical Laboratory Procedures, ed 11. Difco Laboratories, Detroit, 1998.

Eberhard, ML, and Lammie, PJ: Laboratory diagnosis of filariasis. Clin Lab Med 11:4, 1991.

Garcia, LS: Diagnostic Medical Parasitology, ed 4. ASM Press, Washington, DC, 2001.

Goodenough, UW: Deception by pathogens. Am Sci 79:344–355, 1991.

Gryseels, B: Human resistance to *Schistosoma* infections. Parasitol Today 10:380–384, 1994.

Guttierrez, Y: Diagnostic Pathology of Parasitic Infections with Clinical Correlations. Lea & Febiger, Philadelphia, 1990.

Kokoskin, E, et al. Modified technique for efficient detection of microsporidia. J Clin Microbiol 32:1074, 1994.

Luna, VA, et al. Use of the fluorochrome calcofluor white in the screening of stool specimens for spores of microsporidia. Am J Clin Pathol 103:656, 1995.

National Committee for Clinical Laboratory Standards: Use of Blood Film Examination of Parasites. Tentative guideline M15-T. National Committee for Clinical Laboratory Standards, Villanova, PA, 1990.

National Committee for Clinical Laboratory Standards: Protection of Laboratory Workers from Instrument Biohazards and Infectious Disease Transmitted by Blood, Body Fluids, and Tissue. Approved guideline M29-A. National Committee for Clinical Laboratory Standards, Villanova, PA, 1997.

National Committee for Clinical Laboratory Standards: Procedures for the Recovery and Identification of Parasites from the Intestinal Tract. Approved guideline M28-A. National Committee for Clinical Laboratory Standards, Villanova, PA, 1997.

Palmer, J: Modified iron hematoxylin/Kinyoun stain. Clin Microbiol Newslett 13:39 (letter), 1991.

Pinon, JM, et al: Early neonatal diagnosis of congenital toxoplasmosis: value of comparative enzyme-linked immunofiltration assay, immunological profiles, and anti-*Toxoplasma gondii* immunoglobulin M (IgM) or IgA immunocapture and implications for postnatal therapeutic strategies. J Clin Microbiol 34:579–583, 1996.

Rao, LV, et al: Evaluation of immuno-toxoplasma IgG assay in the prenatal screening of toxoplasmosis. Diag Microbiol Infect Dis 27:13–15, 1997.

Ryan, NJ, et al: A new trichrome-blue stain for detection of microsporidial species in urine, stool, and nasopharyngeal specimens. J Clin Microbiol 31:3264, 1993.

Salfelder, K: Atlas of Parasitic Pathology (Current Histopathology Series, Vol 20). Kluwer Academic Publishers, Norwell, MA, 1992.

Sher, A, and Scott, PA: Mechanisms of acquired immunity against parasites. In Warren KS (ed), Immunology and Molecular Biology of Parasitic Infections, ed 3. Blackwell Scientific Publications, Boston, 1993.

Shiff, CJ, et al: The *ParaSight®*-F test: A simple rapid manual dipstick test to detect *Plasmodium falciparum* infection. Parasitol Today 10:494–495, 1994.

Warren, KS (ed): Immunology and molecular biology of parasitic infections, ed 3. Blackwell Scientific Publications, Boston, 1993.

Weber, R, et al: Improved light-microscopical detection of microsporidia spores in stool and duodenal aspirates. N Engl J Med 326:161, 1992.

Wheatley, WB: A rapid staining procedure for intestinal amebae and flagellates. Am J Clin Pathol 2:990–991, 1951.

Wilson, M, et al: Evaluation of six commercial kits for detection of human immunoglobulin M antibodies to *Toxoplasma gondii*. J Clin Microbiol 35:3112–3115, 1997.

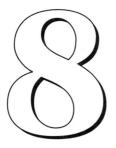

CONTROL AND TREATMENT OF PARASITIC DISEASE

LEARNING OBJECTIVES

ON COMPLETION OF THIS CHAPTER, THE STUDENT WILL BE ABLE TO:

1 Define the terms *epidemiology, epidemic, endemic, pathogenicity,* and *virulence.*
2 List considerations for planning parasitic disease control strategies.
3 Describe methods used to control parasitic disease.
4 List the major objectives of a treatment program.
5 Explain the difference between a radical and a clinical cure for malaria.
6 List the most common parasitic diseases reported in immunocompromised patients.

● Introduction

From the parasite's point of view, the best relationship that it could have with a host is one in which the host would suffer little or no harm because this allows the parasite to survive. Organisms such as *Entamoeba coli* are often called parasites, but they are actually commensals and have a good relationship with their host. In a world where drug treatments are available, parasites that cause diseases are subject to steps taken to control them—a problem, of course, only to the parasite.

Most lay people believe that treating an infected individual controls the parasitic disease and that avoiding an infected individual prevents catching the infection. These people also generally accept the idea that practicing good hygiene and taking medication lessen or prevent infections. Such concepts, in fact, do lead to a decreased incidence of many diseases; however, the actual control of parasitic diseases in nature, as you now know, is far more complicated. In this chapter, you will learn various approaches to controlling specific parasites, preventing spread of disease, and treating infected hosts.

● Defining Terms

Various terms applied to this discussion must be explained to fully understand the problems related to controlling parasitic disease.

1. **Epidemiology** is the study of the relationships of the various factors that determine the frequency and distribution of an infectious process or disease in a community; the results of these studies are used to help control health problems.
2. An **epidemic** is an infectious disease that attacks many people at the same time in the same geographic region. An example is an outbreak of cryptosporidiosis.
3. An **endemic disease** is one that occurs continuously or in expected cycles within a given population, with a certain number of cases expected over a given period. An example is malaria in Africa.
4. **Pathogenicity** is the parasite's ability to produce pathologic changes and disease in or on a host. To be pathogenic, a parasite must be able to colonize a host and grow

and produce toxins that induce a response by the host or directly cause tissue damage. The progression and extent of the infection is related to the number of organisms living within the host, the parasite's virulence, and the extent of the host's response.

5. **Virulence** relates to the ability of pathogenic organisms to thrive in a host, including the abilities of the parasite to attach or adhere to a target tissue or cell, release enzymes or toxins that damage or interfere with normal host functions, resist or evade host defense mechanisms, and reproduce and distribute offspring effectively.

● Controlling Parasitic Disease

Aside from survival within a host, parasites also have another major problem to overcome: transportation from host to host. Various parasites have complex and varied life cycles; therefore, we must find ways to break these cycles if control and possible eradication of disease-causing organisms are to occur.

Several questions must be answered when developing a control strategy for a given parasitic disease:

1. What is the cost/benefit of controlling this parasite?
2. What would happen if nothing were done about the problem?
3. What controllable factors affect the host's ability to respond to the disease?
4. What controllable environmental factors affect the life cycle?
5. Can the life cycle be interrupted without host cooperation?
6. Can and should the host be protected from exposure to the parasite?
7. Is an effective vaccine available?

Treating a disease represents the final and most direct interruption of a parasite's life cycle, but this step is complex and may have adverse repercussions for the host. In addition, we must consider the cultural beliefs, personal hygiene, and dietary habits of the host; the status of national and community affluence, education, sanitation, and medical practices; the availability and impact of drugs; and the use of chemicals on the environment. Finally, ecologic and biological factors, as well as the general health of the actual and potential local domestic and wild reservoir animals, must be evaluated.

Aparasite's life cycle may involve a single host with no free-living stages (e.g., *Enterobius*, which spreads very easily). Other parasites have a very complex life cycle (e.g., *Clonorchis*) involving multiple specific hosts and parasitic stages. *Enterobius vermicularis* solves its transportation problem by releasing environmentally resistant infective eggs that remain infective for many days. Eggs can become airborne, thereby infecting others not directly in contact with the infected host. Reinfection of the host can also occur through hand-to-mouth transfer of eggs. This parasite is endemic in many parts of the world and can cause small local epidemics in family homes and other institutions, such as schools or nursing care facilities, where people are closely associated for extended periods.

Control of pinworm infection attempts to protect a host from exposure to the parasite by relying heavily on preventing the contamination of bed linens. This is done by wearing nonporous close-fitting clothing to bed, sterilizing sheets, and vacuum cleaning rugs and furniture frequently. Also important is attention to details, such as covering toothbrushes and other personal articles to guard against exposure to bathroom dust, which may carry airborne eggs. Sunlight (ultraviolet) kills the larvae, as does dry heat; however, many household and other toxic chemicals do not penetrate the eggshells. Treatment of the entire family or other institutionalized residents may be necessary to prevent further spreading of the infection. Lack of cooperation between the patient and family members may hamper control and treatment.

On the other hand, *Schistosoma* spp., as another example with a more complex life cycle, solve their transportation problem through intermediate forms that live in nonhuman hosts and survive in water. Because this parasite is so virulent and causes significant pathology, it is important to treat infected individuals as well as the environment. Controlling and eradicating this parasite can be accomplished by interrupting the life cycle at several points; that is, it can be done by treating infected people, destroying the snail host, destroying the infective cercariae larvae released into the water from the snail host, or preventing fecal or urine contaminations of the water. With this type of life cycle, control measures depend less heavily on the involvement or cooperation of the local citizenry; instead, control can be handled independently by knowledgeable experts working with the government. It is important, however, to ensure that the local population is adequately informed, particularly if chemicals or sprays are to be used and if hygiene education is required.

Ensuring safe water and limiting snail populations are the two most important and viable measures for controlling schistosomiasis. An example of successful preventive management occurred in Puerto Rico in the mid-1900s. Early in the control campaign, a trial mass chemotherapy treatment of infected individuals led to the death of some people because of drug side effects. Chemotherapy was suspended, and attention was focused on snail control. A molluscan competitor was introduced into ponds, lakes, and rivers in an effort to reduce the numbers of the specific host species. Concurrently, the project managers improved sanitary waste disposal systems, thus reducing the exposure of the snails to sources of infective miracidia. By the mid-1960s, some 15 to 20 years of work began to show success. In most areas of Puerto Rico, the rate of infection in the population fell from 20% to almost 0%. In other parts of the world, however, creation of new dams has led to increases in snails that can serve as hosts for this disease.

Because schistosomiasis is still a major problem in many parts of the world, similar control methods are being tried elsewhere. Chemotherapeutic measures are still being used, however. For example, 1100 primary schoolchildren in suburbs of Bujumbura, Burundi, were treated annually with praziquantel for 3 years. Infection rates declined from almost 20% to 8%. The World Health Organization (WHO) plans to continue this strategy.

Another important control strategy is human behavior modification. Because human infection with schistosomiasis occurs when cercariae penetrate bare skin, wearing wading boots, avoiding fecal contamination of water, and avoiding contact with contaminated water can break the parasite's life cycle. One study found that when people applied niclosamide as a 1% lotion to the skin before entering snail-infested waters, cercariae penetration was prevented. This alternative, if affordable, makes sense when people must use snail-infested water for bathing, clothes washing, or raising of crops such as rice. Most important, by teaching people to use toilets or latrines, infected urine or feces cannot contaminate soil or water supplies.

Barrier protection prevents exposure of humans to various infective forms. Examples include wearing wading boots in water when cercaria might be present, wearing shoes while walking in contaminated soil where hookworm and *Strongyloides* larvae are present, and using mosquito netting for protection from biting mosquitoes. These and other barrier measures are used along with other control strategies.

Chemical Vector Control Strategies

In controlling the spread of other parasitic diseases, chemical measures have had varying degrees of success. Treating the local environment is difficult because dormant stages of parasites, such as eggs and cysts, are generally resistant to toxic substances. Also, for many reasons, communities are increasingly resisting the local use of chemicals. In many cases, when an arthropod is involved, a practical solution is vector control. For instance, sprays and dips reduce flea and tick infestations in livestock and domestic pets even though they do not totally clear the environment. Biodegradable chemicals in water supplies have been used to control black fly larvae, and insecticide sprays are still widely used to control the tsetse fly vector of trypanosomiasis.

Malaria Control Strategies

The WHO sponsored an ambitious program to eradicate malaria worldwide. Early in the program, investigating members of the project found many mosquitoes resting inside houses. Consequently, investigators had the inside walls of some houses and other buildings sprayed with DDT (dichlorodiphenyl-trichloroethane). This initial, aggressive attack dramatically reduced the malaria problem in parts of Africa. Unfortunately, when local follow-up procedures became lax following initial success, the incidence of malaria increased to significantly high levels. In addition, some observers have claimed that the WHO program contributed greatly to the DDT resistance seen in mosquitoes; however, the resistance problem can actually be traced to indiscriminate agricultural use of the chemical.

Another problem hampered WHO's African mosquito attack: Either two insect groups existed (house-dwelling and bush-dwelling), or some of the house-dwelling mosquitoes developed new behavior patterns and became bush-dwelling mosquitoes. Some investigators believed that the DDT house-spraying measures may have selected for the bush-dwelling mosquitoes. However, when the spraying stopped, the house-dwelling mosquitoes reappeared, suggesting still another biological change. Regardless of the reasons for the changes, the DDT experience offers an example of the importance of understanding the complex biology and behavior patterns of insect vectors when choosing control strategies and using every effort to understand the long-term consequences of any intervention strategy.

Of serious ecologic concern is the history of indiscriminate spraying of insecticide prior to human understanding of the biological impact of chemicals such as DDT on all plants and animals in the food chain. Our failure to predict that such spraying would cause selection for insect vectors resistant to chemicals also is a major concern. These human errors should not be allowed to recur.

In March 2000, WHO emphasized the need to find alternatives to DDT in controlling mosquito populations. DDT is now allowed only for indoor residual spraying of homes to reduce malaria transmission in areas where it is endemic. Treaty negotiations are under way to finally eliminate its use altogether. The major problem will be to find suitable and affordable alternatives. An immediate alternative is access to insecticide-treated bed netting, but at the cost of $4 to $5 each, many impoverished people will not be able to afford it.

Vector control strategies can reduce infected arthropod host populations, thus reducing human or animal exposure to the parasite and eventually leading to parasite eradication. Endemic malaria in the United States was finally eradicated in the 1950s, and since then, only imported cases brought from endemic locations by refugees, travelers, and military service personnel have been noted. Because anopheline mosquitoes are still present, however, it is possible that malaria could again become endemic if proper vigilance is not maintained.

Biological and Environmental Control Strategies

A successful control experience occurred in Central America, where a well-planned strategy was used to control *Culicoides* spp. that bred in the Farfan Swamp in the Panama Canal zone. These tiny biting gnats (no-see-ums) flew through normal window screen mesh and forced workers caring for military communications equipment located in the swamp to wear uncomfortable, finely meshed, protective suits. Because temperatures often reached more than 90°F, the obvious problems forced other control measures to be sought. Chemical control of the insect in the swamp began in the early 1950s, but the gnat developed genetic resistance to the insecticide, making other control measures necessary.

The Farfan Swamp, although fed by a freshwater stream, was brackish because seawater backed into it. The endemic *Culicoides* spp. breeds only in salty water; thus, tidal gates were built to keep the seawater out of the swamp. Gradually, the swamp's water became fresh, and by the late 1950s the gnat population had diminished to an acceptable level. Later, in the mid-1960s, a canal dredging operation began dumping its dredge into the swamp, causing the water to become salty again. This change caused the gnat population to grow, and subsequent efforts were then made to halt dumping in the Farfan Swamp. It took about 2 years to clear the salt once again from the swamp water, and consequently, to bring the *Culicoides* back under control.

Various other methods of biological insect and parasitic control have been tried. Elimination of primary screwworm fly myiasis from the southeastern United States was accomplished by releasing numerous male *(Callitroga) Cochliomyia hominivorax* flies that had been sterilized by irradiation. Competitive mating decreased the offspring to below critical mass levels for breeding. Similar successful elimination in the southwestern United States has not been achieved because the insect population entering from Mexico could not be adequately controlled at the border. By contrast, the Florida peninsula effectively isolated its area from invading flies. More recently, the state of California used irradiated flies in its campaign against the Mediterranean fruit fly. Daily, 20,000 irradiated male flies raised in an agricultural research station in Hawaii were shipped to California and released. This helped save the fruit crop and lessened the need for chemical control measures. This example illustrates that combining various strategies can control insect populations.

Other Control Strategies

Serious efforts are also being expended on perfecting other control systems. Immunization has already proved successful against several serious parasites of domestic animals. Brazilian research institutes are preparing a vaccine (2001) *S. mansoni*. The impact of a successful campaign could be huge because this parasite affects as many as 10 million Brazilians. Similar efforts are occurring in Egypt, and phase II clinical trials of a vaccine against *S. haematobium* began in the year 2000 in Senegal and Niger. Malaria vaccine trials in Papua New Guinea and Gambia have shown promising results against *Plasmodium falciparum*. Continuing research will surely lead to other successful vaccines, but the formidable technical and financial problems of producing, distributing, storing, and getting them to affected individuals will be a great and costly challenge.

Other biological methods are also being explored, such as improved insect traps using pheromones; genetic manipulation of insect hosts; introduction of predators for insect, snail, and other host species; introduction of competitive species of nonpathogenic parasites or nonsupportive hosts; and mass treatment of host populations with chemotherapeutic agents. For example, India, which spends 45% of its national health budget controlling malaria, is now looking for less costly alternatives to the millions of dollars spent on pesticides. These include breeding fish that eat mosquito larvae in infested waters and later selling the fish as a cash crop, filling in water-holding pits to create usable land, and planting eucalyptus trees in swamps to soak up water and later using the wood for cooking and construction.

Human Behavior and Culture

Cultural behavior of world populations both helps and hinders the control of parasitic diseases. For instance, the dietary customs of Jewish and Moslem peoples have greatly reduced their exposure to *Taenia solium* and *Trichinella spiralis* infections. Various cleaning and cooking habits and rituals practiced by many peoples around the world have lessened their exposure to parasitic diseases. However, people in many parts of the world, including the United States, still use untreated human waste (known as night soil) to fertilize crops. Some people bathe and wash clothes and cooking utensils in water contaminated with human waste. Such behavior obviously promotes the transmission of parasites. In some wealthy countries, again including the United States, many people are "getting back to nature" or vacationing in health resorts offering natural or untreated water and raw foods. Unfortunately, one side effect to this lifestyle has been an increase in giardiasis and other parasitic diseases.

In contrast, affluence has many benefits. Home freezers contribute to the control of trichinosis because freezing pork for 6 days at $-20°F$ kills encysted larvae. Similarly, freezing other foodstuffs for various periods can prevent other diseases. In addition, use of window screens in more affluent countries is greatly reducing human exposure to disease-carrying vectors. The most valuable invention for preventing the spread of parasitic infections, however, has been the flush toilet; its use, along with waste-water treatment, is always accompanied by decreased disease.

Probably the most effective control measure among those available may also be the hardest one to accomplish—the changing of human behavior through education and the demonstrated rewards of improved health. For example, the WHO campaign to teach people in endemic areas to strain drinking water through T-shirt cotton is successfully reducing the incidence of *Dracunculus* infections.

● Treating Parasitic Disease

It is evident, on paper at least, that various methods can control parasitic diseases. Until widespread control is achieved, however, a need continues for chemotherapeutic intervention for infected individuals. Chemotherapy can support other control efforts when used to treat infected target groups (as has been done in Egypt to combat schistosomiasis) or when used prophylactically to protect people from becoming infected, but it is not necessarily required as a parasitic disease control method. Treatment per se is generally used to alleviate and cure conditions caused by infections. Before treating a given infection with chemotherapy, the physician weighs several factors, including the severity and duration of infection, the health conditions of the host, and the availability and toxicity of the drug treatment. If the toxicity or side effects of a treatment are more hazardous to the patient than the disease itself, treatment may be reasonably withheld. Furthermore, if the chance of reinfection is great, the disease is mild, and the cost or risk of treatment is high, then treatment is questionable.

General Considerations

Once the decision to treat an infection has been made, consideration of the need to treat asymptomatic family members or others closely associated with the infected individual is important. For example, some parasites, such as *Enterobius*, may be spread to others in a family or in an institutional setting; therefore, treatment of other resident individuals may be appropriate. Because *Trichomonas vaginalis* is transmitted sexually, all sexual partners of the infected person should also be treated. However, in other diseases, it is useless to treat others or isolate an infected person if direct transmission is not possible. This is why it is important to understand life cycles.

Some parasitic infections need not be treated because they are at a stage of low worm burdens, are self-limiting and nonpathogenic, and probably will not be transmitted to others. However, some infections require chemotherapy, surgical intervention, or both. At present, cysticercosis and hydatid disease require surgery. Treatment of amebiasis of the liver or appendix requires surgical attention less often because more effective chemotherapeutics are now available.

The objectives of a treatment program should be to stop the parasite's growth, reproduction, and transmission; kill parasites without inducing a harmful host response; and expel parasites from the host. Finding those drugs that are selective for parasitic metabolic systems without adversely affecting human systems has been difficult. Not surprisingly, many drugs are toxic, especially the ones that affect energy metabolism. A variety of drugs currently in use are known carcinogens or teratogens.

Pharmacodynamics

Most drugs commonly used to treat infections affect various metabolic pathways, such as the following:

1. Energy metabolism
2. Cell wall synthesis
3. Protein synthesis
4. Membrane function
5. Nucleic acid synthesis
6. Cofactor synthesis

Several drugs selectively affect neuromuscular systems of the helminths. The selective action of many antiprotozoal drugs results from either preferential absorption of the drug by the parasite or from the ability of the drug to discriminate between isofunctional targets in the host cells versus those in the parasitic cell. However, little is known about the selective action of most antihelminthic chemicals.

Resistance to Treatment

To survive, parasites must react to conditions in their environment, including the pressure exerted by chemotherapeutic agents. Drug resistance develops when pathogenic organisms are able to do the following:

1. Metabolize the drug to an inactive form
2. Alter their permeability to the drug
3. Use a metabolic pathway not affected by the drug
4. Increase enzyme production to overcome the level of the drug being administered
5. Change the drug's binding site target on or inside of the organism

The extent to which each of the drug resistance factors mentioned affects the treatment of parasitic disease is not fully known. Alterations in permeability, drug-binding activity, and enzyme production all have been demonstrated for some parasites, with altered permeability being the single most common resistance mechanism. Parasite changes with respect to binding activity and enzyme production can be genetically passed to offspring.

Table 8–1 (p. 205) contains a partial listing of chemotherapeutic agents commonly in use, along with some of their important side effects. The reader will find a further listing and updating of agents and side effects in the *Medical Letter* cited in the bibliography for this chapter. The following is a brief discussion of the treatments used for selected parasites.

Treatment of Helminths

The correct treatment of helminths relies on the correct identification of the parasite or parasites involved. Generally, albendazole, pyrantel pamoate, and mebendazole are considered the drugs of choice in the treatment of most intestinal nematode infections. Thiabendazole is useful against cutaneous and visceral larval migrans and *Strongyloides stercoralis.* Niclosamide is effective against cestodes. Praziquantel is effective against all *Schistosoma* spp. and other flukes; metrifonate and oxamniquine are suitable alternatives for some schistosomes.

A recent study suggests that artemether, a drug used to treat malaria, can be used prophylactically against immature *Schistosoma mansoni* worms and that, when combined with praziquantel, it is very effective against active *Schistosoma* infections. The researchers point out that this strategy should be used only in areas where malaria is not endemic to preserve the drug's effectiveness against multidrug-resistant *P. falciparum.*

Treatment of Filariasis

Filariasis is treated with diethylcarbamazine; however, some authorities recommend excision of the adult *Onchocerca* worm before treatment because this drug does not kill the adult. An alternative treatment for onchocerciasis begins with a 3-week course of diethylcarbamazine followed by suramin. Suramin kills the adult worm. Furthermore, antihistamines or corticosteroids may be needed to reduce the allergic (Mazzotti) reaction to disintegrating microfilariae. Extreme caution is needed while treating onchocerciasis because the allergic reaction may be fatal.

Treatment of Protozoa

Amebiasis

Treatment of amebiasis caused by *Entamoeba histolytica* depends on the severity of the clinical symptoms and the parasites' locations in the host. Debate over the treatment of asymptomatic carriers continues; however, when treated, the carrier is usually given diloxanide furoate or diiodohydroxyquin. When either mild or severe intestinal symptoms are evident and the patient is passing both trophozoites and cysts, metronidazole (a tissue amoebicide) plus diiodohydroxyquin is the treatment of choice. Extraintestinal amebiasis is treated using metronidazole. Diiodohydroxyquin is also required with a concurrent bowel infection. Because newer drugs are less toxic, emetine is no longer considered the best treatment for extraintestinal amebiasis. However, the higher cost and limited availability of newer drugs in other parts of the world have perpetuated its use.

Flagellates

Giardiasis responds to metronidazole within 5 days in most cases. Albendazole is also effective. Because *Giardia* infections can be acquired by drinking contaminated water, small amounts of water can be purified using iodine solution. A stock solution is made by adding 6 g of iodine crystals to 60 mL (2 ounces) of water, shaking the solution, and letting it stand for 2 hours (the crystals will not dissolve completely). To kill *Giardia,* 25 mL of the stock solution is added to 1 L (5 tsp/quart) of water and allowed to stand for 20 minutes at 20°C (68°F) before drinking. The 25 mL can be replaced in the stock container with clean water after each use until the iodine crystals have dissolved completely. Campers and backpackers who wish to purify stream or river water can use this method as well.

Infections with *T. vaginalis* in people of either sex are effectively treated with the oral medication metronidazole. Pregnant women should not take this drug, however. Topical preparations containing halogenated hydroxyquinolines are useful in relieving the symptoms of vaginitis, but they may not completely eliminate the parasite because the preparation may not reach every organism. Other topical preparations are also available. Sexual partners should be treated simultaneously.

Trypanosomiasis

Early diagnosis and treatment of African trypanosomiasis is important because treatment is difficult after the central nervous system becomes involved. Suramin sodium is the drug of choice early on; however, because it does not cross the blood-brain barrier, melarsoprol is needed for the late disease stages. All drugs for African trypanosomiasis are toxic, and most should be administered during hospitalization. Nifurtimox is most useful when treating *T. cruzi* infections.

Researchers at Johns Hopkins University found that the antibiotic thiolactomycin could inhibit synthesis of the fatty acid myristate, which is needed by *Trypanosoma brucei* to anchor surface proteins to its cell membrane, thus killing the parasite. Although this specific antibiotic is cleared too rapidly from the human bloodstream to be effective, the research does suggest that a new and selective approach to treating this disease needs to be pursued.

Leishmaniasis

Visceral leishmaniasis is treated with antimony sodium stibogluconate (Pentostam), which is administered either intravenously or intramuscularly for 28 days. Oral miltefosine has been successfully administered in India at a dosage rate of 100 mg/day (not to exceed 4 mg/kg per day) for 4 weeks. At the end of a phase II trial, researchers believe they have found the first oral agent that is effective against visceral leishmaniasis.

Cutaneous leishmaniasis is also treated using sodium stibogluconate for 20 days. A 28-day course is needed for mucocutaneous disease. The oral medication dapsone, tested in India, showed an 82% cure rate for cutaneous leishmaniasis.

Treatment of Malaria

The treatment of malaria follows two strategies: clinical cure and radical cure. A clinical cure is accomplished when symptoms are relieved; in case of malaria, symptoms cease because asexually reproducing parasites are eliminated from peripheral circulation. However, this treatment does not necessarily mean that all parasites have been eradicated from the body. Chloroquine phosphate (Aralen) is the drug of choice for treating all species of malaria sensitive to the drug; it produces a clinical cure, but it does not completely eliminate the parasite from the host in those infections caused by relapsing species of malaria. A radical cure (elimination of all parasites from the body, including secondary tissue schizonts) for *Plasmodium vivax* and *Plasmodium ovale* is accomplished using primaquine phosphate as the second course of treatment.

Travelers to endemic areas, including former residents who are returning to their home after living in nonmalarious areas for some time, are advised to begin taking chloroquine phosphate once weekly 1 to 2 weeks before travel. They should continue prophylactic doses throughout their stay in the endemic area and for 4 weeks after they return. In addition, they should take primaquine phosphate for 2 weeks after leaving the area. This prophylactic course normally prevents disease. Because chloroquine phosphate does not prevent liver invasion by the parasite, it is especially important to use primaquine to prevent a relapse with *P. vivax* or *P. ovale*. Individuals deficient in glucose-6-phosphate dehydrogenase (G6PD) should not use primaquine.

Various strains of *P. falciparum* and *P. vivax* have become resistant to chloroquine. Successful treatment of these infections requires the use of alternative antimalarials, such as a combination of pyrimethamine and sulfadoxine. Quinine or quinidine may be used in place of chloroquine phosphate.

For prophylaxis, the Centers for Disease Control and Prevention (CDC) recommends using mefloquine (Lariam) in place of chloroquine phosphate once weekly for travelers in endemic areas of drug-resistant malaria. It should be noted that areas of chloroquine-resistant malaria are no longer limited to East Africa; they now include many locations in Central Africa as well.

An interesting and novel treatment strategy is being tested at the University of Washington in Seattle. Malaria trophozoites break down hemoglobin for protein synthesis and energy, liberating free hemoglobin in the process. The parasite neutralizes the toxic free hemoglobin by synthesizing a quasi-crystalline array known as malaria pigment or hemozoin. Because hemozoin contains iron, it is ferromagnetic. Researchers hypothesized that exposing the parasites to an oscillating magnetic field would disrupt the formation of new hemozoin molecules, leading to an accumulation of the toxic free hemoglobin, which would ultimately kill the parasite. Blood cells infected with *P. falciparum* were exposed to oscillating magnetic fields and the parasitemia was significantly reduced, suggesting that an inexpensive, simple, portable, and noninvasive treatment method for malaria might yet be found.

Treatment of Parasitic Disease in Immuno-compromised Patients

Since the discovery and identification of HIV and its relationship to AIDS and AIDS-related complex (ARC), several opportunistic parasitic infections have been recognized as serious problems for immunocompromised patients. These problems are not limited only to patients with AIDS; they also affect individuals who have compromised immune systems resulting from congenital absence or abnormal development of the immune system, malignancy, irradiation, cytotoxic drug therapy, or other underlying infections. These patients have higher incidence of bacterial, viral, and fungal infections as well as parasitic disease.

The most likely immunocompromised patient population, continuing to grow in number, is the group of patients with AIDS. Commonly affected people in this group in the United States include intravenous drug users, homosexual and bisexual men and their partners, prostitutes, hemophiliacs, people seeking treatment for sexually transmitted diseases, people having multiple sexual partners, people who consider themselves at risk, and children born to infected mothers.

AIDS is not curable currently, but it is generally preventable for adults. Prevention is accomplished by avoiding high-risk practices, such as unprotected sex and drug needle-sharing. All medical care workers must follow the Occupational Safety and Health Administration's rules related to bloodborne pathogens, referred to as the "Universal Precautions,"' with blood or other body fluids. These rules provide a way for medical personnel to avoid becoming infected with any disease-causing organism—not just HIV. If they do not follow these practices, health workers may become infected and may even infect fellow workers or patients.

Most Common Parasites in Immunocompromised People

At least eight parasitic infections are most commonly reported in immunocompromised patients. Seven of these are protozoan, and the other one is caused by *S. stercoralis*. Immunocompetent hosts may harbor *Strongyloides* for years without symptoms other than an unexplained eosinophilia. When the patient becomes compromised, the number of larvae and adults increases rapidly, producing disseminated strongyloidiasis. As *S. stercoralis* rhabditiform larvae become infective filariform larvae, they carry bacteria with them as they invade the intestinal mucosa; bacteremia, pneumonia, and even meningitis can result. *Strongyloides* hyperinfections have also been found in patients with leukemias, lymphomas, fungal infections, leprosy, tuberculosis, and other conditions (e.g., renal disease, asthma). Patients who have high eosinophilia (10% to 50%) and unexplained bacteremia or other problems caused by enteric bacteria should be tested for strongyloidiasis.

The protozoa most commonly encountered in immunocompromised humans include *E. histolytica, Giardia lamblia, Toxoplasma gondii* (encephalitis), *Cryptosporidium parvum, Isospora belli*, and at least seven genera of Microsporidia. The intestinal protozoa usually cause chronic diarrhea and chronic wasting syndrome ("slim disease"). Although *E. histolytica* and *G. lamblia* are not considered opportunistic parasites, they must be mentioned in this list because they can produce rather severe symptoms in immunocompromised hosts. Extraintestinal invasion by *E. histolytica* is more likely to occur in these patients as well.

Cryptosporidium infection is difficult to treat, requiring fluid replacement, nutrition, and antidiarrheal medication. Paromomycin, spiramycin, and eflornithine have provided limited success. *Isospora* infections are treated with trimethoprim-sulfamethoxazole (TMP-SMX) for approximately 1 month.

Microsporidia have been found throughout the body, but the most frequent protozoal infection found in patients with AIDS has been caused by *Enterocytozoon bieneusi*. These patients have chronic diarrhea, fever, and weight loss that mimics other intestinal infections. It is important to thoroughly investigate these symptoms, although there is no satisfactory treatment for these parasites. Albendazole has been helpful in treating some *Encephalito-*

zoon spp. infections. Immunocompetent patients with *E. bieneusi* eye infections usually respond to treatment.

● *Summary*

Treatment of parasitic diseases relies heavily on accurate diagnosis, followed by good judgment on the part of the physician. Certain factors—such as drug effectiveness versus toxicity, the parasite's location and numbers in the host, the length of the treatment course required, the method of the drug's administration, other drugs being administered, and the patient's general condition—must all be considered to provide maximum benefit. If only one drug is available, however, and the patient's condition necessitates treatment, there may be no other choice. Furthermore, certain long treatment schedules may facilitate parasitic resistance to the drug or create cumulative toxicity problems for the patient. Finally, good nutritional management and patient involvement in self-care are important to help the patient overcome infection and promote resistance to subsequent infections.

The CDC can provide detailed information about the treatment and use of various drugs. It also can supply drugs for treating rare diseases. Note that some drugs are teratogenic in animals, and special care should be taken to avoid prescribing them to pregnant women. Teratogens are noted in Table 8–1, as are others that may have more severe effects for pregnant women or young children.

TABLE 8–1 □ CHEMOTHERAPY OF PARASITIC DISEASES

Parasite	Infection	Chemotherapeutic Agent	Adverse Reactions*
Acanthamoeba spp.	Chronic meningoencephalitis Keratitis	Amphotericin B and sulfadiazine or sulfisoxazole Topical propamidine isethionate plus neomycin-polymyxin B-gramicidin ophthalmic solution	**Rash,** photosensitivity, hepatic and renal toxicity, blood dyscrasia, vasculitis
Ancylostoma braziliense or *A. caninum*	Cutaneous larval migrans; or creeping eruption	Albendazole	**GI disturbance**
Ancylostoma duodenale	Hookworm	Albendazole or Mebendazole† or Pyrantel pamoate	**GI disturbance** **GI disturbance** **GI disturbance** dizziness, rash, fever
Ascaris lumbricoides	Roundworm	Albendazole or Mebendazole† or Pyrantel pamoate	**GI disturbance** **GI disturbance** **GI disturbance,** dizziness, rash, fever
Balantidium coli	Balantidiasis	Tetracycline or Metronidazole†	**Anorexia, nausea,** vomiting, renal and hepatic impairment **Nausea, headache,** vomiting, diarrhea, vertigo, insomnia, ataxia
Clonorchis sinensis	Clonorchiasis (Chinese liver fluke)	Praziquantel or Albendazole	Sedation, abdominal discomfort, fever, sweating, nausea, eosinophilia, photosensitivity, urticaria, vomiting and diarrhea **GI disturbance**
Cryptosporidium parvum	Cryptosporidiosis	Paromomycin	Adverse reactions
Dientamoeba fragilis	Dientamoebiasis	Iodoquinol or Tetracycline or Paromomycin	**Iodine toxicoderma,** rash, slight thyroid enlargement, nausea **Anorexia, nausea,** vomiting, renal and hepatic impairment **GI disturbance**
Diphyllobothrium latum	Diphyllobothriasis (fish tape worm)	Niclosamide† or Praziquantel	Nausea, abdominal pain Sedation, abdominal discomfort, fever, sweating, nausea, eosinophilia, photosensitivity, urticaria, abdominal pain, vomiting, and diarrhea
Dracunculus medinensis	Filariasis; guinea worm	Metronidazole† or Thiabendazole 1. Ivermectin† or 2. Niridazole	**Nausea, headache,** vomiting, diarrhea, vertigo, insomnia, ataxia **Nausea, vomiting, vertigo, rash,** leukopenia, color vision disturbance, tinnitus, shock **Allergic and febrile reactions** from worm **Immunosuppression,** vomiting, cramps, dizziness, headache
Echinococcus spp.	Hydatid cyst	Albendazole or Mebendazole†	**GI disturbance**

Continued on following page

TABLE 8–1. ☐ CHEMOTHERAPY OF PARASITIC DISEASES (Continued)

Parasite	Infection	Chemotherapeutic Agent	Adverse Reactions*
Entamoeba histolytica	Amebiasis	Iodoquinol or	**Iodine toxicoderma,** rash, slight thyroid enlargement, nausea
		Paromomycin	**GI disturbance**
	Intestinal disease	Metronidazole† plus	**Nausea, headache,** vomiting, diarrhea, vertigo, insomnia, ataxia
		Iodoquinol or Paromomycin	**Iodine toxicoderma,** rash, slight thyroid enlargement, nausea
	Hepatic disease	Metronidazole† plus	**Nausea, headache,** vomiting, diarrhea, vertigo, insomnia, ataxia
		Iodoquinol or Paromomycin	**Iodine toxicoderma,** rash, slight thyroid enlargement, nausea
Enterobius vermicularis	Enterobiasis (pinworm)	Pyrantel pamoate or	**GI disturbance,** dizziness, rash, fever
		Mebendazole† or Albendazole	**GI disturbance**
Fasciola hepatica	Liver rot: sheep liver fluke	Bithionol or	Photosensitivity skin reaction, vomiting, diarrhea, abdominal pain, urticaria
		Triclabendazole	Approved for veterinary use in United States—only single dose needed
Fasciolopsis buski	Fascioliasis	Praziquantel or	Sedation, abdominal discomfort, fever, sweating, nausea, eosinophilia, photosensitivity, urticaria, abdominal pain, vomiting and diarrhea
		Niclosamide†	Nausea, abdominal pain
Giardia lamblia	Giardiasis	Metronidazole† or	**Nausea, headache, vomiting,** diarrhea, vertigo, insomnia, ataxia
		Quinacrine	Vomiting, vertigo, headache, psychosis, blood dyscrasia, ocular damage, rash, hepatic necrosis
Heterophyes heterophyes	Heterophyiasis, intestinal fluke	Praziquantel	Sedation, abdominal discomfort, fever, sweating, nausea, eosinophilia, photosensitivity, urticaria, abdominal pain, vomiting, and diarrhea
Hymenolepis nana	Dwarf tapeworm	Praziquantel	Sedation, abdominal discomfort, fever, sweating, nausea, eosinophilia, photosensitivity, urticaria, abdominal pain, vomiting, and diarrhea
Isospora belli	Intestinal disease	Trimethoprim-sulfamethoxazole (TMP-SMX) (teratogenic in animals)	Rash, photosensitivity, hepatic and renal toxicity, blood dyscrasia, vasculitis
Leishmania braziliensis complex or *L. mexicana* complex	Leishmaniasis: mucocutaneous	Antimony sodium gluconate (stibogluconate sodium)	**Diarrhea,** muscle pain and joint stiffness, bradycardial colic, rash; contraindicated in pregnancy
L. donovani complex	Leishmaniasis: visceral	Antimony sodium gluconate (stibogluconate sodium) or	**Diarrhea,** muscle pain and joint stiffness, bradycardial colic, rash, contraindicated in pregnancy
		Pentamidine isethionate	**Hypotension-hypoglycemia vomiting, blood dyscrasias, renal damage,** rash, hepatic toxicity

Parasite	Infection	Chemotherapeutic Agent	Adverse Reactions*
L. tropica complex	Leishmaniasis: cutaneous	Antimony sodium gluconate (stibogluconate sodium)	**Diarrhea,** muscle pain and joint stiffness, bradycardial colic, rash; contraindicated in pregnancy
Loa loa	Filariasis: eyeworm	Diethylcarbamazine or Ivermectin[†]	**Allergic and febrile reactions** resulting from death of the worm
Metagonimus yokogawai	Metagonimiasis: intestinal fluke	Praziquantel or	Sedation, abdominal discomfort, fever, sweating, nausea, eosinophilia, photosensitivity, urticaria, abdominal pain, vomiting, and diarrhea
		Trachloroethylene	**Epigastric burning, dizziness, headache,** drowsiness, severe nausea and vomiting (Antabuse-like effect) with alcohol
Microsporium spp.	Tissue parasites	Albendazole	**GI disturbance**
Naegleria fowleri	Primary meningoencephalitis	Amphotericin B	**Chills, sweating, fever, muscle pain, nausea, vertigo**
Necator americanus	Hookworm	Albendazole or Mebendazole[†] or Pyrantel pamoate	**GI disturbance** **GI disturbance** **GI disturbance,** headache, dizziness, rash, fever
Onchocerca volvulus	Filariasis; river blindness	1. Ivermectin[†] 2. Diethylcarbamazine plus suramin[†]	**Allergic and febrile reactions** resulting from death of the worm **Rash, pruritus, paresthesias,** vomiting, peripheral neuropathy, shock
Opisthorchis viverrini	Opisthorchiasis; liver fluke	Praziquantel	Sedation, abdominal discomfort, fever, sweating, nausea, eosinophilia, photosensitivity, urticaria, abdominal pain, vomiting, and diarrhea
Paragonimus westermani	Paragonimiasis; lung fluke	Praziquantel or Bithionol	Sedation, abdominal discomfort, fever, sweating, nausea, eosinophilia, photosensitivity, urticaria, abdominal pain, vomiting, and diarrhea Photosensitivity skin reaction, vomiting, diarrhea, abdominal pain, urticaria
Pediculus humanus var. *corporis* or *capitis*	Body or head lice	1% permethrin or Pyrethrin with piperonyl butoxide or 0.5% malathion lotion or 1% lindane or Ivermectin	Irritation to skin, eyes, and mucous membranes Irritation to skin, eyes, mucous membranes; ragweed-sensitized people should not use Skin rash, itching, nontender tissue swelling
Phthirus pubis	Crab lice	1% permethrin or Ivermectin	Irritation to skin, eyes, and mucous membranes Skin rash, itching, nontender tissue swelling

Continued on following page

TABLE 8–1 ☐ CHEMOTHERAPY OF PARASITIC DISEASES (Continued)

Parasite	Infection	Chemotherapeutic Agent	Adverse Reactions*
*Plasmodium falciparum***	Malignant malaria (chloroquine-susceptible) (Note: Chemoprophylaxis: chloroquine phosphate or mefloquine) (chloroquine-resistant)	Chloroquine phosphate (Note: no primaquine† after infection)	Headache, vomiting, confusion, skin eruptions, retinal injury
		Quinine sulfate and	Cinchonism, hypotension, arrhythmias, blood dyscrasia, photosensitivity, blindness
		Pyrimethamine–sulfadozine (Fansidar) or	**Folic acid deficiency,** blood dyscrasia, rash, vomiting, convulsions, shock
			Rash, photosensitivity, hepatic and renal toxicity, blood dyscrasia, vasculitis
		Doxycycline	**Absolutely contraindicated if patient has sulfonamide intolerance**
		Quinine (parenteral	**Anorexia, nausea,** vomiting, renal and hepatic impairment
	(comatose patient)		**Cinchonism, hypotension, arrhythmias,** blood dyscrasia, photosensitivity, blindness
*Plasmodium malariae***	Quartan malaria	Chloroquine phosphate (Note: no primaquine† after infection)	Headache, vomiting, confusion, skin eruptions, retinal injury
*Plasmodium ovale***	Ovale malaria (radical cure)	Chloroquine phosphate followed by primaquine† phosphate (prevents relapses)	Headache, vomiting, confusion, skin eruptions, retinal injury
Hemolytic anemia in G6PD-deficient patients, neutropenia, nausea, hypertension; **contraindicated in pregnancy**
Plasmodium vivax	Tertian malaria (radical cure)	Chloroquine phosphate followed by primaquine† phosphate (prevents relapses)	Headache, vomiting, confusion, skin eruptions, retinal injury
Hemolytic anemia in G6PD-deficient patients, neutropenia, nausea, hypertension; **contraindicated in pregnancy**
	Chloroquine-resistant	Quinine sulfate plus	**Cinchonism, hypotension, arrhythmias,** blood dyscrasia, photosensitivity, blindness
		Pyrimethamine–sulfadozine (Fansidar) or	**Folic acid deficiency,** blood dyscrasia, rash, vomiting, convulsions, shock rash, photosensitivity, hepatic and renal toxicity, blood dyscrasia, vasculitis
		Doxycycline	**Absolutely contraindicated if patient has sulfonamide intolerance**
Anorexia, nausea, vomiting, renal and hepatic impairment
Sarcoptes scabiei	Mites, scabies	5% permethrin or	Irritation to skin, eyes, and mucous membranes
		Ivermectin	Skin rash, itching, nontender soft tissue swelling
Schistosoma haematobium	Schistosomiasis (bilharziasis); bladder cancer	Praziquantel	Sedation, abdominal discomfort, fever, sweating, nausea, eosinophilia

Parasite	Infection	Chemotherapeutic Agent	Adverse Reactions*
Schistosoma japonicum	Schistosomiasis (bilharziasis); blood fluke	Praziquantel	Sedation, abdominal discomfort, fever, sweating, nausea, eosinophilia
Schistosoma mansoni	Schistosomiasis (bilharziasis); blood fluke, swamp fever	Praziquantel or	Sedation, abdominal discomfort, fever, sweating, nausea, eosinophilia
		Oxamniquine (Vansil)	Headache, fever, dizziness, nausea, insomnia, diarrhea, hepatic enzyme changes
Strongyloides stercoralis	Strongyloidiasis; threadworm	Ivermectin or	Skin rash, itching, nontender soft tissue swelling
		Thiabendazole	**Nausea, vomiting, vertigo, rash,** leukopenia, color vision disturbance, tinnitus, shock
Taenia saginata	Taeniasis; beef tapeworm	Praziquantel or	Sedation, abdominal discomfort, fever, sweating, nausea, eosinophilia, photosensitivity, urticaria, abdominal pain, vomiting, and diarrhea
		Niclosamide†	Nausea, abdominal pain
Taenia solium	Taeniasis; pork tapeworm	Praziquantel or	Sedation, abdominal discomfort, fever, sweating, nausea, eosinophilia, photosensitivity, urticaria, abdominal pain, vomiting, and diarrhea
		Niclosamide†	Nausea, abdominal pain
	Cysticercosis	Albendazole (experimental) or Praziquantel (experimental) or surgery	**GI disturbance** Sedation, abdominal discomfort, fever, sweating, nausea, eosinophilia, photosensitivity, urticaria, abdominal pain, vomiting, and diarrhea
Toxocara canis	Visceral larval migrans	Albendazole or Mebendazole† or Diethylcarbamazine or Thiabendazole	**GI disturbance** **GI disturbance** **GI disturbance** **Nausea, vomiting, vertigo, rash,** leukopenial color vision disturbance
Toxoplasma gondii	Toxoplasmosis (moderate to severe illness)	Pyrimethamine plus	**Folic acid deficiency,** blood dyscrasia, rash, vomiting, convulsions, shock; administer corticosteroids in ocular toxoplasmosis, folinic acid may be added to counteract bone marrow depression
		Sulfadiazine (teratogenic in animals) or	**Rash,** photosensitivity, hepatic and renal toxicity, blood dyscrasia, vasculitis
	(immunosuppressed host)	Spiramycin	**Absolutely contraindicated if patient has sulfonamide intolerance**
		Pyrimethamine plus Sulfadiazine plus	GI disturbance **Folic acid deficiency,** blood dyscrasia, rash, vomiting, convulsions, shock; administer corticosteroids in ocular toxoplasmosis

Continued on following page

TABLE 8–1 □ CHEMOTHERAPY OF PARASITIC DISEASES (Continued)

Parasite	Infection	Chemotherapeutic Agent	Adverse Reactions*
		Folinic acid	**Rash,** photosensitivity, hepatic and renal toxicity, blood dyscrasia, vasculitis **Absolutely contraindicated if patient has sulfonamide intolerance** Folinic acid may be added to counteract bone marrow depression
Trichinella spiralis	Trichinosis	Metronidazole† plus steroids for severe symptoms or Albendazole plus steroids for severe symptoms	**Nausea, headache, vomiting,** diarrhea, vertigo, insomnia, ataxia **GI disturbance**
Trichomonas vaginalis	Trichomoniasis	Metronidazole†	**Nausea, headache, vomiting,** diarrhea, vertigo, insomnia, ataxia
Trichuris trichiura	Trichuriasis; whipworm	Mebendazole†	**GI disturbance**
Trypanosoma cruzi	Chagas' disease	Benznidazole‡ (Nifurtimox§)	Skin allergy, peripheral neuropathy Nausea, dizziness, insomnia, vertigo, neuropathy
Trypanosoma gambiense	West African sleeping sickness	Suramin¶ or	**Rash, pruritus, vomiting, paresthesias,** shock, peripheral neuropathy
	Hemolymphatic disease	Pentamidine isethionate	**Breathlessness, dizziness, headache,** tachycardia, vomiting, itching
	CNS disease	Melarsoprol	**Encephalopathy,** vomiting, neuropathy, rash, myocarditis, hypertension
Trypanosoma rhodesiense	East African sleeping sickness	Suramin¶ or	**Rash, pruritus, vomiting, paresthesias,** shock, peripheral neuropathy
	Hemolymphatic disease	Pentamidine isethionate	**Breathlessness, dizziness, headache,** tachycardia, vomiting, itching
	CNS disease	Melarsoprol or	**Encephalopathy,** vomiting, neuropathy, rash, myocarditis, hypertension
		Tryparsamide and Suramin¶	**Nausea, vomiting** **Rash, pruritus, vomiting, paresthesias,** shock peripheral neuropathy
Wuchereria bancrofti	Filariasis, Bancroft's filariasis	Diethylcarbamazine or Ivermectin¶	**Allergic and febrile reactions** resulting from death of the worm Skin rash, itching, nontender tissue swelling

*Most common adverse reactions are noted in **boldface.**
†Not recommended for pregnant women or children younger than 2 years of age.
‡Available as Rochhagan (Roche, Brazil).
§Nifurtimox is no longer manufactured but is available from CDC in selected cases.
¶Available from CDC Drug Service, Centers for Disease Control and Prevention, Atlanta, GA 30333.
**Several other alternative drugs are available for treating malaria, including mefloquine, Halofantrine, and Artemether. See The Medical Letter for further details.

ABBREVIATIONS: CNS = Central nervous system; G6PD = glucose-6-phosphate dehydrogenase; GI = gastrointestinal.

FOR REVIEW

1. *List three methods used to control parasitic diseases, and explain how each method can lead to disease control.*

2. *Explain how education can help control disease.*

3. *Seven guests had severe diarrhea for several days about 1 week after attending a country club banquet. Laboratory tests confirmed that all patients were infected with Cryptosporidium spp. This situation describes an example of an <u>endemic/epidemic</u>. Circle the correct answer and explain your choice.*

4. *True or False. Malaria has been eradicated in the United States; therefore, there is no danger of it becoming re-established in the future. Explain your answer.*

5. *List the objectives of a patient treatment program, and explain why some asymptomatic individuals should be treated and why some symptomatic patients should not be treated:*

6. *Explain how a radical cure differs from a clinical cure when treating malaria:*

7. *What advice would you give to a traveler who is planning a trip to Africa where chloroquine-resistant malaria is endemic?*

BIBLIOGRAPHY

Abu-Elyazeed, RR, et al: Field trial of 1% niclosamide as a topical antipenetrant to *Schistosoma mansoni* cercariae. Am J Trop Med Hyg 49:403–409, 1993.

Altman, RM, et al: Control of *Culicoides* sand flies, Fort Kobbe Canal Zone in 1968. Mosquito News 30(2):235–240, 1970.

Anderson, RM, and May, RM: Helminthic infections of humans: Mathematical models, population dynamics, and control. Adv Parasitol 24:1–101, 1985.

Bennett, CJ, and Plum, F: Cecil Textbook of Medicine, ed 20. WB Saunders, Philadelphia, 1996.

Brabin, L, and Brabin, BJ: Parasitic infections in women and their consequences. Adv Parasitol 31:1–81, 1992.

Bruce-Chwatt, LJ: History of malaria from pre-history to eradication. In Wernsdorfer, WH, McGregor, SI (eds): Malaria, Principles and Practice of Malariology. Churchill Livingstone, Edinburgh, 1988.

Bundy, DAP, and Guyatt, HL. Schools for health: focus on health, education and the school-aged child. Parasitol Today 12(8):1–16, 1996.

Centers for Disease Control and Prevention: Update: Chloroquine-resistant *Plasmodium falciparum* Africa. Morb Mortal Wkly Rep 32(33):437–438, 1983.

Centers for Disease Control and Prevention: Health Information for International Travel 1999–2000, Chemoprophylaxis and Treatment of Malaria. DHHS, Atlanta 1999, pp. 114–121.

Centers for Disease Control and Prevention: Malaria Surveillance—United States, 1993. Morb Mortal Wkly Rep 46(SS-2), 1997

Crompton, DWT: Hookworm disease: Current status and new directions. Parasitol Today 5:1–2, 1989.

Cox, FEG (ed): Modern Parasitology: A Textbook of Parasitology, ed 2. Blackwell Scientific Publications, Oxford, 1993.

Davies, JB: Sixty years of onchocerciasis vector control: A chronologic summary with comments on eradication, reinvasion and insecticide resistance. Annu Rev Entomol 39:23–45, 1994.

Dogra, J. A double-blind study on the efficacy of oral dapsone in cutaneous leishmaniasis. Trans R Soc Trop Med Hyg 85:212–213, 1991.

Dye, C: The analysis of parasite transmission by bloodsucking insects. Annu Rev Entomol 37:1–19, 1992.

Dye, C: Leishmaniasis epidemiology: The theory catches up. Parasitology 104(suppl):S7–18, 1992.

Evans, DB, and Guyatt, HL. The cost-effectiveness of mass drug therapy for intestinal helminths. Pharmacoeconomics 8(1):14–22, 1995.

Feagin, JE, et al: Magnetic Fields and Malaria. In Holick MF and Jung EG (eds): Biologic Effects of Light: Proceedings of the Biologic Effects of Light Symposium. Kluwer Academic Publishers, Hingham, MA, 1999, pp. 343–349.

Goodwin, LG (ed): Chemotherapy of Tropical Diseases: The Problem and the Challenge. Wiley, Somerset, NJ, 1987.

Greenwood, BM: A malaria control trial using insecticide-treated bed nets and targeted chemo-prophylaxis in a rural area of The Gambia, West Africa. Trans R Soc Trop Med Hyg 87(suppl 2):1–60, 1993.

Gustafsson, LL, and Abdi, YA (eds): Handbook of Drugs for Tropical Parasitic Infections. Taylor & Francis, Bristol, PA, 1987.

Hesein, MH, et al: Who misses out with school-based health programmes? A study of schistosomiasis control in Egypt. Trans R Soc Trop Med Hyg 90(4):362–365, 1996.

Kierszenbaum, F (ed): Parasitic Infections and the Immune System. Academic Press, San Diego, 1994.

Lane, RP: The contribution of sandfly control to leishmaniasis control. Ann Soc Belg Med Trop 71(suppl)1:65–74, 1991.

Liew, FY (ed): Vaccination Strategies of Tropical Diseases. CRC Press, Boca Raton, FL, 1989.

Lin, LB: Bednets treated with pyrethroids for malaria control. In Target GAT (ed): Malaria: Waiting for the Vaccine. Wiley, Chichester, 1991, pp. 67–82.

Mectizan and onchocerciasis: a decade of accomplishment and prospects for the future, the evolution of a drug into a development concept. In Ann Trop Med Parasitol 92(suppl 1):7–10, 2000.

The Medical Letter, Inc: Drugs for parasitic infections. March, 2000, pp. 1–12.

Miller, MJ, and Love, EJ (eds): Parasitic Diseases: Treatment and Control. CRC Press, Boca Raton, FL, 1989.

Pampano, E: A Textbook of Malaria Eradication, ed 2. Oxford University Press, London, 1969.

Pearson, R, and Guerrant, R: Praziquantel: A major advance in anti-helminthic therapy. Ann Intern Med 99:195, 1983.

Physicians Desk Reference, ed 54. Medical Economics, Orasill, NJ, 2000.

Proceedings of a Symposium of the International Atomic Energy Commission: Sterile insect technique and radiation in insect control. June 29–July 3, 1981, United Nations, New York, 1982.

Schultz, MG: Current concepts in parasitology. Parasitic diseases. N Engl J Med 297:1259–1261, 1977.

Schad, GA, and Warren, KS, eds: Hookworm Disease: Current Status and New Directions, 1991.

Soulsby, EJL: Immune Responses in Parasitic Infections: Immunology, Immunopathology and Immunoprophylaxis (4 Vols). CRC Press, Boca Raton, FL, 1987.

Warren, KS: Immunology and Molecular Biology of Parasitic Infections, ed 3. Blackwell Scientific Publications, Oxford, 1992.

Warren, KS and Mosteller, F (eds): Doing More Good Than Harm: The Evaluation of Health Care Interventions, Ann NY Acad Sci 703, 1993.

WHO Expert Committee on Malaria, Twentieth Report. World Health Organization, 2000.

World Health Organization. Management of severe malaria: a practical handbook. World Health Organization, 2000.

World Health Organization: Tropical Disease Research, Thirteenth Report. World Health Organization, 1997.

FINAL EXAMINATION

Using separate sheets of paper, answer the following questions. Allow 90 minutes to complete this text. **Except when indicated, all questions are worth 1 point each.** A satisfactory score is 80% or more. Answers are given in the next section.

1. State the scientific name for the parasites illustrated below. **(5 points)**

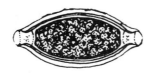

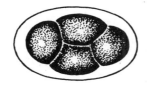

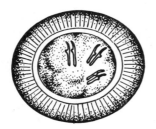

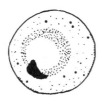

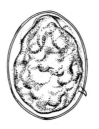

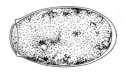

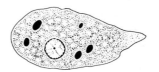

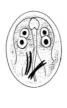

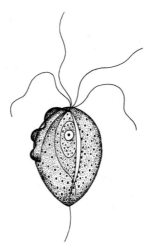

2. Draw the life cycle for each parasite given below. (**10 points**)

    a. *Ascaris lumbricoides*   d. *Enterobius vermicularis*
    b. *Diphyllobothrium latum*   e. *Leishmania donovani*
    c. *Trypanosoma cruzi*

3. A patient was treated with immunosuppressant drugs during a kidney transplant and subsequently exhibited symptoms of two parasitic infections. Which were they? (**2 points**)

    a. *Ascaris lumbricoides*   d. *Strongyloides stercoralis*
    b. *Toxoplasma gondii*   e. *Plasmodium falciparum*
    c. *Schistosoma mansoni*

4. Which one of the following parasites is *not* found most prevalently in North or South America?

    a. *Trypanosoma cruzi*   d. *Mansonella ozzardi*
    b. *Leishmania braziliensis*   e. *Paragonimus westermani*
    c. *Necator americanus*

5. For each parasite given, select its most common body location in humans. Choices may be used more than once. (**5 points**)

    _____ a. *Schistosoma mansoni*   1. Blood
    _____ b. *Clonorchis sinensis*   2. Liver
    _____ c. *Trichura trichiura*   3. Intestine
    _____ d. *Leishmania braziliensis*   4. Striated muscle
    _____ e. *Trypanosoma b. rhodesiense*   5. Skin
    _____ f. *Echinococcus granulosus*   6. Lymph nodes
    _____ g. *Endolimax nana*   7. Heart muscle
    _____ h. *Plasmodium vivax*   8. Eye
    _____ i. *Strongyloides stercoralis*   9. Bladder veins
    _____ j. *Loa loa*   10. Intestinal veins
                                     11. Subcutaneous tissue
                                     12. Macrophages

6. The intermediate host for *Taenia saginata* is:

    a. Pig   d. Bear
    b. Cow   e. Sheep
    c. Human

7. Which of the following are the diagnostic morphologic characteristics for *Entamoeba histolytica*? (Choose all that apply.)

    a. Centrally located karyosome   e. Large karyosome with a faintly
    b. A micronucleus and macronucleus   visible nuclear membrane
    c. Large glycogen vacuole   f. Ingested red blood cells
    d. Flagella

8. Which of the following require no intermediate host? (Choose all that apply.)

    a. *Hymenolepis nana*   d. *Trichuris trichiura*
    b. *Giardia lamblia*   e. *Schistosoma mansoni*
    c. *Strongyloides stercoralis*

9. Which cestode produces an operculated egg?

    a. *Taenia saginata*   d. *Echinococcus granulosus*
    b. *Hymenolepis nana*   e. *Taenia solium*
    c. *Diphyllobothrium latum*

10. A stained blood smear reveals giant platelets and many reticulocytes containing Schüffner's dots, large ring forms, and schizonts with 12 to 24 merozoites. You would name this as:

    a. *Plasmodium vivax*
    b. *Plasmodium falciparum*
    c. *Plasmodium ovale*
    d. *Plasmodium malariae*
    e. *Babesia* spp.

11. When purged specimens are to be examined for amoebae, which of the following should be used to obtain the specimen?

    a. Barium salts
    b. Castor oil
    c. Fleet Phospho-Soda
    d. Mineral oil

12. A stained fecal smear reveals mononucleate flagellates with a comma-shaped posterior, and lemon-shaped mononucleate cysts with a clear, nipplelike bleb at one end. You would name this as:

    a. *Trichomonas hominis*
    b. *Chilomastix mesnili*
    c. *Trichomonas vaginalis*
    d. *Giardia lamblia*
    e. *Endolimax nana*

13. Infection with *Brugia malayi* is best diagnosed by:

    a. Zinc-sulfate flotation concentration
    b. Cellophane tape test
    c. Xenodiagnosis
    d. Trichrome staining of a fecal smear
    e. Knott concentration test

14. All but one of the following are methods of human infection with *Toxoplasma gondii*. Which of the following is *not* a method of toxoplasmosis infection?

    a. Mosquito bite
    b. In utero transmission
    c. Ingestion of oocyst
    d. Ingestion of pseudocyst in meat
    e. Ingestion of trachyzoite in milk

15. Which of the following conditions is *not* a zoonotic infection?

    a. Scabies
    b. Swimmer's itch
    c. Tropical eosinophilic lung
    d. Visceral larval migrans
    e. Cutaneous larval migrans

16. Patient traveled last summer to Africa and has a spiking fever every third day. Stained blood smears reveal the following:

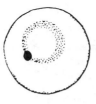

The parasite causing this infection is:

    a. *Plasmodium vivax*
    b. *Plasmodium malariae*
    c. *Plasmodium falciparum*
    d. *Plasmodium ovale*

17. Cercariae of this parasite penetrate the skin of humans, thereby causing infection.

    a. *Fasciolopsis buski*
    b. *Heterophyes heterophyes*
    c. *Schistosoma japonicum*
    d. *Paragonimus westermani*

18. These two infections were found by stool examination of a child who had a history of eating dirt. **(2 points)**
   a. *Trichinella spiralis*
   b. *Ascaris lumbricoides*
   c. *Paragonimus westermani*
   d. *Trichuris trichiura*
   e. *Taenia solium*

19. Recovery in human feces of a 7-mm-long gravid proglottid containing eight lateral uterine branches indicates infection with:
   a. *Hymenolepis nana*
   b. *Diphyllobothrium latum*
   c. *Echinococcus granulosus*
   d. *Taenia saginata*
   e. *Taenia solium*

20. This parasite was found in the blood smear of a patient who had a recent summer vacation in New England and reported many insect and tick bites.
   a. *Plasmodium vivax*
   b. AIDS virus
   c. *Phthirus pubis*
   d. *Babesia* spp.

21. Pinworm disease can be best diagnosed by using:
   a. The formalin-ethyl acetate concentration method
   b. The cellophane tape test
   c. A direct fecal smear preparation
   d. None of these

22. A small, operculated egg with a light bulb shape was found in the feces of a patient with liver abnormalities.
   a. *Fasciola hepatica*
   b. *Paragonimus westermani*
   c. *Fasciolopsis buski*
   d. *Clonorchis sinensis*

23. Mature trophozoites and young schizonts in blood smear show a distinct tendency toward band formation and the red blood cells are not enlarged.
   a. *Plasmodium vivax*
   b. *Plasmodium malariae*
   c. *Plasmodium falciparum*
   d. *Plasmodium ovale*

24. Found in the feces of a patient complaining of abdominal distress and diarrhea.
   a. *Giardia lamblia*
   b. *Trichomonas vaginalis*
   c. *Chilomastix mesnili*
   d. *Trichomonas tenax*

25. Only one of the following parasites produces eggs that are immediately infective to humans, and the eggs infect a person directly via ingestion. Which is it?
   a. *Schistosoma mansoni*
   b. *Enterobius vermicularis*
   c. *Trichuris trichiura*
   d. *Clonorchis sinensis*
   e. *Taenia saginata*

26. Match the arthropod vectors with the appropriate organism. **(5 points)**
   _____ a. Mosquito (*Culex* spp.)
   _____ b. Black fly (*Simulium* spp.)
   _____ c. Mango fly (*Chrysops* spp.)
   _____ d. Crustacean (*Cyclops* spp.)
   _____ e. Tsetse fly (*Glossina* spp.)

   1. *Loa loa*
   2. *Onchocerca volvulus*
   3. *Trypanosoma b. rhodesiense*
   4. *Diphyllobothrium latum*
   5. *Wuchereria bancrofti*

27. Which of the following intestinal protozoa is *not* identified as a causative agent of diarrhea?
   a. *Entamoeba histolytica*
   b. *Dientamoeba fragilis*
   c. *Giardia lamblia*
   d. *Balantidium coli*
   e. *Entamoeba coli*

28. Identified from the bloody sputum of an immigrant from the Far East:

   a. *Fasciola hepatica*   c. *Paragonimus westermani*
   b. *Clonorchis sinensis*   d. *Fasciolopsis buski*

29. Control of a flea infestation is different from control of lice. Why?

   a. Fleas are much more resistant to insecticides
   b. Fleas reproduce off the host, laying eggs in the environment
   c. Fleas are larger than lice
   d. Fleas do not need a blood meal

30. In clinical cases of *Wuchereria bancrofti,* the most favorable time to find parasites in the blood is:

   a. Early morning   c. Late afternoon
   b. Middle of the night   d. Any time

31. Match the disease with the causative parasite. **(4 points)**

   _____ a. Creeping eruption
   _____ b. Visceral larval migrans
   _____ c. Tropical eosinophilia
   _____ d. Eosinophilic meningitis

   1. *Dirofilaria* spp.
   2. *Anisakis* spp.
   3. *Angiostrongylus* spp.
   4. *Toxocara* spp.
   5. *Ancylostoma caninum*

32. All of the following except one are best diagnosed by identification in a blood smear. Which one is *not?*

   a. *Trypanosoma b. gambiense*   d. *Onchocerca volvulus*
   b. *Babesia microti*   e. *Wuchereria bancrofti*
   c. *Plamodium falciparum*

33. All of the following, except one, infect humans by entrance of the infective stage through the skin. Which one has a different route of entrance?

   a. *Schistosoma japonicum*   d. *Necator americanus*
   b. *Strongyloides stercoralis*   e. *Heterophyes heterophyes*
   c. *Ancylostoma duodenale*

34. Match the following with the appropriate question. **(10 points)**

   1. *Entamoeba histolytica*   4. *Iodamoeba bütschlii*
   2. *Entamoeba coli*   5. *Dientamoeba fragilis*
   3. *Endolimax nana*

   _____ a. Which amoeba trophozoite feeds on red blood cells?

   _____ b. Which amoeba has a nucleus with a heavy chromatin ring and an eccentrically located karyosome?

   _____ c. Which amoeba has a nucleus with an even chromatin ring and a centrally located karyosome?

   _____ d. Which amoeba has up to four nuclei in a round cyst?

   _____ e. Which amoeba cyst contains a glycogen vacuole?

   _____ f. Which amoeba has a nucleus with a large karyosome and a chromatin ring that is not visible?

   _____ g. Which amoeba does not form cysts?

   _____ h. Which amoeba causes intestinal ulcers and bloody dysentery?

   _____ i. Which amoeba can invade the liver and cause pathology in that organ?

   _____ j. Which amoeba forms the smallest cyst?

35. The trichrome stain is used to identify:
    a. Blood protozoa
    b. Helminth eggs in feces
    c. Intestinal protozoa
    d. Antibodies to tissue parasites

36. Below are listed sources of error that may affect a quality smear stained for parasites. Identify which one is *not* a source of error.
    a. Blood smear too thick
    b. Blood smear too new
    c. Stain buffer has wrong pH
    d. Wrong timing during staining

37. The head of the scolex of *Diphyllobothrium latum:*
    a. Is armed with hooks
    b. Has a retractable rostellum
    c. Has four suckers
    d. Has two sucking grooves

38. Egg has a large lateral spine.
    a. *Schistosoma haematobium*
    b. *Clonorchis sinensis*
    c. *Fasciola hepatica*
    d. *Schistosoma mansoni*

39. Which of the following is the best transport preservative for protozoa or flagellate trophozoites?
    a. Zinc sulfate
    b. Formalin and ethyl acetate
    c. Polyvinyl alcohol
    d. Iodine

40. The cysticercus larva form is found where noted as part of the life cycle of which parasite?
    a. On aquatic vegetation; *Fasciola hepatica*
    b. In fish muscle; *Diphyllobothrium latum*
    c. In pork muscle; *Taenia solium*
    d. In mosquitoes; *Dracunculus medinensis*

41. Which of these Platyhelminthes infect humans through ingestion of undercooked fish? (You may choose more than one answer.) **(5 points)**
    a. *Clonorchis sinensis*
    b. *Paragonimus westermani*
    c. *Diphyllobothrium latum*
    d. *Heterophyes heterophyes*
    e. *Schistosoma mansoni*
    f. *Echinococcus granulosus*

42. *Babesia* spp. is transmitted to humans by:
    a. The bite of an infected tick
    b. The bite of an infected fly (*Chrysops* spp.)
    c. Ingestion of a cyst
    d. The bite of an infected mosquito (*Anopheles* spp.)

43. Name two zoonotic infections caused by: **(6 points)**
    a. Nematodes
    b. Protozoa
    c. Platyhelminthes

44. Which of the following causes primary amebic meningoencephalitis?
    a. *Entamoeba histolytica*
    b. *Babesia* spp.
    c. *Naegleria* spp.
    d. *Sarcocystis* spp.
    e. *Acanthamoeba* spp.

45. Because you are responsible for parasite control on an island, you chemically treat the small freshwater lake for snails, but you accidently dump in too much chemical and kill every living thing in the lake. Your action breaks the life cycle and controls the spread of which of the following parasites? (Choose all correct answers.) **(5 points)**

    a. *Fasciolopsis buski*
    b. *Taenia solium*
    c. *Schistosoma mansoni*

    d. *Diphyllobothrium latum*
    e. *Hymenolepsis nana*

46. Which of the following requires two different intermediate hosts in its life cycle?

    a. *Clonorchis sinensis*
    b. *Schistosoma mansoni*
    c. *Trichuris trichiura*

    d. *Loa loa*
    e. *Echinococcus granulosus*

47. Which of the following exhibits diurnal periodicity?

    a. *Wuchereria bancrofti*
    b. *Brugia malayi*

    c. *Loa loa*
    d. *Onchocerca volvulus*

48. Below is shown the final centrifuge tube appearance for two different concentration techniques. Indicate where the parasites are found in each tube and state what concentration technique each tube represents. **(5 points)**

A.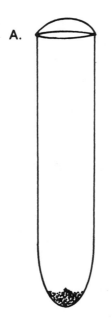

B.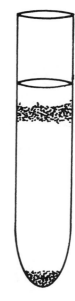

TEST QUESTIONS ANSWER KEY

CHAPTER 1

1. b	6. a
2. d	7. d
3. c	8. b
4. c	9. a
5. c	10. c

11. a = 3; b = 5; c = 1; d = 2; e = 4

12. a. **Vector.** Any arthropod or other living carrier that transports a pathogenic microorganism from an infected to a noninfected host.

   b. **Host.** The species of animal or plant that harbors a parasite and provides some metabolic resources to the parasitic species.

   c. **Proglottid.** One of the segments of a tapeworm; each contains male and female reproductive organs when mature.

   d. **Definitive host.** Animal in which a parasite passes its adult existence, sexual reproductive phase, or both.

   e. **Operculum.** The caplike cover on certain helminth eggs.

CHAPTER 2

1.

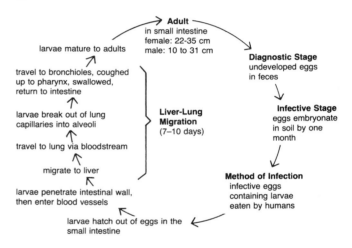

2. a. *Wuchereria bancrofti*
   b. *Culex* or *Anopheles* spp. mosquito
   c. Blood specimen, stained thick and thin smears; concentrate the specimen by centrifugation; serology also helpful

3. a. **Cutaneous larval migrans.** A disease caused by the migration of larvae of *Ancylostoma* spp. (dog or cat hookworm) or other helminths under the skin of humans. Larval migration is marked by thin, red papular lines of eruption. Also termed creeping eruption.

   b. **Diurnal.** Occurring during the daytime.

   c. **Diagnostic stage.** A developmental stage of the pathogenic organism that can be detected in human body secretions, discharges, feces, blood, or tissue by chemical means or microscopic observation as an aid in diagnosis.

   d. **Infective stage.** The stage of a parasite at which it is capable of entering the host and continuing development within the host.

   e. **Prepatent stage.** The time elapsing between initial infection with the parasite and reproduction by the mature parasite.

4. d

5. b

6. a

7. d

8. b

9. c

10. c

11. b

12. c

13. c, c, d, a

14. c & a, d, e, b & a

15. d

16. b

CHAPTER 3

1. a. **Hexacanth embryo.** A tapeworm larva having six hooklets; also termed onchosphere; found in all *Taenia* spp. eggs.

   b. **Hermaphroditic.** Having both male and female reproductive organs within the same individual. All tapeworms have both sets of reproductive organs in each segment of the adult (i.e., all adult tapeworms are hermaphroditic).

   c. **"Armed" scolex.** Crown of hooks on anterior end of a tapeworm; causes attachment to the wall of the intestine of a host by means of suckers and hooks (e.g., *Taenia solium*).

   d. **Proglottid.** One of the segments of a tapeworm (all adult tapeworms form proglottids). Each proglottid contains male and female reproductive organs when mature.

   e. **Hydatid cyst.** A vesicular structure formed by *Echinococcus granulosus* larvae in the intermediate host; contains fluid, brood capsules, and daughter cysts in which the scolices of potential tapeworms are formed.

2. a. 5 (4)
   b. 4
   c. 7
   d. 2, 1
   e. 10 (4)

3. a. *Hymenolepis nana*

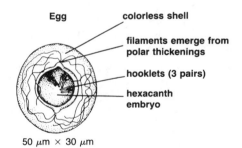

50 μm × 30 μm

   b. *Diphyllobothrium latum*

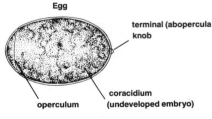

75 μm × 45 μm

c. *Taenia saginata*

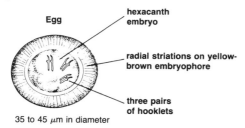

Egg

hexacanth embryo

radial striations on yellow-brown embryophore

three pairs of hooklets

35 to 45 μm in diameter

d. *Taenia solium*

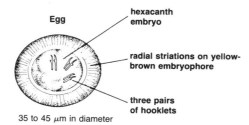

Egg

hexacanth embryo

radial striations on yellow-brown embryophore

three pairs of hooklets

35 to 45 μm in diameter

e. *Echinococcus granulosus*

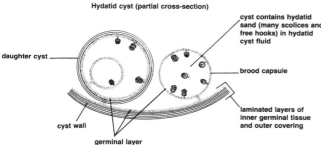

Hydatid cyst (partial cross-section)

cyst contains hydatid sand (many scolices and free hooks) in hydatid cyst fluid

daughter cyst

brood capsule

laminated layers of inner germinal tissue and outer covering

cyst wall

germinal layer

4. a. 5
   b. 4
   c. 1
   d. 7
   e. 6
   f. 2
   g. 3

5. a	12. a
6. c	13. c
7. c	14. b
8. b	15. e
9. b	16. d
10. c	17. b
11. b	18. a

CHAPTER 4

1. 1 Egg
   2 Miracidium
   3 Sporocyst
   4 Redia
   5 Cercaria
   6 Metacercaria
   7 Adult

2. d. Possible contact with sheep-transmitted, sheep-dog-transmitted, and freshwater fish–transmitted parasites
   a. No contact with pigs. No contact with snails or fish hosts of Oriental lung fluke
   b. No contact with snails or host *S. mansoni* or hosts of *C. sinensis*
   c. No contact with snail hosts of *S. japonicum*
   e. No contact with snails or fish hosts of *H. heterophyes*

3. a. 1. *Fasciolopsis buski* (large intestinal fluke) ingestion
      2. *Clonorchis sinensis* (Chinese liver fluke)
      3. *Schistosoma mansoni* (Manson's blood fluke)
   b. 1. Human eats metacercariae on uncooked water plant.
      2. Human eats metacercariae on uncooked fish.
      3. Cercariae penetrate skin.

4. Method of infection with blood flukes (schistosomes) is by penetration of the skin by cercariae in fresh water. Prevention of infection with blood flukes therefore requires prohibiting human feces or urine from contaminating fresh water, controlling the snail population, not entering contaminated water without protection, treating carriers with drugs, and educating the public.

   Prevention of infection with intestinal flukes requires cooking all fish and crustaceans thoroughly, washing water plants such as watercress and water chestnuts thoroughly, educating people about methods of infection and about not contaminating fresh water with human waste, treating carriers, and controlling the snail population.

5. b	11. a
6. b	12. b
7. a	13. e
8. d	14. a
9. b	15. a
10. b	

CHAPTER 5

1. a. 4
   b. 7
   c. 14
   d. 8
   e. 11
   f. 5, 1, 2
   g. 2
   h. 9, 10
   i. 1
   j. 3
   k. 6
   l. 12

2. *Entamoeba histolytica* is morphologically identical to *Entamoeba dispar* except *E. histolytica* trophozoites will have ingested RBCs; *E. dispar* never ingests RBCs. Further confirmation can be made using immunologic procedures.

3. In trophozoite: Study differential characteristics of size, consistency, and inclusions (bacterial or RBCs) in cytoplasm, directional versus random motility, shape of pseudopodia, or staining characteristics of nuclear structures. In cysts: Study differential characteristics of size, number of nuclei, nuclear structure, shape of chromatoid bodies, or vacuoles.

4. a. **Trophozoite.** The motile stage of a protozoa that feeds, multiplies, and maintains the colony within the host.
   b. **Cyst.** The immotile stage protected by a cyst wall formed by the parasite. In this stage, the protozoa is readily transmitted to a new host.
   c. **Sporozoite.** The form of *Plasmodium* that develops inside the sporocyst, invades the salivary glands of the mosquito, and is transmitted to humans.
   d. **Schizogony.** Asexual multiplication of *Apicomplexa;* multiple intracellular nuclear division precedes cytoplasmic division.
   e. **Carrier.** A host harboring and disseminating a parasite but exhibiting no clinical signs or symptoms.
   f. **Oocyst.** The encysted form of the ookinete; occurs on the stomach wall of the *Anopheles* spp. mosquitoes infected with malaria.
   g. **Pseudocyst.** A cystlike structure formed by the host during an acute infection with *Toxoplasma gondii.* The cyst is filled with tachyzoites in normal hosts; may occur in brain or other tissues. Latent source of infection that may become active if immunosuppression occurs.
   h. **L.D. body (Leishman-Donovan body).** Each of the small ovoid amastigote forms found in tissue macrophages of the liver and spleen in patients with *Leishmania donovani* infection.
   i. **Paroxysm.** The fever-chills syndrome in malaria. Spiking fever corresponds to the release of merozoites and toxic materials from the parasitized RBC, and shaking chills occur during schizont de-

velopment. Occurs in malaria cyclically every 36 to 72 hours, depending on the species.
   j. **Atrium.** An opening; in a human, refers to the mouth, vagina, and urethra.

5. a. Bite of *Phlebotomus* spp.
   b. Ingestion of cyst in contaminated water or food
   c. Infected feces of *Triatoma* spp. rubbed into bite or conjunctiva
   d. Ingestion of oocyst, trophozoite, or pseudocyst; congenital transmission
   e. In men, sexual intercourse; in women, contamination with infectious material from vagina
   f. Ingestion of cyst in contaminated water or food
   g. Tick bite
   h. Bite of *Anopheles* mosquito; contaminated blood injection
   i. Bite of *Glossina* spp.
   j. Bite of *Phlebotomus* spp.

6. *P. vivax*

Trophozoite (single ring)

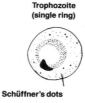

Schüffner's dots

Note: Single ring, one third diameter of an RBC; invades only immature RBCs so that large bluish cells are parasitized. RBC shows red-stained Schüffner's dots which become visible between 15 and 20 hours following invasion of the cell.

P. malariae

Trophozoite (single ring)

Note: Trophozoite forms band across RBC during early schizogony.

P. falciparum

Trophozoites

small ring forms

RBC vacuole

accolé form

red nucleus   blue cytoplasm

7. d	17. a
8. d	18. d
9. b	19. b
10. d	20. a
11. e	21. e
12. e	22. d
13. c	23. a
14. b	24. d
15. a	25. b
16. d	

CHAPTER 6

1. a. 5
   b. 6
   c. 1
   d. 3
   e. 2
2. a. 5
   b. 1, 2, 3, 4, 5, 7
   c. 4
   d. 6
   e. 5
   f. 3
   g. 3
   h. 1
   i. 7
   j. 2
3. All flea stages develop to maturity in the environment rather than on the host, as is the case with lice. Therefore, treatment for fleas must include treating the host and chemically treating the rooms of the house. For lice, primary treatment is to the infected individual, although personal items such as combs, bedding, and towels must also be disinfected.
4. Annoyance, allergic reaction, blood loss, toxins or venom in bites, secondary bacterial infections, transmission of a variety of microorganisms by mechanical or biological methods, loss of food crops, loss of animal productivity, and myiasis.

5. d	13. a
6. b	14. b
7. a	15. c
8. e	16. d
9. c	17. b
10. e	18. b
11. c	19. d
12. d	

CHAPTER 7

1. False—1 or 2 is sufficient for helminths, 3 to 6 for suspected amebiasis or giardiasis.
2. True
3. False—not all intestinal protozoa form cysts; trophozoites die and hookworm eggs may hatch if specimen is not rapidly preserved.
4. True
5. False—oil enemas make examination impossible.
6. False—other species of parasites may also be present.
7. Low light for contrast; unstained amoebae are translucent.
8. First thing in the morning before washing or defecation because generally pinworms deposit eggs at night.
9. Formalin-ethyl acetate; sedimentation of parasite stages. Zinc sulfate; flotation, based on differential specific gravity of parasite and the liquid medium. For procedures, see pages 167 to 171.
10. 1.18 to 1.20; hydrometer
11. Schistosome eggs, infertile ascaris eggs, operculated eggs
12. Ether or ethyl acetate
13. Thin: little distortion, but hard to find the parasites
    Thick: distortion, but easier to find the parasites
14. Place slide in distilled water until hemoglobin color disappears from slide.
15. Cytoplasm is light blue-green or pink for *E. histolytica*, more purplish for *E. coli*. Karyosomes stain ruby red.
16. Disodium phosphate and monosodium phosphate, pH 7.0
17. Microsporidia spores (1 to 2 μm) stain red with modified acid-fast stains. Final identification must be confirmed using modified trichrome stain, fluorescent antibody, or other antibody techniques.
18. a. Antibody methods use patient serum to detect circulating antibody against the parasite in question. Results can confirm exposure to the parasite and, in some cases (e.g., toxoplasmosis), can help determine the stage of the infection.
    b. Antigen methods are used to detect and identify particular parasites found in clinical specimens, such as feces or urine. A wide range of methods are used for both groups including EIA, ELISA, and IIF. DNA probes and polymerase chain reaction techniques are also used.

19. a. 2, 4
    b. 1, 5
    c. 6
    d. 4
    e. 7
    f. 4
    g. 7
    h. 4

20. a

21. d

22. c

23. b

24. b

25. a

FINAL EXAMINATION

1. *Trichuris trichiura*
   Necatur americanus (or *Ancylostoma braziliense*)
   Taenia solium or *Taenia saginata*
   Ascaris lumbricoides
   Plasmodium vivax
   Schistosoma japonicum
   Entamoeba histolytica
   Paragonimus westermani
   Giardia lamblia
   Trichomonas vaginalis

2. a. Diagram 2–4 (p. 19)
   b. Diagram 3–3 (p. 50)
   c. Diagram 5–8 (p. 108)
   d. Diagram 2–2 (p. 15)
   e. Diagram 5–9 (p. 110)

3. b, d

4. e

5. a = 10; b = 2; c = 3; d = 12, 5, 11; e = 1; f = 2;
   g = 3; h = 1, (2); i = 3; j = 8, 1

6. b

7. a, f

8. a, b, c, d

9. c

10. a

11. c

12. b

13. e

14. a

15. a

16. b

17. c

18. b, d

19. e

20. d

21. b

22. d

23. b

24. a

25. b

26. a = 5; b = 2; c = 1; d = 4; e = 3

27. e

28. c

29. b

30. b

31. a = 5; b = 4; c = 1; d = 3

32. d

33. e

34. a = 1; b = 2; c = 1; d = 1; e = 4; f = 3; g = 5; h = 1;
    i = 1; j = 3

35. c

36. b

37. d

38. d

39. c

40. c

41. a, c, d

42. a

43. a. *Ancylostoma* spp., *Angiostrongylus* spp., *Anisakis* spp., *Capillaria philippinensis, Dirofilaria* spp., *Gnathostoma* spp., *Gongylonema pulchrum, Thelazia* spp., *Toxocara* spp.
    b. *Trypanosoma* spp., *Sarcocystis* spp., *Leishmania* spp., *Toxoplasma gondii, Babesia* spp.
    c. *Fasciola hepatica,* swimmer's itch, *Echinococcus granulosus, Hymenolepis diminuta, Dipylidium caninum,* sparganosis, cysticercosis

44. c

45. a, c, d

46. a

47. c

48. a. Parasites at the top of the fluid: flotation method
    b. Parasites at the bottom of the tube: sedimentation method

CASE STUDY ANSWER KEY

CHAPTER 2

CASE 2–1

1. The physician evidently suspected *Enterobius vermicularis* (pinworm) infection when ordering the cellophane tape test. This procedure is correct for identification because the female worm leaves the anus and releases eggs outside the intestine.

2. Pinworm infection is acquired by ingesting infective eggs that are found in dust, bed linens, and other surfaces where airborne eggs have landed. Infected individuals may reinfect themselves by ingesting eggs after scratching the perianal region (autoreinfection). Occasionally, eggs may hatch in the perianal region, where larvae may migrate back into the rectum and large intestine to become adults (retroinfection).

3. Careful cleaning of the local environment and concurrent treatment of all residents will eliminate this infection.

4. *Dientamoeba fragilis* may be transmitted along with *Enterobius vermicularis*.

CASE 2–2

1. *Ascaris lumbricoides*, the large intestinal roundworm

2. When infective eggs are swallowed, they hatch in the stomach and small intestine. Larvae penetrate the intestinal mucosa and move to the liver via the portal blood vessels. The blood then carries larvae through the heart to the lungs. After further maturation, they migrate into the bronchioles, are coughed up to the pharynx, and are swallowed to return to the intestine where they become adults.

3. *Trichuris trichiura* (whipworm) can be harbored along with *Ascaris lumbricoides* because infection is also acquired by ingesting infective eggs from contaminated soil.

4. A fecal concentration method should be performed to confirm the infection and to rule out other parasites.

5. Adult worms are active migrators, especially when provoked by fever, some drugs, or anesthesia. The worms' migration can trigger vomiting, or the worms may exit out of the patient's mouth, nose, or anus. It is important to treat the *Ascaris* infection first because drugs used to treat other infections, including parasites, may only stress the ascarid, leading to serious consequences related to its migratory behavior.

CASE 2–3

1. *Brugia malayi* (Malayan filaria)

2. This parasite exhibits nocturnal periodicity, meaning that microfilaria are found in the blood in the late afternoon and evening hours. If blood was drawn in the morning, parasites would not be seen, and the diagnosis would be missed.

3. The primary mosquito vector is found in the genus *Mansonia*. Other vectors include *Anopheles* spp. mosquito.

4. *Wuchereria bancrofti* and *Brugia malayi* cause obstruction of the lymphatics, which may lead to lymph edema of the feet, ankles, and inguinal area, resulting in swelling of the lower extremities and scrotum in men. Elephantiasis is more severe in *W. bancrofti*. When swelling is seen in *B. malayi*, it is usually found below the knee or in the elbow. In this case, the anemia and renal symptoms are related to other causes.

CASE 2–4

1. *Ascaris lumbricoides, Ancylostoma duodenale, Necator americanus,* and *Strongyloides stercoralis* are all nematode parasites that have a lung phase in their life cycle.

2. *Strongyloides stercoralis* (threadworm)

3. The adult worm lives in the small intestine; eggs hatch in the intestine, releasing noninfective larvae that are either shed in feces or mature to become infective larvae. Infective larvae penetrate skin (from contaminated soil) or the intestinal lining directly (autoreinfection). In both cases, larvae are carried to the lung, where they break out of the capillary into the alveoli. Larvae are coughed up and swallowed, completing the life cycle. Long-standing infections are maintained by the patient's immune system and

the autoreinfection phase of the life cycle. When the immune system becomes compromised by disease processes (e.g., HIV infection) or intentionally, as in this case, the autoreinfection cycle becomes more active, and disease symptoms increase.

4. More severe lung symptoms and invasion of the central nervous system can occur in these patients if treatment is not successful.

CASE 2–5

1. *Trichinella spiralis* (trichinosis)

2. Periorbital edema and eosinophilia are classic signs associated with this disease.

3. Tissue biopsy of skeletal muscle, especially the gastrocnemius (outer lower leg muscle), or serology should be used to confirm the diagnosis.

4. Complete cooking of pork or, in this case, bear meat is critical. The U.S. Department of Agriculture regulations for conventional oven cooking state that *"all part of pork muscle tissue must be heated to a temperature not lower than 137°F (58.3°C)."* Contaminated pork roasts cooked in microwave ovens may still have viable larvae because of uneven heating by this cooking method. Freezing the meat in a home freezer for 20 days or more at −15°C is usually sufficient to kill encysted larvae. *Trichinella nativa*, although rarely encountered, resists freezing; therefore, freezing cannot be relied on to destroy all *Trichinella* spp. larvae.

CHAPTER 3

CASE 3–1

1. *Diphyllobothrium latum* (broadfish tapeworm)

2. The pleurocercoid larva encysted in muscle tissue of freshwater fish is infective for humans if raw fish is ingested. When the pleurocercoid reaches the intestine, the tapeworm's scolex emerges and attaches to the intestinal mucosa. Maturation and growth lead to the formation of tapeworm segments. Other parasites that have encysted infective forms in fish muscle include *Clonorchis sinensis*, *Heterophyes heterophyes*, and *Metagonomus yokogawai*. The zoonotic nematode infection caused by *Capillaria philippinensis* is acquired by ingesting infective larva encysted in freshwater fish.

3. Infections are usually asymptomatic, but individuals (especially Scandinavians) with long-standing infections may have abdominal distress and, in rare cases, develop pernicious anemia because of the tapeworm's utilization of the patient's vitamin B_{12}.

4. After the patient is treated with drugs, feces may be screened to recover the scolex. Recovery of the scolex implies a successful cure. Current therapies no longer demand that this procedure be performed in all cases.

CHAPTER 4

CASE 4–1

1. *Paragonimus westermani* (the Oriental lung fluke)

2. The physician ordered the examination because the patient's travel history included Japan, an endemic area for this parasite. Crayfish, an intermediate host in *Paragonimus westermani*'s life cycle, were eaten by the patient, possibly exposing the patient to this parasite. The mature fluke lives in the lung and releases eggs, which are coughed up by the patient. Sputum should be examined for the presence of eggs. Groups of eggs may resemble iron filings macroscopically; therefore, it is important to examine any reddish brown, bloody areas found in the specimen.

3. Snails serve as the first intermediate host, and crabs or crayfish serve as the second intermediate host in this life cycle. Humans become infected after eating the undercooked intermediate host.

4. **Eggs** may also be recovered in **feces** if the patient has swallowed infected sputum. Diagnosis may be made or confirmed when eggs are observed in feces.

CHAPTER 5

CASE 5–1

1. *Trichomonas vaginalis*

2. This trophozoite is transferred from host to host by sexual intercourse. Cysts are not formed by this parasite.

3. Men are generally asymptomatic but may have urethral discharges containing trophozoites.

4. All sexual partners should be treated to prevent reinfection.

CASE 5–2

1. *Cryptosporidium parvum.* Oocysts are round and measure 4 to 6 μm in diameter.

2. Immunocompetent adults have abdominal symptoms, anorexia, and 5 to 10 frothy bowel movements per day. The diarrhea is self-limiting, usually lasting about 2 weeks. The disease may last longer in infants and young children who suffer more than adults because the multiple episodes (less than 10 per day) of diarrhea often lead to severe dehydration and weight loss. Treatment is directed toward rehydrating the patient and maintaining electrolyte balance. Immunocompetent patients do not receive chemotherapeutic agents, but paromomycin is used to suppress relapses in AIDS patients.

3. Children in day-care centers are at greater risk of infection because toys often become fecally contaminated by infected toddlers who do not know how to practice good hygiene. These toys may be touched or mouthed

by other children who then become infected. Furthermore, day-care workers who do not practice good hygiene when changing diapers of infected children may then spread the disease to others through food handling or other items used by the children.

4. When the diarrhea is completely resolved, the child may return to day care.

CASE 5–3

1. *Plasmodium vivax* (tertian malaria)

2. When present, Schüffner's dots suggest *Plasmodium vivax* or *P. ovale*. Geographic clues also suggest the type of parasite involved in the infection. In this case, *P. vivax* is probable because *P. ovale* is found most commonly in Africa. Other characteristics include invasion of reticulocytes (bluish appearance of RBCs is noted), ameboid trophozoites, and 18 to 24 merozoites in the mature schizont.

3. The patient acquired this infection from the bite of an infected *Anopheles* spp. mosquito.

4. The patient could have avoided this infection by sleeping under an insecticide-treated bed net, by using insect repellents, and by taking chloroquine phosphate as a prophylactic before, during, and after returning from the endemic area.

CASE 5–4

1. *Giardia lamblia*

2. The boys probably acquired the infection by drinking the treated water because *G. lamblia* cysts are resistant to chlorine. Filtration and iodine treatment of stream water provide better protection against this parasite.

3. *Giardia* does not appear consistently in the feces. Periods of high excretion often alternate with periods of low excretion; therefore, it may be necessary to collect several specimens over an extended period to diagnose this disease.

4. Entero-Test, duodenal aspirates, and immunologic methods are other ways used to detect this parasite.

CASE 5–5

1. *Entamoeba histolytica*

2. *E. histolytica* is identified by the following:
   Size—trophozoite and cyst = 10 to 20 μm
   Nucleus—cyst = 1 to 4 nuclei; small centrally located karyosome with fine spokelike chromatin radiating outward to the nuclear membrane in both cysts and trophozoites
   Chromatoid bars with rounded ends in cysts
   Ingested RBCs in trophozoite—differentiates *E. histolytica* from *E. dispar*, which does not ingest RBCs

3. *E. histolytica* may invade the liver, causing abscesses, and, less commonly, may invade the brain, skin, or other tissues.

4. This infection was probably acquired either by drinking contaminated water or by eating contaminated food.

WORD PUZZLE
ANSWER KEY

CHAPTER 1

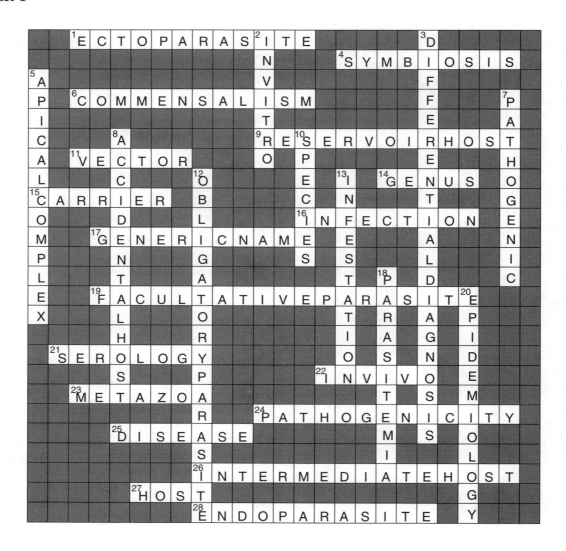

CHAPTER 2

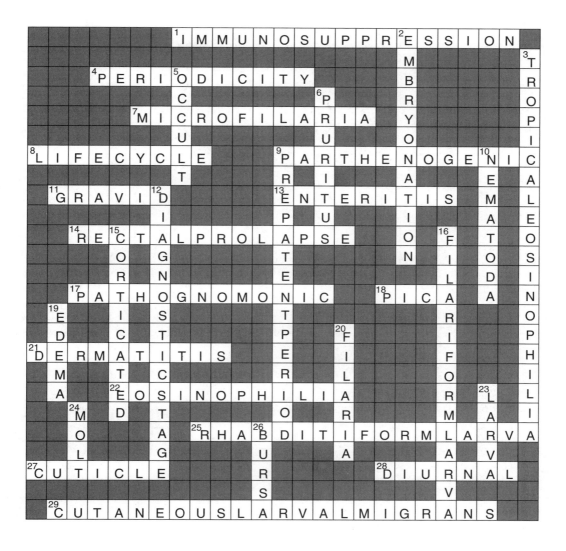

```
V  M  R  G  A  R  M  H  O  F  T  L  L  E  G  R  A  V  I  D  E  S  W  C  R
D  A  H  E  Q  V  N  C  L  R  I  L  C  K  T  L  O  M  H  Q  O  A  S  X  A
O  Y  E  E  M  R  O  E  A  P  L  N  I  Y  Y  P  R  U  R  I  T  U  S     D
I  C  B  T  P  F  A  I  D  U  A  A  U  N  C  S  L  A  N  R  U  I  D  E
R  R  D  R  Q  V  S  F  L  S  E  T  T  R  J  E  E  U  R  R  P  S  K  H  E  L
E  E  I  I  A  P  K  Z  N  S  M  O  H  I  G  G  O  P  A  C  I  P     A  Y  C
P  E  F  T  B  I  L  R  Y  T  E  O  R  V  E  G  O  A  N  S  R  L  E  R  C
N  P  O  I  S  O  H  O  I  S  D  D  R  J  P  C  I  N  R  Q  E  H  Q  J  A  E
O  I  R  S  O  H  R  T  S  L  Y  I  I  S  P  O  N  O  M  R  H  O  X  L  F
I  N  A  A  P  A  I  A  D  Y  P  A  O  A  U  R  F  M  L  L  T  X  I  F  I  L
T  G  D  P  P  O  N  R  A  E  T  Y  G  D  E  S  T  E  O  A  G  R  F  I
A  R  O  O  L  I  T  O  A  N  O  R  I  Y  N  I  Z  O  I  C  N  R  D  A  I
B  U  L  N  A  T  Y  L  G  U  C  M  D  C  O  C  M  N  C  T  I  V  W  P
U  P  A  A  I  S  C  R  I  F  C  X  C  A  N  N  S  I  E  U  A  I  C  A  S
C  T  M  T  S  C  E  B  F  Q  P  S  K  U  T  U  H  T  T  L  M  T  O  K  A  Z
N  I  E  C  O  E  R  M  O  R  G  G  O  Q  R  L  I  C  N  I  Y  C  M  E  N  L
I  O  E  E  R  R  B  E  R  N  Y  M  O  V  A  T  T  E  L  C  R  I  I  D  L
H  N  D  R  V  M  E  R  C  J  L  Y  L  R  O  X  V  I  F  H  S  S  T  E  A
E  S  D  C  Q  H  Q  C  E  L  E  P  H  A  N  T  I  A  S  I  S  Y  E  M  U  E  S  Y  D  T  I  U  G
U  V  M  W  Y  C  X  N  M  E  L  U  S  P  A  C  L  A  C  C  U  B        A  S  C
S  R  D  O  I  R  E  P  T  N  E  T  A  P  E  R  P  U  F  J  M  B  I  G  H
P  S  N  A  R  G  I  M  L  A  V  R  A  L  L  A  R  E  C  S  I  V  R  T  E
P  B  J  A  S  R  U  B  I  N  F  E  C  T  I  V  E  S  T  A  G  E  F  X  O
```

CHAPTER 3

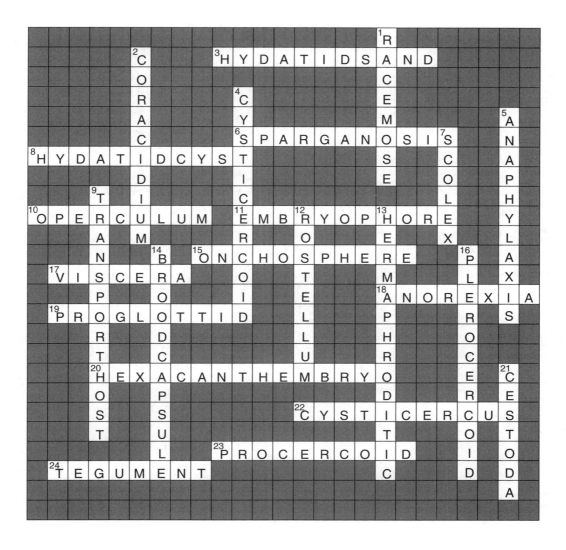

```
V  S  H  I  Y  I  L  P  C  K  V  S  A  T  E  E  E  G  S  V
C  M  T  Z  O  U  U  Y  C  O  I  I  S  E  C  F  A  B  O  V
Y  U  E  R  G  X  R  E  R  E  X  R  O  S  E  M  I  A  C  J  M
S  L  G  R  D  N  C  E  L  O  T  U  T  C  E  E  X  K  L  X  P
T  L  U  A  J  B  Y  H  R  M  O  S  R  I  E  R  U  J  M     D
I  E  M  K  Q  H  Z  O  P  D  G  O  P  K  D  C  A  L  P     E
C  T  E  B  P  Z  P  N  A  S  N  O  E  A  R  I  I  R  V     S
R  S  N  A  Q  S  G  D  E  A  O  D  F  E  C  B  U  F  N     O
C  O     N  H  N  H  P  K  L  H  T  H  P  I  X  D  W  M     M
O  R  A  H  A  S  N  I  P  U  D  I  O  C  R  E  C  O  R  P  E
I  A  E  R  O  H  P  O  Y  R  B  M  E  M  N  M  F  F  O  T  C
D  T  X  H  Y  D  A  T  I  D  S  A  N  D  O  D  S  B  R  A
R  D  M  S  S  U  C  R  E  C  I  T  S  Y  C  M  L  I  R  B
O  Z  R  W  D  I  T  T  O  L  G  O  R  P  Z  X  D  M     X
Y  C  O  H  E  X  A  C  A  N  T  H  E  M  B  R  Y  O  F  T
S  C  O  L  E  X  B  H  Y  D  A  T  I  D  C  Y  S  T  S  V
L  P  K  A  S  P  A  R  G  A  N  O  S  I  S  X  Y  X  Z  S
O  S  C  I  T  I  D  O  R  H  P  A  M  R  E  H  H  V  N  V
X  Z  U  H  V  D  I  O  C  R  E  C  O  R  E  L  P  L  D  B
```

CHAPTER 4

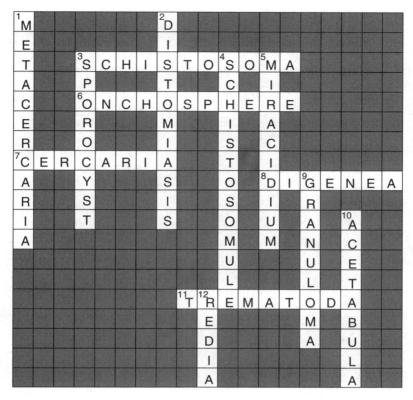

CHAPTER 5

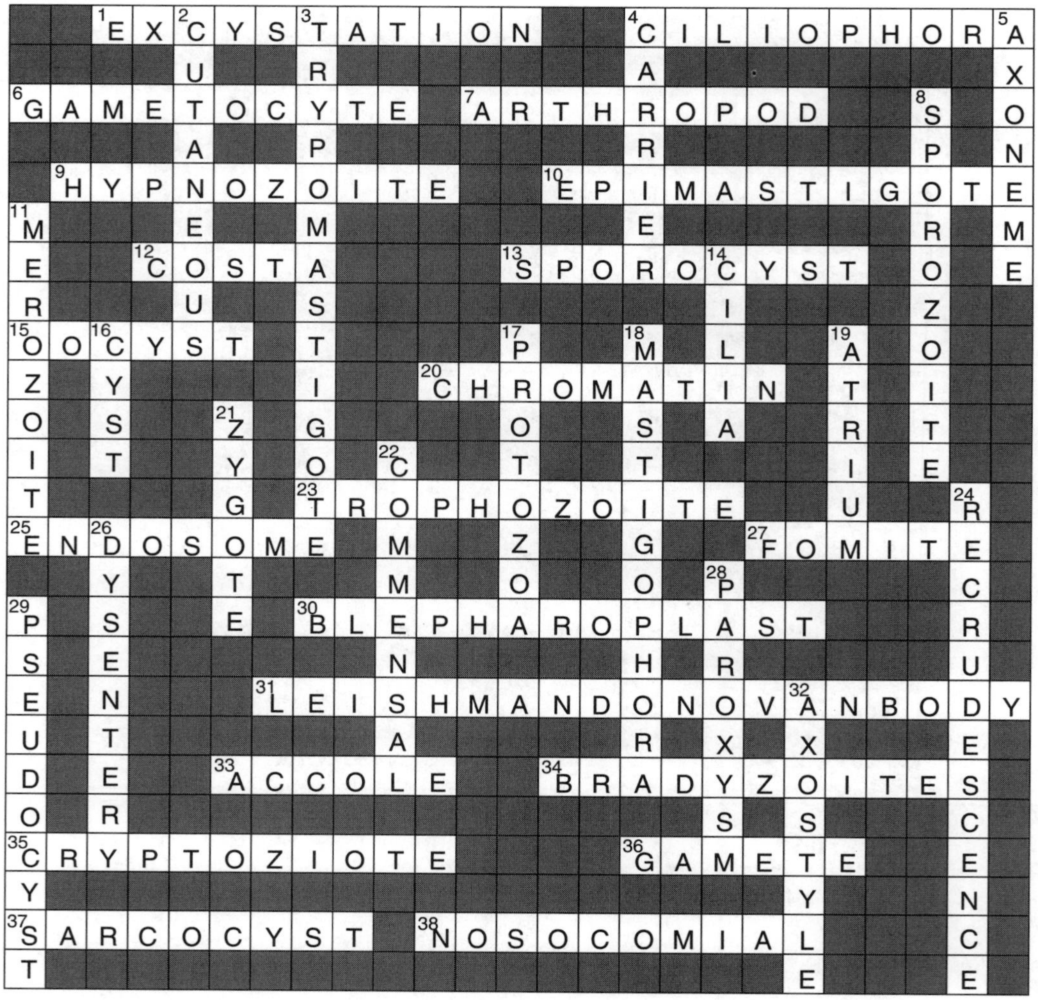

Crossword puzzle solution grid:

- 1 Across: EXCYSTATION
- 4 Across: CILIOPHORA
- 6 Across: GAMETOCYTE
- 7 Across: ARTHROPOD
- 9 Across: HYPNOZOITE
- 10 Across: EPIMASTIGOTE
- 12 Across: COSTA
- 13 Across: SPOROCYST
- 15 Across: OOCYST
- 20 Across: CHROMATIN
- 23 Across: TROPHOZOITE
- 25 Across: ENDOSOME
- 27 Across: FOMITE
- 30 Across: BLEPHAROPLAST
- 31 Across: LEISHMANDONOVANBODY
- 33 Across: ACCOLE
- 34 Across: BRADYZOITES
- 35 Across: CRYPTOZIOTE
- 36 Across: GAMETE
- 37 Across: SARCOCYST
- 38 Across: NOSOCOMIAL

Down answers (letters shown in grid):
- 2 Down: CYSTAQUEUM (C-Y-S-T-A-U-E-U-M)
- 3 Down: TROPHOMASTIGOT
- 5 Down: AXONEME
- 8 Down: SPOROZOITE
- 11 Down: MERIZOITE / MERIDODOCYST
- 14 Down: CYST
- 16 Down: CYSTE
- 17 Down: PROTOZOO
- 18 Down: MASTGO
- 19 Down: ARITEE
- 21 Down: ZYGOTE
- 22 Down: CTMM
- 24 Down: RECRUDESCENCE
- 26 Down: DYSENTER
- 28 Down: PRHR
- 29 Down: PSEUDOPODORY
- 32 Down: ANBODY

```
F  O  M  I  T  E  T  I  O  Z  O  T  P  Y  R  C  S  U  P     C
K  G  A  T  S  O  C  Y  E  T  I  O  Z  O  R  E  M  S     N  C  P
Q  E  T  A  C  H  Y  Z  O  I  T  E  S  A  O  U  U  Y     I  P  P
E  T  O  G  I  T  S  A  M  A  T  A  T  O  L  O  N  M     M  A  P  F
A  E  T  N  W  T  M  L  O  Q  J  X  S  C  L  E  U  I     O  R  N
I  M  N  V  N  E  A  Z  M  V  Y  Y  E  N  G  I  O  Q     R  M  O
L  A  T  Q  O  R  S  O  V  C  S  G  A  O  R  Y  S  B     H  I
I  G  E  E  Z  G  N  R  T  A  T  Z  T  T  L  W  C     A  T
C  S  T  O  H  C  E  P  Y  C  H  T  J  R  Y  N  L     L  A
E  E  B  G  I  N  M  Y  C  J  S  D  E  S  Y  O  T     L  L
T  I  U  O  S  M  O  H  S  T  R  Y  F  L  C  T  E     E  L
I  Z  S  T  S  Y  C  O  D  U  E  S  P  Y  O  S  N     G  E
O  Z  M  S  Y  X  O  R  A  P  G  O  X  T  R  M  I     A  G
Z  Y  H  A  J  R  E  I  R  R  A  C  N  S  O  P  A     L  A
O  D  I  M  T  S  Y  C  O  C  R  A  S  O  S  G  T     F  L
P  A  R  O  H  P  O  G  I  T  S  A  M  X  R  T  N     X  F
R  R  Y  R  E  T  N  E  S  Y  D  S  F  A  I  M     O  E
T  B  H  P  A  P  I  C  O  M  P  L  E  X  A  K  B     N  T
B  I  F  X  O  P  A  R  O  H  P  O  I  L  I  C  Z     N
```

CHAPTER 6

Across:
1. GAMETE
10. GAMETE
11. MEROZOITE
12. NOSOCOMIAL
14. LEISHMANDONOVANBODY
16. PHYLUM
17. KINETOPLAST
19. ENDOPLASM
21. OOCYST
23. TERM
26. EXCYSTATION
27. FOMITE
28. ENDOSOME
29. EXFLAGELLATION
30. PROMASTIGOTE

Down:
1. GAMETOGON
2. EPIMASTIGOTE
3. LARVA
4. THS
5. ANY
6. FLAGELLUM
7. CLASS
8. HYPNOZOITE
9. MASTIGOTE
13. ACYCLT
15. HGARD
16. PARR
18. INFESTATION
20. KAY
22. PAREITES
24. MEROGONY
25. COMBLKY

```
H  W  A  Y  F  K  U  P  N  I  T  I  H  C  B  V  O  C  N  M
A  R  R  A  S  U  I  L  P  U  A  N  T  V  I  V  S  A  S  X
G  F  T  Q  M  U  L  U  T  I  P  A  C  H  B  I  O  K  E  I  P
A  O  H  W  D  O  I  N  Z  W  L  I  P  M  S  C  N  M  T  R  E
E  C  R  Y  G  H  A  I  I  A  H  M  M  A  V  Z  R  C  A  B  J
C  Y  O  P  Q  E  G  N  U  L  N  R  Y  R  I  A  Z  V  B  E  J
A  F  P  T  H  R  H  T  P  C  M  C  P  C  H  O  T  S  E  T  M
T  N  D  A  T  E  M  P  O  R  A  R  Y  H  O  S  T  N  Q  R  E  I
S  F  A  R  P  V  D  K  O  P  U  G  D  N  S  T  N  J  T  R  M  J
U  O  U  M  U  T  U  C  S  K  I  I  H  I  K  C  I  R  E  V  N  I
R  W  F  F  N  I  J  F  R  G  V  U  L  F  Q  D  L  G  V  N  J  A
C  S  F  Q  Q  N  O  T  E  L  E  K  S  O  X  E  A  D  N  I
F  W  W  A  T  C  E  S  N  I  C  M  B  O  W  D  X  V  S  B  I  A
O  L  D  J  L  K  P  Y  Y  J  K  P  A  R  G  C  Y  P  R  I  S
L  S  I  S  O  H  P  R  O  M  A  T  E  M  N  E  H  Q  V  P  F
D  D  C  F  X  U  X  M  A  S  I  S  Y  D  C  E  T  B  C  E
A  M  B  Q  I  G  A  K  G  B  G  M  U  I  D  I  N  E  T  C
M  D  D  W  Q  D  O  E  N  T  O  M  O  L  O  G  Y  V  C  T
B  U  W  J  D  C  S  I  S  O  L  U  C  I  D  E  P  Z  I  H
```

INDEX

An "f " following a page number indicates a diagram or an illustration. A "t" following a page number indicates a table. A number in **boldface** indicates a color plate number.